NATIONAL ACADEMIES *Sciences Engineering Medicine*

NATIONAL ACADEMIES PRESS
Washington, DC

Blueprint for a National Prevention Infrastructure for Mental, Emotional, and Behavioral Disorders

Marcella Alsan, Marthe R. Gold,
Alina B. Baciu, and Alexis Wojtowicz, *Editors*

Committee on a Blueprint for a National
Prevention Infrastructure for Behavioral
Health Disorders

Board on Population Health and
Public Health Practice

Health and Medicine Division

Consensus Study Report

NATIONAL ACADEMIES PRESS 500 Fifth Street, NW Washington, DC 20001

This activity was supported by contracts between the National Academy of Sciences and the Centers for Disease Control and Prevention under Contract No. 75D30121D11240, Task Order No. 75D30123F00025; the National Institutes of Health under Contract No. HHSN263201800029I, Task Order No. 75N98023F00016; and the Substance Abuse and Mental Health Services Administration, under Contract No. 75S20123P00005. Any opinions, findings, conclusions, or recommendations expressed in this publication do not necessarily reflect the views of any organization or agency that provided support for the project.

International Standard Book Number-13: 978-0-309-73092-1
International Standard Book Number-10: 0-309-73092-9
Digital Object Identifier: https://doi.org/10.17226/28577
Library of Congress Control Number: 2025938404

This publication is available from the National Academies Press, 500 Fifth Street, NW, Keck 360, Washington, DC 20001; (800) 624-6242; http://www.nap.edu.

Copyright 2025 by the National Academy of Sciences. National Academies of Sciences, Engineering, and Medicine and National Academies Press and the graphical logos for each are all trademarks of the National Academy of Sciences. All rights reserved.

Printed in the United States of America.

Suggested citation: National Academies of Sciences, Engineering, and Medicine. 2025. *Blueprint for a national prevention infrastructure for mental, emotional, and behavioral disorders*. Washington, DC: National Academies Press. https://doi.org/10.17226/28577.

The **National Academy of Sciences** was established in 1863 by an Act of Congress, signed by President Lincoln, as a private, nongovernmental institution to advise the nation on issues related to science and technology. Members are elected by their peers for outstanding contributions to research. Dr. Marcia McNutt is president.

The **National Academy of Engineering** was established in 1964 under the charter of the National Academy of Sciences to bring the practices of engineering to advising the nation. Members are elected by their peers for extraordinary contributions to engineering. Dr. John L. Anderson is president.

The **National Academy of Medicine** (formerly the Institute of Medicine) was established in 1970 under the charter of the National Academy of Sciences to advise the nation on medical and health issues. Members are elected by their peers for distinguished contributions to medicine and health. Dr. Victor J. Dzau is president.

The three Academies work together as the **National Academies of Sciences, Engineering, and Medicine** to provide independent, objective analysis and advice to the nation and conduct other activities to solve complex problems and inform public policy decisions. The National Academies also encourage education and research, recognize outstanding contributions to knowledge, and increase public understanding in matters of science, engineering, and medicine.

Learn more about the National Academies of Sciences, Engineering, and Medicine at **www.nationalacademies.org**.

Consensus Study Reports published by the National Academies of Sciences, Engineering, and Medicine document the evidence-based consensus on the study's statement of task by an authoring committee of experts. Reports typically include findings, conclusions, and recommendations based on information gathered by the committee and the committee's deliberations. Each report has been subjected to a rigorous and independent peer-review process and it represents the position of the National Academies on the statement of task.

Proceedings published by the National Academies of Sciences, Engineering, and Medicine chronicle the presentations and discussions at a workshop, symposium, or other event convened by the National Academies. The statements and opinions contained in proceedings are those of the participants and are not endorsed by other participants, the planning committee, or the National Academies.

Rapid Expert Consultations published by the National Academies of Sciences, Engineering, and Medicine are authored by subject-matter experts on narrowly focused topics that can be supported by a body of evidence. The discussions contained in rapid expert consultations are considered those of the authors and do not contain policy recommendations. Rapid expert consultations are reviewed by the institution before release.

For information about other products and activities of the National Academies, please visit www.nationalacademies.org/about/whatwedo.

COMMITTEE ON A BLUEPRINT FOR A NATIONAL PREVENTION INFRASTRUCTURE FOR BEHAVIORAL HEALTH DISORDERS

MARCELLA ALSAN, (*Cochair*), Harvard University Kennedy School of Government
MARTHE R. GOLD, (*Cochair*), City University of New York Medical School
RINAD BEIDAS, Northwestern University Feinberg School of Medicine
CAMILLE C. CIOFFI, University of Oregon; Influents Innovations; Oregon Research Institute
JOSEPH P. GONE, Harvard University
KYLE LYNN GRAZIER, University of Michigan School of Public Health
JEFFREY HOM, San Francisco Department of Public Health
MARGARET KUKLINSKI, University of Washington
DAVID MANDELL, University of Pennsylvania School of Medicine
VELMA MCBRIDE MURRY, Vanderbilt University
ANAND PAREKH, Bipartisan Policy Center
LISA SALDANA, Chestnut Health Systems, Lighthouse Institute
PAULA SMITH, University of Utah
LONNIE SNOWDEN,[1] University of California Berkeley School of Public Health
EMILY WANG, Yale University
DONALD (DON) WARNE, Johns Hopkins University

Study Staff

ALINA B. BACIU, Study Director
ALEXIS WOJTOWICZ, Program Officer
MADELEINE M. DEYE, Research Associate (*from January 2024*)
ELLA CASTANIER, Senior Program Assistant (*from October 2024*)
RACHEL RILEY SORRELL, Senior Program Assistant (*until August 2024*)
MISRAK DABI, Senior Finance Business Partner (*until October 2024*)
CHRISTIE BELL, Senior Finance Business Partner (*from October 2024*)
ROSE MARIE MARTINEZ, Senior Board Director
REBECCA MORGAN, Senior Research Librarian

---

[1] Deceased January 25, 2025.

NAM Fellow

SEBASTIAN TONG, National Academy of Medicine James C. Puffer/
American Board of Family Medicine Fellow, University of
Washington, Seattle

Consultants

ALANA ROSENBERG, Yale University
ANNE HARRINGTON, Harvard University
LUCINDA LEUNG, National Academy of Medicine Emerging Leader in
Health and Medicine Scholar, University of California, Los Angeles
TAMI MARK, RTI

Reviewers

This Consensus Study Report was reviewed in draft form by individuals chosen for their diverse perspectives and technical expertise. The purpose of this independent review is to provide candid and critical comments that will assist the National Academies of Sciences, Engineering, and Medicine in making each published report as sound as possible and to ensure that it meets the institutional standards for quality, objectivity, evidence, and responsiveness to the study charge. The review comments and draft manuscript remain confidential to protect the integrity of the deliberative process.

We thank the following individuals for their review of this report:

NATHANIEL COUNTS, Kennedy Forum
DANIEL MAX CROWLEY, The Pennsylvania State University
KRISTEN DILLON, Health Resources and Services Administration
SHERRY GLIED, New York University
HEATHER J. GOTHAM, Stanford University
RITA K. KUWAHARA, Association of Asian Pacific Community Health Organizations
HEDWIG (HEDY) E. LEE, Duke University
MICHELLE LEMMING, Texoma Health Foundation
ALAN I. LESHNER, American Association for the Advancement of Science (Retired)
MYRA PARKER, University of Washington
BERNICE A. PESCOSOLIDO, Indiana University
MELISSA PFAFF, Leavitt Partners

JONATHAN PURTLE, New York University
ZILI SLOBODA, Applied Prevention Science International, Inc.
MARYLOU SUDDERS, Commonwealth of Massachusetts (Formerly)
ROSE WEAHKEE, Indian Health Service

Although the reviewers listed above provided many constructive comments and suggestions, they were not asked to endorse the conclusions or recommendations of this report nor did they see the final draft before its release. The review of this report was overseen by **GEORGE J. ISHAM,** HealthPartners Institute, and **ERIC B. LARSON,** University of Washington. They were responsible for making certain that an independent examination of this report was carried out in accordance with the standards of the National Academies and that all review comments were carefully considered. Responsibility for the final content rests entirely with the authoring committee and the National Academies.

Acknowledgments

The committee wishes to thank and acknowledge the many individuals and organizations that contributed to the study process and development of this report. To begin, the committee would like to thank the study sponsors, the Centers for Disease Control and Prevention, National Institutes of Health, and Substance Abuse and Mental Health Services Administration of the National Institutes of Health, for their support of this work.

The committee is grateful to the individuals who presented to the committee: Kym Ahrens, Deepa Avula, Kari Benson, Kirsten Beronio, Brenda Blasingame, Joshua Breslau, Rahil Briggs, Pamela Buckley, Sarah Chilenski, Namkee G. Choi, David M. Clark, Zeke Cohen, Nathaniel Counts, Chinazo Cunningham, Jonah C. Cunningham, Patsy Cunningham, Erin Day, Nancy J. Donovan, Rev. Que English, Abigail Fagan, Diana Fishbein, Lisa Gennetian, Amy Goldstein, Anne Harrington, Brian Hepburn, Jody Heymann, Rani Hoff, David Hughes, Jeanette Ickovics, Christopher Jones, Angela Kimball, Amy Lansky, Stephanie Lee, Shari M. Ling, Sally Manninen, Sarah Mariani, Greta Massetti, Kristine McCoy, Katie McLaughlin, Benjamin Miller, Robert Morrison, Michael Mumper, Joe Neigel, Jonathan Purtle, Therese S. Richmond, Zili Sloboda, Tequila Terry, Sue Thau, Robert Ursano, Nora Volkow, Sara Whaley, Reginald D. Williams II, and David Willis.

The committee thanks Tami Mark, the consultant on this report, for her expertise and writing of Appendix C, which greatly enhanced the following work.

The committee also thanks the dedicated staff at the National Academies of Sciences, Medicine, and Technology, particularly the study staff in the Board on Population Health and Public Health Practice (BPH): Alina

Baciu, Alexis Wojtowicz, Madeleine Deye, Ella Castanier, Crysti Park, and Rose Marie Martinez. The committee also thanks Samantha Chao, Monica Feit, Annalee Gonzales, Lori Brenig, Leslie Sim, and Taryn Young (Health and Medicine Division Executive Office), Amber McLaughlin and Sam Gerard (Health and Medicine Division Communications), Rebecca Morgan and Colleen Willis (Research Center), Nicole Cohen (Office of Congressional and Government Affairs), and Megan Lowry (Office of News and Public Information). The committee also thanks BPH staff Amy Geller, Nicholas Murdock, Aimee Mead, and Stephanie Puwalski for their additional support.

The committee thanks NAM Puffer/ABFM Fellow Sebastian Tong and NAM Emerging Leader Lucinda Leung, along with consultants Alana Rosenberg and Alexandra Halberstam.

National Academies staff are grateful for helpful and timely background information, examples, and insights shared by Heidi Christensen, Terry Cross, Heather Gotham, Holly Hagle, Katie Johnson, Grace Kindt, Jane Koppelman, Katya Miltimore, Jessica Roark, Joshua Sharfstein, Tyler Winkelman, and Rachel Witmer.

Finally, the National Academies staff thank the committee's indispensable executive assistants and support staff for their help with scheduling committee meetings and calls: Mayra Blakey, Bree-Lyn Cash, Grace Kim, Loretta Grey Cloud, Susie Carey, Patricia Gomez, Ana Rodriguez, Salisha Marryshow Batson, and Aubry Dunaway.

In Memoriam

The committee would like to dedicate this report to honor the life and work of Lonnie Snowden. Dr. Snowden was a valued member of the committee and passed away January 25, 2025.

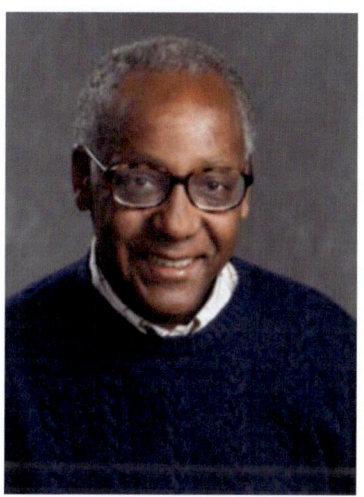

Lonnie Snowden, Ph.D., was a professor at University of California, Berkeley and director of the University of California, Berkeley–University of California, San Franscico Center for Mental Health Services Research. Dr. Snowden was an expert in psychology and mental health care access, and championed work examining the disparities in access to mental health care between Black and White Americans. His 1982 book *Reaching the Underserved: Mental Health Needs of Neglected Populations* was seminal in the field of health care access research and emphasized critical gaps in service delivery for marginalized groups. With over 160 publications, his work has been recognized with numerous awards, including the 2002 Surgeon General's Exemplary Service Award, the 2012 Berkeley Citation, and the 2021 Presidential Citation from the American Psychological Association.

Contents

PREFACE   xxi

ACRONYMS AND ABBREVIATIONS   xxiii

GLOSSARY   xxvii

SUMMARY   1
    The Committee and Its Charge, 2
    The Current and Proposed Prevention
        Infrastructure for MEB Disorders, 3
    Evidence-Based Preventive Interventions, 6

1 INTRODUCTION   19
    Charge to the Committee, 20
    Context for the Study, 21
    The Prevention Ecosystem, 27
    The Committee's Approach, 30
    How to Use This Report, 38
    Report Overview, 41
    References, 41

2 THE EVIDENCE BASE ON PROGRAMS   45
    Research to Translation Pipeline, 46
    Prevention Approaches, 49
    Implementation Science, 57

Research Needs to Improve the Evidence Base on Interventions and Their Implementation, 62
References, 71

3 WORKFORCE, TRAINING, AND TECHNICAL ASSISTANCE 79
The Workforce and Current Challenges, 80
Prevention Workforce Needs, 82
Building the Prevention Worforce Pipeline, 88
Competencies and Training, 93
References, 105

4 DATA AND DATA SYSTEMS TO SUPPORT THE INFRASTRUCTURE 113
Types of Data Sources, 115
Overview of Existing Data Sources, 119
Federal and National Data Initiatives and Guidelines, 125
Data Issues (Challenges and Opportunities), 135
Helping Communities Work with Data, 141
References, 145

5 GOVERNANCE AND PARTNERSHIPS 153
Federal Governance Structure, 156
State Governance Structure, 167
Tribal Governance, 169
Regional and Local Governance Structure, 171
References, 176

6 FUNDING FOR THE PREVENTION OF MENTAL, EMOTIONAL, AND BEHAVIORAL (MEB) DISORDERS 181
Value of Prevention in Behavioral Health, 183
Federal Funding for Prevention of MEB Disorders, 184
Meeting the Need for Sufficient and Sustainable Funding, 201
Other, Nongovernmental Funding Opportunities, 202
References, 209

7 THE EVIDENCE BASE ON POLICIES 217
Economic Policies and MEB Health, 219
Social Policies that Promote MEB Health, 221
Environmental Policies that Promote MEB Health, 230
Including MEB Health Outcomes in Policy Research, 236
References, 238

APPENDIXES

A	Committee and Staff Biosketches	251
B	Clearinghouses of Preventive Interventions	263
C	Mental Health and Substance Use Disorder Prevention Financing Landscape Analysis	267
D	Public Session Agendas	311
E	Related Reports of the National Academies of Sciences, Engineering, and Medicine	319
F	Calculations for Recommendation 6-1	345

Boxes, Figures, and Tables

BOXES

S-1 Statement of Task (*abridged*), 3

1-1 Statement of Task, 22

2-1 A Note About Adverse Childhood Experiences (ACEs), 48
2-2 Evidence-Based Program: Nurse-Family Partnerships, 51
2-3 Evidence-Based Program: Good Behavior Game, 53
2-4 Boys and Girls Clubs of Washington State Association's Promising Out-of-School Program, 54
2-5 Evidence-Based Program: Family Spirit, 55
2-6 PEARLS: A Promising Preventive Intervention for Older Adults, 56
2-7 Promising Approach: Web-Based Apps, 57
2-8 Eight Steps for Implementation of Preventive Interventions in Communities, 60

3-1 A United Kingdom (U.K.) Model for Building an Infrastructure, 83
3-2 Training Frontline Workers from Other Sectors: Sample Strategies, 86
3-3 Evidence-Based Program Case Example: Familias Unidas, 96
3-4 Implementation Considerations for the Workforce, 101

4-1 Elmo and the State of America's Well-Being, 119
4-2 Using Qualitative Data to Inform Selection of Preventive Strategies, 131
4-3 Implementation Considerations Related to MEB Health Data, 133

5-1 Recommendations from Federal Plan for Equitable Long-Term Recovery and Resilience for Social, Behavioral, and Community Health, 160
5-2 Mental, Emotional, and Behavioral Health Elements in Three Departmental "Learning Agendas", 162
5-3 Endorsing a Recommendation on Community Input and Expertise (NASEM, 2023), 173
5-4 Implementation Considerations in Governance and Partnerships for MEB Disorder Prevention, 176

6-1 Solving the Wrong Pockets Problem, 185
6-2 Insights on Funding from State, Local, and Federal Leaders, 207
6-3 Implementation Considerations in MEB Disorder Prevention Funding, 208

7-1 Community-Led Prevention to Reduce Violence on Chicago's South Side, 232
7-2 8 Steps to Support Implementation of Policies for Mental, Emotional, and Behavioral (MEB) Disorder Prevention, 237

FIGURES

S-1 The prevention infrastructure for MEB disorders, 5

1-1 A depiction of the prevention infrastructure for MEB disorders, 36

2-1 Traditional translational pipeline from preintervention, efficacy, effectiveness, and dissemination and implementation studies, 46
2-2 Prevention spectrum for mental, emotional, and behavioral disorders, 48

4-1 Adapted depiction of the public health approach to inform local data systems, 114
4-2 Eight steps toward implementation to promote MEB health equity, 144

5-1 Tribal behavioral health agenda foundational elements, 170

TABLES

1-1 The Prevention Ecosystem in Which the MEB Prevention Infrastructure Is Embedded, 29

1-2 Timeline of Milestones in the History of MEB Health in the United States, 31

2-1 Examples of General Cost Estimates for Selected Interventions, 62

4-1 Examples of Sources and Types of Administrative Data Relevant to MEB Health, 116

4-2 Select Types and Examples of Data Relevant to MEB Health by Life Stage, 120

5-1 Governance Arrangements and Partnerships in Example Accountable Communities for Health, 172

6-1 SAMHSA Breakdown of Spending on Treatment Services for Substance Use Disorders and Mental Health in 2015, 186

7-1 A Map to the Chapter Contents, 218

Preface

The costs associated with our nation's substance use and mental health crises are high, measured in lost and altered lives of children, parents, siblings, and friends and in lost workers, human potential, and the economic productivity of the nation. Groups marginalized on the basis of their race, ethnicity, tribal affiliation, rural status, and low-income status are particularly affected.

The data tell us that the behavioral health (BH) and well-being of people living in the United States is declining. This report marshals evidence that the BH crises individuals and communities face is often preventable. The committee's report is intended to outline a prevention infrastructure that can safeguard the mental, emotional, and behavioral (MEB) health of everyone by promoting protective factors and decreasing risk factors.

Community coalitions around the country have been working for decades to prevent MEB disorders and related challenges. Often, this work is done by volunteers on thin budgets through sheer force of will. Achieving MEB health requires greater resources and infrastructure than our society provides for these activities. The committee finds that effective program interventions are available at every level—from equipping individuals with skills, to strengthening parenting effectiveness, to training teachers and agricultural extension workers, to informing policy makers with the best evidence for policy. The report underscores how improved funding, workforce, data systems, and governance and partnerships can support the implementation of evidence-based programs and policies. Social, economic, and environmental policies enhance protective factors for everyone—and this is needed against a backdrop of challenges that contribute to MEB disorders directly or indirectly. We touch on two examples here. Anxiety, depression, and trauma can result from the community devastation and housing and employment loss caused by extreme weather events. Similar large-scale effects, frequently reinforced, are seen from community firearm violence—which is far more often the cause rather than the outcome of BH disorders. (We note that Recommendation 7-3 for universal prevention interventions of firearm violence as a risk factor for MEB disorders was limited from discussing gun control by the contract that supports this study.)

We all are united in a hope to have our country, our communities, and our children thrive. When they thrive, so does the nation. A strong and sustained infrastructure to prevent MEB disorders and promote well-being is critical to making that hope a reality.

Marcella Alsan and Marthe R. Gold, Cochairs
Committee on a Blueprint for a National Prevention
Infrastructure for Behavioral Health Disorders

Acronyms and Abbreviations

ACA	Affordable Care Act
ACE	adverse childhood experience
ACL	Administration for Community Living
ACF	Administration for Children and Families
ACO	accountable care organization
ACT	Assertive Community Treatment
ADAI	Addictions, Drug & Alcohol Institute
AIAN	American Indian and Alaska Native
AOT	assisted outpatient treatment
ASPE	Assistant Secretary for Planning and Evaluation
ASTHO	Association of State and Territorial Health Officials
AWARE	Advancing Wellness and Resiliency in Education
BCYF	Board on Children, Youth, and Families
BRFSS	Behavioral Risk Factor Surveillance System
CADCA	Community Anti-Drug Coalitions of America
CAPTA	Child Abuse Prevention and Treatment Act
CBO	community-based organization
CDC	Centers for Disease Control and Prevention
CHIP	Children's Health Insurance Program
CHSI	community health status indicators
CHW	community health worker
CMHS	SAMHSA Center for Mental Health Services

CMS	Centers for Medicare & Medicaid Services
COI	conflict of interest
CPWI	Community Prevention and Wellness Initiative
CSAP	SAMHSA Center for Substance Abuse Prevention
CTC	Communities That Care
CSAT	Center for Substance Abuse Treatment
CUA	cost-utility analysis
CVI	community violence intervention
D&I	dissemination and implementation
DFC	Drug-Free Communities
DOJ	Department of Justice
DOL	Department of Labor
DSM-V	*Diagnostic and Statistical Manual of Mental Disorders, 5th Edition*
EBPRC	Evidence-Based Practices Resource Center
EITC	Earned Income Tax Credit
ELTRR	Equitable Long-Term Recovery and Resilience
EPSDT	early and periodic screening, diagnostic and treatment
ERPO	extreme risk protection order
GTO	Getting to Outcomes
HHS	Department of Health and Human Services
HRSN	health-related social need
HRSA	Health Resources and Services Administration
HSI	Health Services Initiative
HYS	Healthy Youth Survey
IC&RC	International Certification & Reciprocity Consortium
IDEA	Individuals with Disabilities Education Act
IRS	Internal Revenue Service
IS	implementation science
LAUNCH	Linking Actions to Unmet Needs in Children's Health
LGBTQ+	Lesbian, Gay, Bisexual, Transgender, Queer (or Questioning), and other sexual identities
MAPP	Mobilizing for Action Through Planning and Partnership
MCO	managed care organization
MEB	mental, emotional, and behavioral

MHSP	mental health services professional
MHTTC	Mental Health Technology Transfer Center
NASADAD	National Association of State Alcohol and Drug Agency Directors
NASMHPD	National Association of State Mental Health Program Directors
NHATS	National Health and Aging Trends Study
NIAAA	National Institute on Alcohol Abuse and Alcoholism
NIDA	National Institute on Drug Abuse
NIDCR	National Institute for Dental and Craniofacial Research
NIH	National Institutes of Health
NIHB	National Indian Health Board
NIMH	National Institute of Mental Health
NIMHD	National Institute on Minority Health and Health Disparities
NNIP	National Neighborhood Indicators Project
NREPP	National Registry of Effective Prevention Programs
NSDUH	National Survey of Drug Use and Health
NSLP	National School Lunch Program
ONDCP	Office of National Drug Control Policy
PLACES	Population Level Analysis and Community Estimates
PROSPER	Promoting School-community-university Partnerships to Enhance Resilience
PSSF	Promoting Safe and Stable Families
PTSD	posttraumatic stress disorder
PTTC	Prevention Technology Transfer Center
QPR	Question, Persuade, Refer
RCT	randomized controlled trial
ROI	return on investment
SAMHSA	Substance Abuse and Mental Health Services Agency
SBHC	school-based health center
SBIRT	screening, brief intervention, and referral to treatment
SDOH	social determinants of health
SDRG	Social Development Research Group
SMI	serious mental illness
SNAP	Supplemental Nutrition Assistance Program

SSI	Supplemental Security Income
SUD	substance use disorder
TANF	Temporary Assistance for Needy Families
TFAH	Trust for America's Health
UC	University of California
UM	University of Michigan
VHA	Veterans Health Administration
WIC	Supplemental Nutrition Program for Women, Infants, and Children

Glossary

Community:	"Any configuration of individuals, families, and groups whose values, characteristics, interests, geography, or social relations unite them in some way."[2]
Health equity:	Concept "that everyone has a fair and just opportunity to be as healthy as possible. This requires removing obstacles to health such as poverty, discrimination, and their consequences, including powerlessness and lack of access to good jobs with fair pay, quality education and housing, safe environments, and health care. For the purposes of measurement, health equity means reducing and ultimately eliminating disparities in health and its determinants that adversely affect excluded or marginalized groups."[3]

---

[2] National Academies of Sciences, Engineering, and Medicine. 2017. Communities in Action: Pathways to Health Equity. Washington, DC: The National Academies Press. https://doi.org/10.17226/24624. pg 1. Adapted from Draft manuscript from Melanie C. Dreher, Rush University Medical Center, provided to staff on February 19, 2016, for the Committee on Community-Based Solutions to Promote Health Equity in the United States. Available by request from the National Academies of Sciences, Engineering, and Medicine's Public Access Records Office. For more information, email PARO@nas.edu.

[3] Braveman, P., E. Arkin, T. Orleans, D. Proctor, J. Acker, and A. Plough. 2018. What Is Health Equity? *Behavioral Science & Policy* 4(1):1-14. https://doi.org/10.1177/237946151800400102, p. 2.

Health disparities:	"Avoidable differences in health or in its key determinants that adversely affect marginalized or excluded groups."[4]
Implementation:	"Systematic, scientific approach to ask and answer questions about how we get 'what works' to people who need it, with greater speed, fidelity, efficiency, quality and relevant coverage."[5]
Indicated prevention:	Targets those already using or engaged in other high-risk behavior (for substance use disorder) or at increased risk of mental illness.
Infrastructure:	"Systems, competencies, frameworks, relationships, and resources that enable [state and local governments and agencies, along with communities, community-based organizations, and their partners,] to perform core functions" central to preventing MEB disorders and promoting health and well-being.[6]
Mental, emotional, and behavioral disorders:	Encompasses both those disorders diagnosable using *Diagnostic and Statistical Manual of Mental Disorders*, 5th Edition (DSM-V) criteria and the problem behaviors associated with them, such as violence, aggression, self-injury, suicide, and antisocial behavior. It includes mental illness and substance use disorders along with a somewhat broader range of concerns associated with problem behaviors and conditions. This committee, like the 2019 committee, chose to use the definition of MEB disorders developed by the authors of the 2009 National Academies report: "the term 'mental, emotional, and behavioral disorders' . . . encompasses both disorders diagnosable using Diagnostic and Statistical Manual of Mental Disorders, 4th Edition (DSM-IV) criteria and the problem behaviors associated with them, such as violence, aggression, and antisocial behavior.

---

[4] Braveman, P., E. Arkin, T. Orleans, D. Proctor, J. Acker, and A. Plough. 2018. What is Health Equity? *Behavioral Science & Policy*:4(1):1-14. https://doi.org/10.1177/237946151800400102, p. 3.

[5] University of Washington. 2024. Step 4: Select Research Methods. https://impsciuw.org/implementation-science/research/select-research-methods/#:~:text=A%20broad%20and%20inclusive%20definition,efficiency%2C%20quality%20and%20relevant%20coverage (accessed January 13, 2025).

[6] Adapted from https://www.naccho.org/programs/public-health-infrastructure (accessed January 13, 2025).

	Many mental, emotional, and behavioral disorders of youth exist on a continuum. . . . The term . . . encompasses mental illness and substance abuse, while including a somewhat broader range of concerns associated with problem behaviors and conditions in youth."[7]
Mental, emotional, and behavioral (MEB) health and well-being:	Defined as the opposite of MEB disorders, a broad construct that encompasses good MEB health and the related concepts associated with measures of subjective well-being, such as flourishing, thriving (the upper end of the Cantril's ladder scale of well-being), and life satisfaction.
Prevention:	Strategies offered before the onset of a disorder that are intended to prevent or reduce the risk for its development.
Primary prevention:	Interventions before the onset of a disorder that are intended to prevent or reduce the risk for its development.
Primordial prevention:	Refers to interventions that address root causes and social factors of MEB disorders.
Program, intervention, approach:	All sometimes used to refer to organized plans for bringing about particular improvements in a public health, and none are used consistently to refer to a single defined method. We use the terms interchangeably unless the context calls for a particular meaning, which we make clear through surrounding text.
Policy:	Refers to public policy—the actions taken by government entities at the city, county, state, or federal levels to pursue social improvements; these actions may include formal rules, legislative actions, administrative programs, targeted funding initiatives, or other mechanisms.
Secondary prevention:	Refers to early detection of disease before it is symptomatic to reduce severity.
Selective prevention:	Refers to targeting those at higher-than-average risk.
Tertiary prevention:	Refers to interventions aimed at reducing severity or worsening of significant adverse outcomes.
Universal prevention:	Refers to interventions targeted at the general population.

---

[7] National Research Council and Institute of Medicine. 2009. Preventing mental, emotional, and behavioral disorders among young people: Progress and possibilities. Washington, DC: The National Academies Press. https://doi.org/10.17226/12480, p. xv.

Summary

Substance use disorder and overdose, suicide, and youth mental illness are major public health crises that cost the United States in lives, human potential, productivity, and resources. Government agencies at the federal, state, tribal, and local levels work together with health care entities, academic institutions, communities, and community-based organizations to respond to these crises largely with treatment and recovery services. Mental, emotional, and behavioral (MEB) disorders are mental and substance use disorders and associated problem behaviors, even if they do not meet diagnostic criteria of the *Diagnostic and Statistical Manual of Mental Disorders, 5th ed.* Less attention and fewer resources are dedicated to delivering services specifically devoted to preventing such disorders and promoting MEB health and overall well-being. Greater support for prevention could minimize the pain and suffering associated with MEB disorders, and, critically, reduce the burden on overtaxed treatment and recovery systems.

This report provides a blueprint to develop the infrastructure to deliver programs that reduce risk factors (characteristics associated with a higher likelihood of negative outcomes) and promote protective factors (characteristics that can reduce the negative impact of a risk factor and promote better outcomes) for MEB disorders across the life course and in an array of settings. The committee's charge was to outline the components and requirements of a well-functioning infrastructure to support the delivery of evidence-based programs at federal, state, tribal, and local levels.

The committee focused on the following infrastructure components and has organized its analysis accordingly:

- Evidence-based programs that are continually evaluated and well-disseminated, with easily accessed details about their effectiveness (including generalizability to other populations) and implementation (Chapter 2);
- A workforce that is sufficiently trained to deliver those strategies, representative of the populations served and able to provide linguistically and culturally appropriate services, fairly paid, and supported with opportunities for career advancement (Chapter 3);
- Data systems that are sufficient for informing needs assessments (including for collecting data about subpopulations to monitor inequities across racial, ethnic, tribal, low-income, and rural communities), selecting strategies, and supporting evaluation and accountability (Chapter 4);
- Governance structures at the federal, state, tribal, and local levels that maximize strategies to ensure shared leadership through cross-sector and community partnerships (Chapter 5);
- Funding that is adequate and sustainable (Chapter 6);
- Evidence-based policies that create and strengthen the social, economic, and environmental conditions necessary for MEB disorder prevention and undergird population health (Chapter 7); and
- Implementation that prioritizes collaborating and co-creating with affected sub-populations (through communities) at each step in the process (discussed in all chapters).

THE COMMITTEE AND ITS CHARGE

At the request of the National Institutes of Health, Substance Abuse and Mental Health Services Administration (SAMHSA), and Centers for Disease Control and Prevention (CDC), the National Academies of Sciences, Engineering, and Medicine convened a committee with expertise in prevention science, implementation science, health and human services research, public health research and policy, the criminal-legal system, substance use and mental health research, economics and finance, and in addressing health disparities (see Appendix A for biographical information of each committee member). The committee's abridged Statement of Task[1] is found in Box S-1.

---

[1] The complete Statement of Task is provided in Chapter 1.

> **BOX S-1**
> **Statement of Task**
> *(abridged)*
>
> The National Academy of Sciences, Engineering, and Medicine will convene an ad hoc committee to develop a blueprint, including specific, actionable steps for building and sustaining an infrastructure for delivering prevention interventions that target risk factors for behavioral health disorders. In conducting its work, the committee will
>
> 1. Identify best practices for creating a sustainable behavioral health prevention infrastructure with attention given to different levels of geography (national and state), prevention (universal, selective, indicated), and settings (from schools to other community settings), and different components (e.g., workforce, data);
> 2. Identify funding needs and strategies, along with existing and potential new sources;
> 3. Identify specific research gaps germane to the widespread adoption of evidence-based behavioral health prevention interventions (from implementation knowledge to economic analyses); and
> 4. Make actionable recommendations about federal and state policies to develop and support infrastructure components.

THE CURRENT AND PROPOSED PREVENTION INFRASTRUCTURE FOR MEB DISORDERS

The committee identified a fragmented and unevenly developed infrastructure to deliver interventions for preventing MEB disorders. It is currently supported by government agencies at all levels (local, state, tribal, federal), academic networks for training and technical assistance, multiple national associations and research societies, and other components. And it is embedded in existing systems: behavioral health (BH),[2] public health, and human services agencies and organizations, along with other sectors of society from community and grassroots organizations to the education system to employers. The committee found the infrastructure currently provides more structures and supports for substance use prevention compared

---

[2] "Behavioral health" and "mental health" are used in this report when reflecting existing agencies or organizations or referring to outcomes discussed in specific studies, while the committee uses "MEB disorders" to encompass the frequently siloed issues of "mental health/illness" and "substance use disorders."

to mental health promotion and disorder prevention and more interventions for children, youth, and young adults than middle and older adults. It does not focus sufficiently on reducing disparities in MEB outcomes associated with social position or other socially defined circumstances—disparities that can begin early in life and increase along the life course. Nor does it focus adequately on expanding fair opportunities for everyone "to attain their full potential for health and well-being."

Therefore, changes to approaching the evidence base and implementation, the workforce, measurement and data, governance, funding and payment, and social policy will be needed. The infrastructure can be nurtured, strengthened, coordinated, and robustly funded to close gaps and provide the interventions needed in every community and across life stages, with a focus on greater support for areas of greatest need. The infrastructure can also be built as a learning prevention framework where each component is invested in furthering ongoing processes of both doing and improving the knowledge of what works. Some characteristics of the learning health care system may apply to the infrastructure for the prevention of MEB disorders, although the focus here is more on communities and less on individuals and on systems beyond health care delivery. Applicable characteristics include data-driven learning that feeds back into the infrastructure, continuous improvement, collaboration and transparency, and seeking guidance by underrepresented groups across every component of the infrastructure.

Prevention research can be improved with more specific support for improving existing interventions and developing new ones with a focus on generalizability, external validity, and implementation science. Dedicated prevention specialists or coordinators exist in many communities, yet they are often left with limited resources to identify needs and lack the evidence-based practices to implement them. Workers in a range of settings and workforces—in schools, primary care, criminal-legal settings, community centers, in congregations, and others—may view preventing MEB disorders as ancillary or incidental to their main mission, but they are well positioned to contribute. However, billing constraints can restrict health insurance reimbursement for integrated behavioral health and primary health care services or MEB preventive care delivery in nonclinical settings. Additionally, funding for public health communication and other strategies that target the entire community is grant-dependent and not sustained.

Figure S-1 illustrates the envisioned infrastructure operating at peak capacity to support the delivery of preventive interventions. The top of the figure identifies the existing systems and infrastructures that constitute a foundation for MEB disorder prevention, while the gears reflect the major components needing support and refinement to successfully work together to deliver interventions along the life course and in a variety of settings.

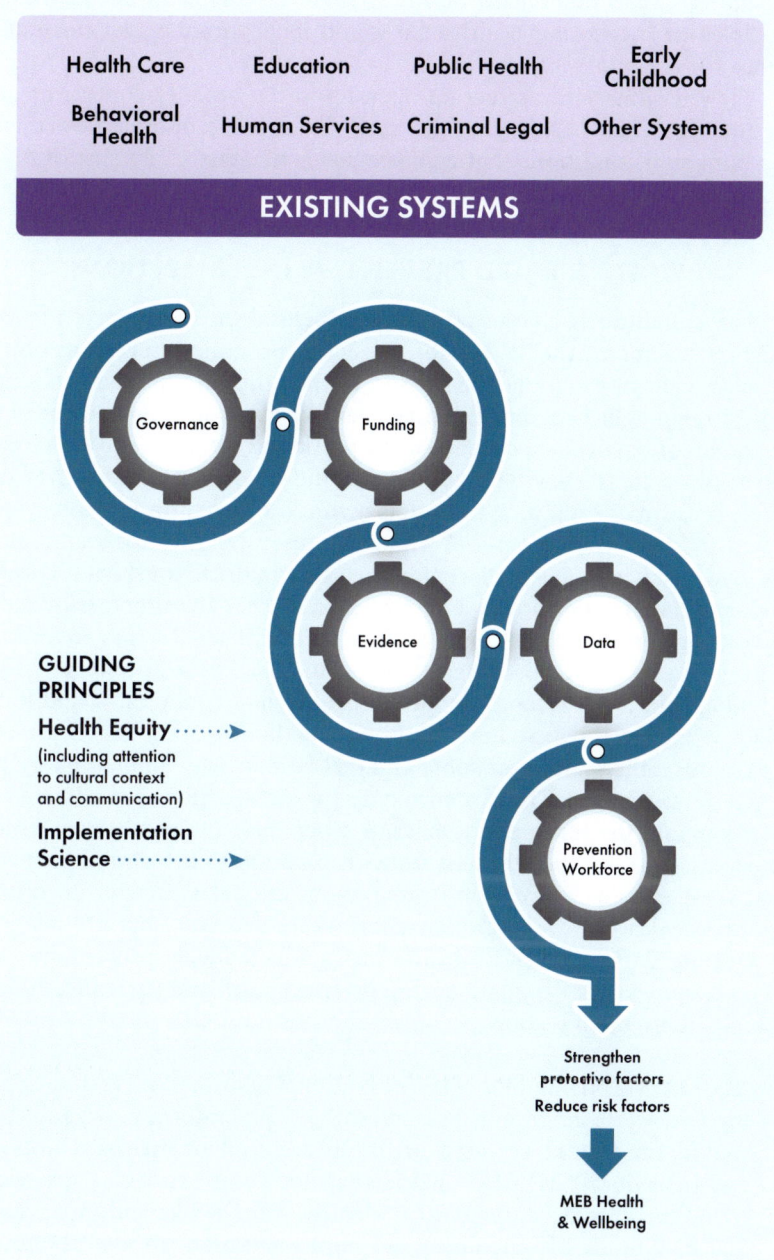

FIGURE S-1 The prevention infrastructure for MEB disorders.
NOTE: MEB = mental, emotional, and behavioral.

To improve MEB outcomes, the infrastructure must embrace the guiding principles of promoting health equity and incorporating implementation science for the interventions and the infrastructure.

The envisioned infrastructure operates in the broader context of policies (not included in the graphic) that shape the economic, social, and environmental conditions that enhance protective factors against or create risk factors for MEB disorders.

EVIDENCE-BASED PREVENTIVE INTERVENTIONS

The committee's charge was largely focused on the aspects of infrastructure to support the delivery of preventive programs and not a comprehensive review of programs themselves. Despite this, the committee found it useful to highlight program examples developed for different stages of the life course of particular populations or particular settings. These examples help to illustrate the flexibility required of the infrastructure to deliver such a wide breadth of programs and offers a window into future research needs related to gaps in interventions and their dissemination to communities. The evidence base is particularly targeted for children, youth, and families. These interventions positively affect many MEB health outcomes by reducing risk factors and promoting protective factors. These factors are relevant at every level of the socioecological model, that is, the intrapersonal (genetic or biological), interpersonal (family), institutional, community, and public policy. While some risk and protective factors (biological or genetic) may be fixed, many others are modifiable and can be positively influenced by preventive interventions. The evidence base for interventions for adults is not as strong, and the reach and impact of all of these interventions is limited for several reasons, including issues with generalizability and implementation. These existing prevention strategies—as critical aspects of the prevention and health promotion infrastructure—are necessary but not adequate for meeting population MEB health needs and reducing preventable poor MEB outcomes that originate during preconception and early life, and can increase along the life course.

> **RECOMMENDATION 2-1:** The National Institutes of Health, Centers for Disease Control and Prevention, and philanthropic organizations should fund more research on the prevention of mental, emotional, and behavioral (MEB) disorders that addresses research gaps related to intervention development (to identify what works and the certainty and magnitude of outcomes) and implementation (to identify how to deliver and sustain interventions with fidelity). This research should prioritize interventions that target MEB health inequities, are needed

for different age groups, and are co-created with the populations they are intended to serve.

Funders can use existing taxonomies,[3] develop new ones, pursue strategies to systematically and consistently identify research needs, and set priorities so appropriate proposals are funded and research needs are addressed. In requests for proposals, funders can emphasize the need for

- Interventions that can be tailored for different contexts, settings, and age ranges, for an array of participants from those who are easily engaged to those who have been historically excluded, underrepresented, or experienced language access barriers;
- Co-design, co-production, or co-creation of intervention and implementation approaches between investigators, community members, and/or future participants in research proposals and projects; and
- Implementation plans for interventions that prove successful.

In addition to further research needed to improve knowledge about interventions themselves, more can be done to improve the dissemination of this knowledge across communities. Dozens of clearinghouses are available in various government agencies and private organizations, but they vary in quality (inconsistent or inadequate criteria, etc.) and sustainability (fluctuating funding sources and ability to be updated with new information). The vast number of options, lack of clarity about how programs are evaluated, and how generalizable they are in any given community can be a hindrance for those wanting to implement preventive interventions. One well-known example is SAMHSA's National Registry of Evidence-Based Programs and Practices, which evaluated interventions but was suspended in 2017 and replaced by the Evidence-Based Practices Resource Center, a static and nonevaluative database. SAMHSA is currently exploring other options in this area. An easily accessible, trustworthy, centralized repository of programs addressing MEB disorder prevention with transparent criteria, evaluations, and regular updates would greatly serve communities, coalitions, and other invested constituents.

RECOMMENDATION 2-2: The Substance Abuse and Mental Health Services Administration (SAMHSA) should manage and maintain a centralized and dynamic evidence clearinghouse for mental, emotional, and

---

[3] See, for example, the clinical prevention foundational issues, analytic framework, and dissemination and implementation taxonomies for identifying research gaps at https://nap.nationalacademies.org/resource/26351/ or the Reconnecting Youth Evidence Gap Map at https://reconnectingyouth.mdrc.org/egm (accessed March 10, 2025).

behavioral health that promotes standardization of criteria for inclusion and evaluation. The clearinghouse should include information about intervention effectiveness, guidance for implementation, and a focus on prevention strategies that address the needs of diverse communities.

To support uptake of effective interventions and integrate practice-based evidence, SAMHSA should also

a. Develop clearinghouse navigation tools to help implementers find relevant strategies, ensure implementation quality, and increase the likelihood of impact; and
b. Work with state and other grantees to develop a mechanism to integrate evaluation of implementation, new knowledge, and community experience.

Possible criteria for inclusion within this centralized and dynamic clearinghouse could include:

1. Quality of the evidence: reliability and internal validity;
2. Generalizability of results to specific and new subpopulations, settings, and geographic locations (external validity); and
3. Pre-implementation, implementation, and cost considerations.

Clearinghouse usability considerations include having straightforward search functions and being tailorable for different needs, concise, and jargon-free.

The Workforce for Prevention of MEB Disorders

The committee found that the MEB disorder prevention workforce is poorly characterized compared to the traditional behavioral health (BH) workforce of graduate degree–trained and licensed practitioners working largely in clinical settings. The extant prevention workforce includes workers with prevention science, public health, and related training; frontline workers from other sectors and systems (e.g., day care providers, teachers, clergy); and direct service practitioners (e.g., community health workers, community health representatives) drawn from and representative of the community. Developing and supporting an effective workforce will require review of competencies, training and certification needs, strategies for developing a pipeline and pathways to professional development, opportunities to expand and support to implement evidence-based programs (and contribute to the development of practice-based evidence) in a variety of settings, and fair pay and labor protections.

Several changes are needed to better characterize and enumerate the prevention workforce, and a SAMHSA office devoted to the MEB disorder prevention workforce could provide a point of coordination and support for all workforce matters, including better integration of prevention related to mental health and substance use.

RECOMMENDATION 3-1: In consultation with Substance Abuse and Mental Health Services Administration (SAMHSA), the Health Resources and Services Administration should describe and enumerate the workforce for mental, emotional, and behavioral (MEB) health promotion and prevention of MEB disorders. SAMHSA should add the newly defined roles to its behavioral health workforce estimates and reports.

RECOMMENDATION 3-2: The Department of Labor should use the most up-to-date description of the prevention workforce for mental, emotional, and behavioral disorders as the basis for updates to the Standard Occupational Classifications for behavioral and public health jobs.

RECOMMENDATION 3-3: The Substance Abuse and Mental Health Services Administration should establish a Coordinating Office on the Mental, Emotional, and Behavioral Prevention Workforce or designate a lead office to coordinate prevention to delineate core competencies, develop a strategic plan, review agency programs and grants for workforce linkages, coordinate with the Centers for Disease Control and Prevention and accrediting and licensure bodies, and strengthen academic-community partnerships.

This enhanced coordination could be accomplished through collaboration between the Center for Substance Abuse Prevention and a new Center for Mental Health Promotion or a new joint Center for Prevention of Behavioral Disorders (see options supporting Recommendation 5-1). If creating a new office is not feasible, SAMHSA leaders working on behavioral health workforce issues would need to coordinate and address the various components for an effective prevention workforce.

Broader dissemination of effective strategies could be facilitated through better coordination with SAMHSA and the CDC among the departments and agencies that serve specific populations (e.g., older adults, K–12 students).

RECOMMENDATION 3-4: The Substance Abuse and Mental Health Services Administration and Centers for Disease Control and Prevention should work with the Administration for Community Living, Administration for Children and Families, U.S. Department of Education, and Department of Justice to incorporate strategies for training on prevention of mental, emotional, and behavioral disorders for frontline personnel in those settings.

Data

Communities and their partners working to promote MEB health need several types of data: demographics, risk and protective factors (including social determinants of health [SDOH] metrics), MEB outcomes, substance use patterns and consequences, prevention resources (e.g., people, organizations, community assets), and community readiness. For population-level data, additional funding and sustained federal support for a small area local data repository is needed to help community prevention implementers integrate data from various sources and use them to plan, implement, and evaluate their efforts.

> RECOMMENDATION 4-1: The Centers for Disease Control and Prevention (CDC) should sustain, enhance, and regularly update Population Level Analysis and Community Estimates (PLACES) as a data tool that communities can access for locally relevant, granular (i.e., census tract and ZIP code) data and the ability to compare themselves to peers. CDC should enhance PLACES in collaboration with the Substance Abuse and Mental Health Services Administration to add measures relevant to mental, emotional, and behavioral health and population well-being, and support functionalities to PLACES that allow community partnerships to layer their own data on PLACES data for their planning and evaluation efforts.

> RECOMMENDATION 4-2: The Substance Abuse and Mental Health Services Administration, Centers for Disease Control and Prevention, and other federal agencies that provide resources for community-based prevention of behavioral disorders should include specific support for data infrastructure in all relevant grant programs, including funding for acquiring relevant data, data integrity and privacy, new data collection, data sharing, collaboration with relevant public- and private-sector partners, and obtaining training and technical assistance as needed.

Federal agencies and others have explored measures of subjective well-being, and the committee asserts that they can be used in tracking MEB health. A measure of population well-being would provide a more expansive way to track progress of programs and policies, complementing specific national measures, such as overdose and suicide deaths, and framing a positive high-level target for the prevention infrastructure.

RECOMMENDATION 4-3: To identify and adopt measures of population well-being that allow the nation to track progress and report on mental, emotional, and behavioral health, the Office of the Assistant Secretary of Health, National Center for Health Statistics, and the Substance Abuse and Mental Health Services Administration should convene and collaborate with relevant partners.

The measure(s) would be disaggregated by socioeconomic factors; race; and ethnicity, age, and geography.

Relevant partners may include the Health and Human Services (HHS) Office of the National Coordinator of Health Information Technology and national public health organizations, such as the Association of State and Territorial Health Officials and the National Indian Health Board.

Governance

The governance structure for prevention of MEB disorders is fragmented, with separate lines of oversight and funding for mental health and substance use disorder (SUD) and far less attention to prevention compared to reactive responses to needs for treatment and recovery. The White House has an Office of National Drug Control Policy that, though originating in the War on Drugs, has evolved to oversee a broad-based array of efforts oriented toward both treatment and prevention. But this is a SUD silo, as linkages to mental health (MH) are minimal.

SAMHSA, like the broader BH enterprise, is asymmetrical in its organizational structure, with greater attention to preventing substance use than other MEB disorders, reflected by the existence of the Centers for Substance Use Prevention and SUD Treatment compared with the singular Center for Mental Health Services, which supports treatment and prevention work with emphasis on serious mental illness.

RECOMMENDATION 5-1: To strengthen capacity and coordination to promote mental, emotional, and behavioral (MEB) health and population well-being, governance structures for prevention should be added at each level in the Executive Branch.

a. The White House could establish a central point for MEB prevention capacity and coordination. There are two options for doing this: appointing a special assistant on MEB disorder prevention to the president who serves on the Domestic Policy Council or establishing a new office on MEB prevention in the White House. Either the special assistant or the new office would coordinate with the Office of National Drug Control Policy and the Office of Management and Budget and convene all executive branch departments with a role in prevention, perhaps through an interagency task force. An office would require more resources than a special assistant but could support a more robust portfolio of efforts to streamline and enhance coordination throughout the Executive Branch. There is a history of interagency task forces spearheaded or called for by an administration to help implement a strategic objective. The relevant executive branch departments include Health and Human Services (HHS), Department of Education, Department of Veterans Affairs, Department of Defense,[4] U.S. Department of Agriculture, Department of Justice, Department of Labor, and Department of Treasury;

b. The HHS Behavioral Health Coordinating Council (or similar intra-departmental entity) could establish a workgroup on promoting MEB health and preventing MEB disorders and adopt strategies to engage individuals with lived experience; and

c. Congress could expand the Substance Abuse and Mental Health Services Administration's (SAMHSA's) ability to support state, tribal, and local MEB disorder prevention efforts by either establishing a Center for Prevention of Behavioral Disorders that integrates the agency's prevention activities or by establishing a Center for Mental Health Promotion (equal to and working closely with the existing Center for Substance Abuse Prevention). In addition, the SAMHSA administrator, who is also the Assistant Secretary for Mental Health and Substance Use, should appoint a prevention advisor to support and report on state efforts to prioritize prevention.

Funding

The committee estimates that federal prevention funding for MEB disorders is approximately $4.57 billion—allocated to several HHS agencies, the Department of Education, and other federal departments and agencies. This funding is not adequate to deliver necessary preventive interventions to all communities. For example, prevention-specific parts of the budgets of SAMHSA and the Administration for Children and Families (ACF) have not kept up with inflation, and the Community Mental Health Services Block Grant has no prevention set-aside, unlike the Substance Use Prevention, Treatment, and Recovery Services Block Grant.

Descriptions of major programs often pair the words "prevention and treatment," which suggests that prevention funding is more robust than it is.

---

[4] DoD's prevention integration initiative is illustrative of high-level attention to prevention in domains external to HHS. https://www.prevention.mil/ (accessed October 1, 2025).

Most of the funding for behavioral health services is directed toward treatment and addressing the opioid crisis; more is needed to support primary prevention. Increasing funding for prevention could be focused on the four agencies that provide the most support for prevention of MEB disorders. More dependable funding could support implementation of evidence-based programs (EBP); help strengthen the workforce; facilitate greater access to data to inform prevention work and show improved outcomes; and nurture greater coordination and collaboration in governance and partnerships at the state and local levels. The approaches to funding could range from transformative—for example, investing holistically in MEB prevention during the impactful period from birth to 18 years of age—to narrow—such as inflation adjusting and modestly increasing capacity.

> **RECOMMENDATION 6-1:** To secure adequate, sustainable, and locally responsive funding for the mental, emotional, and behavioral disorder prevention infrastructure, Congress should consider a range of funding options that includes:
>
> a. Providing $14 billion in new funding to the Department of Health and Human Services for interventions on early life risk factors for mental, emotional, and behavioral (MEB) disorders for all children birth to 18 years old.
> b. At a time of funding constraints, providing $1.8 billion in new funding to the Administration for Children and Families, Centers for Disease Control and Prevention, Health Resources and Services Administration, and Substance Abuse and Mental Health Services Administration would help to increase capacity for MEB disorder prevention.

Investing $14 billion across federal agencies delivering mental, emotional, and behavioral health preventive services to children and youth (up to 18 years old) would include but is not limited to the Administration for Children and Families (ACF), CDC, Health Resources and Services Administration (HRSA), and SAMHSA. Fourteen billion dollars is based on an estimate of $218 per child to provide MEB prevention services to the approximately 74 million U.S. children from birth to 18 years old. Such a commitment could ensure that all children in every community have access to the package of interventions they need to address risk factors and support positive trajectories to MEB health (e.g., reducing risk for, incidence, and severity of depression, anxiety, suicide, and substance use disorders, including alcohol use disorder, and improving general mental health and resilience along the life course as children grow up).

In a setting of fiscal constraints, a more modest $1.8 billion in new funding could be allocated to the four key federal agencies responsible for prevention of MEB disorders, which includes adjusting for inflation for specific ACF and SAMHSA programs and expanding the capacity of specific MEB health-relevant programs in CDC and HRSA. As shown in Appendix F, this amounts to a 40 percent increase from $4.57 billion to $6.37 billion. New funding would allow greater capacity of service delivery in settings along the life course, from preconception through older adulthood.

Detailed calculations describing each of the options above are provided in Appendix F. These increases can be achieved partly by restoring the Prevention and Public Health Fund to its original amount of $2 billion to support SAMHSA and CDC prevention programs.

Medicaid reimbursement is a crucial source of funding for BH services, but barriers exist related to staffing, setting, benefits, and eligibility. Specifically, some types of workers, community settings, and population-level preventive interventions are difficult or impossible to pay with Medicaid dollars. Medicaid does not pay for population-level preventive interventions, such as public health communication campaigns. However, its amendments, authorities, flexibilities, and waivers offer opportunities for greater adaptability and experimentation. Interventions to prevent MEB disorders and promote MEB health could be supported through a range of approaches that create more sustainable, coordinated, and adequate funding beginning with greater flexibility and innovation in federal sources.

RECOMMENDATION 6-2: The committee recommends that the Centers for Medicare & Medicaid Services should

a. Encourage states to use Medicaid 1115 waivers to implement evidence-based approaches for prevention of mental, emotional, and behavioral (MEB) disorders. Potential approaches could focus on school-based strategies and the work of multisector partnerships in other community settings (e.g., accountable communities for health, faith-based, aging services) that are implementing population-based universal interventions (e.g., environmental change, media campaigns).
b. Prioritize specific quality metrics relevant to prevention of MEB disorders, e.g., screening for alcohol misuse, depression, and anxiety in all value-based purchasing programs under Medicaid and Medicare.
c. Facilitate reimbursement of non-licensed non-clinical MEB prevention workers (e.g., prevention specialists, community health workers) considered qualified to deliver such interventions.

Opportunities to generate additional resources to support the promotion of MEB health include public sector incentives and public–private partnerships. One potential source of funding is health system community benefit resources, which most tax-exempt hospital and health systems spend in a manner that does not further their population health improvement goals and is not aligned with the spirit of providing a community benefit. Innovative mechanisms have also been tested in a variety of states and jurisdictions.

> RECOMMENDATION 6-3: Congress should adopt and support the implementation of new or innovative funding mechanisms to generate sustainable and sufficient resources for promoting mental, emotional, and behavioral (MEB) health and for prevention, particularly primary, of MEB disorders by:
>
> a. Offering incentives, such as tax credits, for large-scale social impact investing that supports universal prevention.
> b. Directing the Internal Revenue Service (IRS) to provide guidance on how tax-exempt hospitals can use community benefit funding to support MEB disorder prevention in communities where behavioral disorders are priority health needs within the mandated Community Health Needs Assessment. Specifically, the IRS should modify Lines 3, 6, 7, and 8 of Part II of IRS Schedule H (Form 990) that is used to monitor community benefit spending to specifically include MEB disorder prevention.

> RECOMMENDATION 6-4: State and territorial legislatures and tribal councils, respectively, should adopt and support the implementation of new or innovative funding mechanisms to generate sustainable and sufficient resources for promoting mental, emotional, and behavioral (MEB) health, and prevention, particularly primary, of MEB disorders.

Such mechanisms could include the following:

- Enact new or revise current excise taxes to earmark funding to MEB health promotion programs:
    - New potential sources of funding include sales of recreational cannabis and social media advertising taxes; and
    - Revision of alcohol excise taxes to bring them up to inflation-adjusted levels.
- Establish prevention and wellness funds, which are pools of resources raised to support community prevention efforts;
- Establish children's cabinets and equivalent mechanisms to more effectively coordinate multiagency funding toward a shared mission; and
- Use bonds, including social impact bonds (also known as pay-for-success financing), to support MEB prevention interventions.

Too often, savings that accrue from effective implementation of MEB health interventions are not directly realized by the programs that invest in them. This fails to provide policy makers with an accurate accounting on their return on investment.

> RECOMMENDATION 6-5: The Assistant Secretary for Planning and Evaluation should work with relevant experts to develop a comprehensive economic model that tests the downstream effects of investments in mental, emotional, and behavioral (MEB) disorder prevention. The model should include a range of inputs (e.g., quality early care and education), beneficiary federal agencies (e.g., Department of Health and Human Services/Centers for Medicare & Medicaid Services), and private-sector entities (employers/payers) that will reap the savings from enhancing mental, emotional, and behavioral health at a population level and eliminating MEB health disparities.

The Congressional Budget Office could refer to the model in informing the work of policy makers.

Evidence-Based Prevention Through Policy

The committee found that evidence-based social and economic policies influence trajectories toward MEB disorders, such as linkages between poverty and risk factors for poor MEB outcomes or economic stability bolstered by the Earned Income Tax Credit reducing psychological distress. New evidence on the importance of policy has been emerging in the areas of mass incarceration and exposure to firearm violence, two issues that uniquely affect U.S. children and disproportionately affect racial and ethnic minority communities.

Policies that are shown to have positive effects are not always sustained. For example, free school meals are associated with better MEB health and well-being in children and improved educational outcomes, but the pandemic-era waiver that provided free school meals for all students was ended and only a few states opted to support a continuation of it.

> RECOMMENDATION 7-1: In keeping with the Foundations for Evidence-Based Policymaking Act of 2018, federal and state policy makers should use the best available evidence to sustain, restore, develop, or de-implement social and economic policies, considering the direct or indirect effects of such policies on mental, emotional, and behavioral health and population well-being.

Incarceration constitutes a risk factor for MEB disorders for both the individuals incarcerated and their families, with a detrimental impact on the

MEB health of millions of children and adults in the United States. Incarceration also catalyzes additional trajectories toward poor outcomes, such as loss of parental custody and risk of criminal activity and substance use. Research indicates that there are many opportunities to intervene before incarceration, such as civil court, drug courts, and community programming for youth, overseen by the juvenile criminal legal system. Also, efforts to reduce exposure of youth to incarceration have been shown to yield better MEB outcomes and decrease recidivism.

> RECOMMENDATION 7-2: Federal, state, and county officials should enact evidence-based policies to divert from the criminal legal system and reduce reliance on incarceration where appropriate, while simultaneously building a robust community prevention infrastructure, thus enabling protective factors that support mental, emotional, and behavioral health.

Exposure to firearm violence is a major cause of MEB disorders. The 2024 U.S. Surgeon General Advisory asserted that "beyond the profound consequences of surviving a firearm-related injury, those who do not experience direct bodily harm often grapple with mental health consequences related to firearm violence exposure, including community members, children and adolescents, and families."[5] Firearm violence disproportionately affects youth residing in rural communities and Black youth who experience higher rates of exposure to assaults, police shootings, and community violence. Black individuals are nearly 14 times more likely to die from firearm homicide than White individuals, and their inpatient admission rates for firearm-related injuries are nine times higher. Additionally, more than 7 out of every 10 veteran deaths by suicide (already significantly higher rates than non-veterans) are by firearm. Firearm violence erodes MEB health, directly contributing to poor MEB outcomes including suicide, depression, and anxiety, especially for youth and heavily affected communities.

> RECOMMENDATION 7-3: Federal, state, and local policy makers should implement evidence-based policies to prevent firearm violence—a risk factor for mental, emotional, and behavioral disorders—including but not limited to safe and secure gun storage, community violence interventions, and lethal means safety counseling.

Research undertaken or supported by different federal agencies has demonstrated the possibility of positive effects of policies on MEB health. Examples include housing vouchers and rental assistance, urban green spaces, and the Medicaid Early and Periodic Screening, Diagnostic, and

---

[5] https://www.hhs.gov/sites/default/files/firearm-violenceadvisory.pdf, p. 14 (accessed November 20, 2024).

Treatment benefit. However, MEB outcomes are not consistently included as a policy target, which represents a missed opportunity to learn whether and to what extent policies are effective at preventing MEB disorders.

> **RECOMMENDATION 7-4:** The Department of Health and Human Services (through the National Institutes of Health, Centers for Disease Control and Prevention, and Centers for Medicare & Medicaid Services) and the relevant research entities in the Departments of Defense, Education, Housing and Urban Development, Justice, and Veterans Affairs should direct more targeted funding to research that assesses mental, emotional, and behavioral health and population well-being outcomes related to specific policies directed at social, economic, and environmental factors. Studies should include direction and strength of associations as well as an assessment of causality.

Examples for how the guiding principle of health equity and implementation science can be operationalized in the infrastructure are discussed in each chapter and include:

- Shared governance with communities and people with lived experience;
- Assurance that the evidence about programs is generalizable and represents the communities where they will be implemented and new knowledge generated feeds back into the evidence base;
- A workforce that reflects the community is culturally and linguistically competent; and
- Distribution of funding to support MEB health promotion efforts that targets the communities and subpopulations that bear the highest burden of risk factors and poor outcomes.

Implementation scientists, organizations that provide technical assistance, and others engaged in the translation of knowledge are helping to close the research-to-practice gap and inform best practices for pre-implementation, implementation, and sustainment of evidence-based interventions across settings and communities where prevention services are being delivered.

With resources and data, expertise, leadership and partnerships, and several evidence-based and promising approaches to draw on, the nation can do better in intervening across different settings and along the life course to promote MEB health and prevent MEB disorders. This report provides a blueprint for doing so.

1

Introduction

The central aim of a national prevention infrastructure[1] for mental, emotional, and behavioral (MEB) disorders is to promote people thriving at all stages of life and across all settings in society. Achieving this calls for concerted effort at all levels of government and in community-based multisector partnerships with the objective of creating and sustaining the conditions for infants, children, adolescents and emerging, working, and older adults to experience MEB health and well-being.

Throughout this report, "MEB disorders" is used to describe disorders diagnosable using *Diagnostic and Statistical Manual of Mental Disorders, 5th Edition (DSM-V)* criteria and behaviors associated with them, including violence, aggression, self-injury, suicide, and antisocial behavior. As such, the term "MEB disorders" encompasses mental illness, substance use disorders, and a "broader range of concerns associated with problem behaviors and conditions" (NASEM, 2019, p. 16). Promoting MEB health and well-being in the United States is a focus of a wide range of government and private-sector entities and dedicated prevention workers across a variety of community settings. MEB disorders are at the heart of several ongoing national crises, and the rising prevalence affects every population group, community, and neighborhood in urban, rural, and suburban areas. Treatment and harm reduction are needed to help those who are suffering

---

[1] Infrastructure here refers to "systems, competencies, frameworks, relationships, and resources that enable state and local governments and agencies, along with communities, community-based organizations, and their partners, to perform core functions" central to preventing MEB disorder and promoting health and well-being (NACCHO, n.d.).

or in imminent danger of harm, but to reduce incidence—to keep problems from happening in the first place—primary prevention and health promotion are essential.[2]

The good news is, many MEB disorders can be prevented, and the benefit of doing so is indisputable, measured in lives and resources saved (TFAH, 2009). Unfortunately, despite proven benefits to prevention, a fragmented, unevenly developed, and inadequately funded infrastructure along with deficits in implementation (e.g., to move proven interventions into practice) impede prevention efforts at the federal, state, local, and tribal levels.

Other National Academies of Sciences, Engineering, and Medicine (National Academies) reports have focused on evidence-based approaches for promoting MEB well-being in young people (of note, the report series that includes *Reducing Risks for Mental Disorders* [IOM, 1994], *Preventing Mental, Emotional, and Behavioral Disorders Among Young People* [NRC and IOM, 2009], and *Fostering Healthy Mental, Emotional, and Behavioral Development in Youth* [NASEM, 2019]). This report builds on that foundation by putting forward guidance to support the dissemination, implementation, and sustainment of effective prevention strategies throughout the life course by building a more robust infrastructure. That infrastructure comprises governance and partnerships; funding; data systems; workforce, training, and technical assistance; and the evolving evidence base for both programs to be implemented in a range of settings, and policies that influence the prevalence and distribution of protective and risk factors for MEB health. Risk factors are "characteristics at the biological, psychological, family, community, or cultural level that precede and are associated with a higher likelihood of negative outcomes" and protective factors are "positive countering events" and "characteristics associated with a lower likelihood of negative outcomes or that reduce a risk factor's impact" and generally support healthy outcomes (SAMHSA, 2019). Protective and risk factors may be fixed or variable/modifiable. Variable risk factors include but are not limited to income level and adverse childhood experiences.

This chapter describes the committee's charge and the committee's approach, explains the urgency for action, outlines the prevention ecosystem, and offers a timeline of the history of prevention for MEB disorders and other important milestones.

CHARGE TO THE COMMITTEE

In August 2023, the Health and Medicine Division of the National Academies launched this study at the request of the National Institutes of Health (NIH), Substance Abuse and Mental Health Services Administration (SAMHSA), and Centers for Disease Control and Prevention

---

[2] That is, on interventions intended to prevent and mitigate risk factors for MEB disorders.

(CDC).[3] The committee appointed by the National Academies was asked to create an actionable blueprint to develop, support, and sustain a national infrastructure focused on preventing mental illness and SUDs (see Box 1-1 for the complete statement of task). The National Academies accordingly convened this authoring committee, which has expertise in prevention science, implementation science, health and human services research, public health research and policy, the criminal-legal system, substance use and mental health (MH) research, economics and finance, and developing interventions to address behavioral health disparities (see Appendix A for biographical information of each committee member).

This report serves as the committee's response to the charge. It outlines a path forward for leadership and governance on multiple levels to grow and sustain the infrastructure to prevent MEB disorders. It reviews the landscape of how preventive programs are funded and delivered, who implements them, what policies support and sustain them, and what implementation strategies and other technical assistance are required. Finally, it offers recommendations—for improving and strengthening each of these infrastructure components—to Congress, federal agencies, including the report sponsors, and other partners, including national organizations that represent different categories of public health leaders in state, local, and tribal contexts.

CONTEXT FOR THE STUDY

The Need for Action Now

The United States continues to experience worsening MEB outcomes that affect individuals, families, communities, schools, congregations, and workplaces. These include the increase between 2013 and 2021 in youth reporting persistent feelings of sadness or hopelessness in the past year and the increase between 2013 and 2021 in youth seriously considering attempting suicide (CDC, 2024b). Other noteworthy figures include the increase in the overdose death rate between 1999 and 2022 (NIDA, 2024) and the increase in the age-adjusted suicide rate in 2021 and 2022, largely led by males 75 years and older (Zilkha et al., 2024). One recent bright spot has been the decline in

---

[3] The following centers, institutes, and offices supported the study: **CDC:** National Center for Injury Prevention and Control, Office of the Director; **NIH:** Division of Program Coordination, Planning, and Strategic Initiatives Office of Disease Prevention, Office of Behavioral and Social Science Research, National Cancer Institute Office of the Director, National Institute for Dental and Craniofacial Research Office of the Director, National Institute of Mental Health Office of the Director, National Institute on Alcohol Abuse and Alcoholism Office of the Director, National Institute on Drug Abuse Office of the Director, National Institute of Nursing Research Division of Extramural Science Programs, National Institute on Minority Health and Health Disparities Office of the Director, National Center for Complementary and Integrative Health Office of the Director; and **SAMHSA** Center for Substance Abuse Prevention Office of the Director.

> **BOX 1-1**
> **Statement of Task**
>
> The National Academy of Sciences, Engineering, and Medicine will convene an ad hoc committee to develop a blueprint, including specific, actionable steps for building and sustaining an infrastructure for delivering prevention interventions targeting risk factors for behavioral health disorders. In conducting its work, the committee will
>
> 1. Identify best practices for creating a sustainable behavioral health prevention infrastructure. Review the landscape of behavioral health prevention at different levels (e.g., national and state, including evidence-based prevention services); where different levels of these prevention services (e.g., universal, selected, and indicated services) could be delivered (e.g., within the community, health care settings, justice systems, schools, human services settings); the workforce needed (investment and their training); and the data systems necessary to track prevention needs, outcomes, and program delivery. Informed by this review, the committee will identify the optimal characteristics and components of a sustainable behavioral health prevention infrastructure. For this infrastructure, the committee should consider embedding prevention services within existing systems and settings, establishing an independent prevention delivery system to which existing systems and settings can refer individuals and families for the receipt of prevention services, and/or other possible approaches

the rate of opioid overdose deaths beginning in the second half of 2022 and continuing into 2024 (NIDA, 2024) and sustained decline in 2024 (CDC, n.d.-a).

The effects of increases in MEB disorders include staggering loss of life and significant mental, social, and economic costs for individuals, families, communities, and the nation as a whole (Abramson et al. 2024). In addition to the overall burden for all of the United States, specific sub-populations as described below, such as Black and American Indian and Alaska Native, experience a disproportionate burden of MEB disorders (Dawes et al., 2024; Morales et al., 2020).

Highlighting the Scope of the Problem

- Suicide is the 11th leading cause of death overall (48,100 deaths in 2021), the second leading cause among people ages 10–14 and

by which behavioral health prevention programs can be delivered and sustained.
2. Identify funding needs and strategies. Review current funding sources for prevention, identify ways those funding sources could be better deployed (including ways to facilitate the integration of funding streams at the state level to be more impactful), and identify new or emerging funding sources that could be redirected and deployed in a coordinated effort to support the prevention infrastructure (e.g., use of opioid settlement funds).
3. Identify specific research gaps germane to the widespread adoption of evidence-based behavioral health prevention interventions. Identify key policy and implementation knowledge gaps and the resulting research opportunities that could provide the information needed to support the adoption and sustainment of a national prevention infrastructure for behavioral health. Research gaps are expected to be identified in the realms of policy research and health services research (e.g., dissemination and implementation, economic analyses).
4. Make actionable recommendations. Recommend how federal and state policies could be expanded or implemented to develop and sustain the prevention infrastructure system, including those that improve financing for evidence-based prevention and support workforce development, data interoperability, and evidence-based policy making. Recommendations for research necessary to fill the prevention services research gaps should also be identified.

25–34, and the third leading cause for ages 15–24 (NIMH, n.d.). Suicide deaths have been increasing since the pandemic-related funding and government supports were removed, only to return to prepandemic levels. The U.S. suicide death rate is the highest among 10 peer nations (Gunja et al., 2023).

- In urban areas, White non-Hispanic people have the highest suicide rates (Ivey-Stephenson et al., 2017); in rural areas, non-Hispanic American Indian and Alaska Native (AIAN, per the U.S. Census Bureau) people have the highest rates (CDC, n.d.-b).
- The drug overdose rate in adolescents was 2.40 per 100,000 in 2010 (518 deaths) and increased to 5.49 (1,146 deaths) in 2021 (Friedman et al., 2022).
- Deaths related to alcohol have increased by 29.3 percent from 2016–2017 to 2020–2021 (Esser et al., 2024).

- Firearms are the leading cause of death among children, and more than three-quarters of adults experience stress associated with fear of a mass shooting; 51 percent of children aged 14–17 report fears of a school shooting (OSG, 2024).
- Survey data collected between July 2021 and December 2022 indicate that among adolescents aged 12–17, 21 percent reported symptoms of anxiety in the past 2 weeks and 17 percent reported depression symptoms, and that over the decade between 2011 and 2021, adolescents reporting feelings of sadness and hopelessness increased from 28 to 42 percent (Panchal, 2024).
- The economic cost of mental illness is an estimated $282 billion annually (Abramson et al., 2024).
- The economic cost of opioid use and overdose deaths during 2017 was $1,021 billion (Luo et al., 2021).
- Easy access to firearms makes suicide attempts much more likely to succeed, and half of suicide deaths are from firearms (Miller et al., 2013).

Highlighting the Scope of the Problem in Populations that Experience Disproportionate Burdens

- Between 2020 and 2021, the age-adjusted rate of drug overdose deaths rose more than 14 percent. In 2021, AIAN people had the highest overall rate (56.6 per 100,000), followed by non-Hispanic Black (44.2) and White (36.8) people (Spencer et al., 2022).
- "Native Hawaiian or Other Pacific Islander and non-Hispanic AIAN people experienced the largest percentage increases in drug overdose death rates from 2020 through 2021, with rates increasing by 47 percent and 33 percent, respectively" (Spencer et al., 2022, p. 3).
- In 2022, the suicide rate in AI/AN people was 91 percent higher than that of the general population, and suicide is the second leading cause of death for non-Hispanic AI/AN people ages 10–34 (CDC, 2024a; HHS, n.d.).
- In 2022, suicide was the leading cause of death for Asian American youth ages 15–24 years. In 2023, Asian American adults were 50 percent less likely to have received mental health treatment than non-Hispanic White adults (OMH, 2024).

The COVID-19 pandemic revealed the precarity of many U.S. families, schools, and communities, and the moment of national crisis offered opportunities to enact policies that have had far-reaching effects, such as the expansion of the Child Tax Credit White House Executive Order 13985: Advancing Racial Equity and Support for Underserved Communities, and American Rescue Plan Act,[4] which provided vital support for early childhood care and education, and Elementary and Secondary School Emergency Relief Fund, which gave state education agencies $122.8 billion in grants to support schools. These policy actions stabilized systems under strain and offered a glimpse of what is possible in strengthening systems of care (ACF, 2021; Randi, 2021).

Although the public- and private-sector institutions, facilities, services, funding, and workforce for addressing the MEB crises are largely focused on treatment (i.e., intervening after problems arise), the foundations for an effective prevention infrastructure may be found at every level of government and in most communities. Promoting well-being is a key aspect of preventing MEB conditions across the life course and the multifaceted solution that this report addresses is infrastructure.

Comparing the United States to Peer Nations

The United States compares unfavorably to most of its peer nations regarding MEB health and well-being and on multiple measures of health, from life expectancy at birth to infant mortality. The economic insecurity many people face from the lack of effective social policy has negative effects on MEB well-being. Examples include the lack of paid parental leave, which has been linked with postpartum depression; and the lack of paid sick leave—dramatically highlighted by the COVID-19 pandemic—which makes the United States an extreme outlier compared to approximately four-fifths of the world and most high-income countries, and affects medical recovery and caregiving (Heymann et al., 2020; Hidalgo-Padilla et al., 2023).

International comparisons on MH needs indicate that U.S. people experience high MH needs (37 percent, second only to Australians at 41 percent). Also, they are the most likely to forgo needed MH services because of cost (18 percent, compared to 16 percent of Australians, 13 percent of Canadians, 9 percent of New Zealanders and Britons, and 8 percent of Swiss) (Gunja et al., 2024). Before the need for treatment arises, many other wealthy nations have implemented strategies to promote well-being and prevent MEB disorders. These include public health campaigns and population-level interventions, such as the Netherlands' "Well-being at School" national program that integrates preventive interventions,

---

[4] American Rescue Plan Act of 2021, Public Law 117-2, 117th Cong., 1st sess. (March 11, 2021).

teacher and parent education, and school policy changes (Williams, 2024). A Commonwealth Fund report found that "[s]ome countries have begun to recognize that MEB issues are often rooted in or exacerbated by societal problems such as racism, workplace stress, and unemployment. To promote well-being, leaders have sought to ameliorate such systemic factors while also offering support to those coping with their effects" (Hostetter and Klein, 2021). For example, Australia has launched and funds "headspace centers" that are overseen by a nonprofit and provide both MH services and a variety of social supports, such as helping young people find jobs. This is a nonstigmatizing, community-based approach to supporting the MH and well-being of young people.

Although U.S. public- and private-sector institutions, facilities, services, funding, and workforce for addressing these crises are largely focused on treatment, the foundations for an effective prevention infrastructure may be found at every level of government and in most communities and will be strengthened by the recommendations made by this report.

Why Well-Being?

Well-being is a more holistic way to consider the outcomes of an effective prevention infrastructure, and the report generally mentions MEB health and well-being as a broad label. In the context of health measurement, well-being is a broad construct (see the World Health Organization definition of health as "a state of complete physical, mental and social well-being and not merely the absence of disease or infirmity of health") (WHO, 2024). There are measures of objective and subjective well-being, and the discussion is focused on the latter. Well-being has been defined as "how people think, feel, and function—at a personal and social level—and how they evaluate their lives as a whole" (Pronk et al., 2021, p. 243) and "a relative state where one maximizes his or her physical, mental and social functioning in the context of supportive environments to live a full, satisfying, and productive life" (Kobau et al., 2010).

MEB health refers to key components of well-being that reflect progress in whether individuals and communities are able to flourish and thrive (Rule et al., 2024). Multiple indicators of MH support this picture. One example is the United States's poor performance on the World Happiness Index (Helliwell, 2024), which describes well-being in the United States to have steadily dropped, placing the United States 23rd in international standings. Of particular concern is the finding that the well-being of younger U.S. people has declined the most of any age group (Helliwell, 2024), indicating that the nation's resiliency and strength is in serious jeopardy.

Value of Prevention

The best-known public health typology of prevention levels is primordial, primary, secondary, and tertiary.[5] The typology frequently used in the context of MEB health—universal, selective, and indicated—refers to targeting preventive interventions to the entire population, groups at increased risk, and individuals showing early signs of exposure/subclinical condition respectively.

Despite significant efforts to support those suffering with MEB disorders, that work has largely been done at the secondary and tertiary prevention levels. Far greater attention and funding is needed for primordial and primary prevention, and implementing prevention requires partnering with all affected communities to build the capacity and secure and deploy the resources needed to implement evidence-driven programming. In addition to greater resources shifted toward preventive services, a strategic investment will focus especially on communities that are under-resourced and/or have historically experienced disinvestment. This is critical to not only prevent disorder, disability, reduced quality of life, and unnecessary deaths but to promote well-being. Investing in the implementation, infrastructure, and programs to support the scale-up of prevention has a clear return on investment not only from a cost-savings perspective but also in disability-adjusted life years averted. For example, a study modeling the return on investment on preventing and treating adolescent MH disorders and suicide using a package of evidence-based interventions across 36 countries that account for 80 percent of the burden measured in disability-adjusted life years showed $23.6 return per $1 spent over 80 years (Stelmach et al., 2022).[6]

THE PREVENTION ECOSYSTEM[7]

Within the U.S. Department of Health and Human Services (HHS), NIH includes several institutes, centers, and offices with missions relevant

---

[5] That is, on interventions intended to prevent and mitigate risk factors for MEB disorders. Primordial prevention – interventions that address social conditions and root causes of disorders; primary prevention = interventions to reduce risk factors and promote protective factors to prevent the onset of disease; secondary prevention = interventions that identify disease before it is symptomatic to treat early and reduce severity; tertiary prevention = interventions to prevent significant adverse consequences once a disease has been established.

[6] In addition to MEB health investments, evidence-based prevention programs to increase physical activity, prevent smoking, and improve nutrition can yield $5.60 in savings on every $1 spent (TFA, 2008).

[7] While prevention research, science, and practice sometimes does not always distinguish between MEB and physical health outcomes, the focus of this description is on entities that address MEB disorder prevention.

to prevention; SAMHSA has a Center for Substance Abuse Prevention and preventive functions within the Center for Mental Health Services, and CDC's National Center for Injury Prevention and Control operates the agency's behavioral health (BH) coordinating unit. Several other federal agencies also conduct prevention-related research or provide services (see Chapter 2 for a sample of clearinghouses of evidence-based prevention programs managed by federal agencies). The Indian Health Service Division of Behavioral Health includes a focus on primary prevention of MEB disorders. The state and local levels have BH agencies or public health agencies with BH units. There are also national associations (e.g., the National Association of State Alcohol and Drug Abuse Directors, the National Association of State Mental Health Directors, CADCA, formerly known as the Community Anti-Drug Coalitions of America), research groups, such as the Society for Prevention Research, and the academic networks of Prevention Technology Transfer Centers (and to a lesser extent the Mental Health Technology Transfer Centers, which were shuttered in September 2024),[8] as well as the prevention research centers, etc. This rich ecosystem (see Table 1-1) is better developed for the substance use components of the prevention end of the continuum, and it will take better coordination, more robust and sustainable funding, and more integrated governance of prevention functions at the federal level and with state and tribal partners to move toward a stronger prevention infrastructure.

A Brief History and Milestones

The United States was not always so predominantly focused on treatment of MEB disorders. In the interwar period leading into the Second World War, the approach to MH was focused on mental hygiene in workers so that society could nurture a productive workforce. As the medical field advanced, however, the focus shifted to the individual level, and medical breakthroughs and exposés on horrid conditions within institutions for the mentally ill led to the closure of many of them (Harrington, 2023). The Community Mental Health Act of 1963 represented a change that, in theory, brought treatment into the community, shifting it out of state hospitals. But states and the federal government did not create enough or adequately resource community capacity to take care of deinstitutionalized patients or respond to the considerable needs of people with serious mental illness (IOM, 1991).

Although the onus is not on individual practitioners, the following quote highlights a recognition of the broad context in which MEB disorders arise: "[P]sychiatrists must . . . distinguish between those areas in which [system and structural] social forces rather than psychiatric illness are at

---

[8] See https://mhttcnetwork.org/ for more info (accessed October 14, 2024).

TABLE 1-1 The Prevention Ecosystem in Which the MEB Prevention Infrastructure Is Embedded

Part of Ecosystem	Sample Relevant Entities
Governance and funding: federal and tribal	U.S. Department of Health and Human Services: Substance Abuse and Mental Health Services Administration (SAMHSA), National Institutes of Health (NIH), Centers for Disease Control and Prevention (CDC), Indian Health Service, Centers for Medicare & Medicaid Services, Health Resources and Services Administration, and the Administration for Children and Families, and Administration for Community Living
	U.S. Departments of Veterans Affairs; Defense; Education; Agriculture; Justice
	White House Office of National Drug Control Policy
Governance and funding: state	Single state agency for substance use, MH, or substance use & MH
	State public health agency
	State Medicaid
Governance, funding, and partnerships: local	Coalitions (e.g., on substance use disorder/Drug Free Communities; violence prevention)
	Accountable communities for health
	Other community entities, such as community health needs assessment advisory groups. Could include other types of partnerships or networks in a variety of systems/settings or associated with individual agencies
Knowledge creation	NIH (multiple institutes and centers, e.g., National Institute on Drug Abuse, National Institute of Mental Health, Office of Disease Prevention, National Institute on Alcohol Abuse and Alcoholism, National Institute on Minority Health and Health Disparities); CDC; research entities in other federal government departments
	Academic institutions
	Other evidence-based intervention developers
	Practice-based research networks and partnerships
Knowledge translation, technical assistance for service delivery	SAMHSA-funded Prevention Technology Transfer Centers
	NIH Clinical and Translational Service Awards program and AHRQ Healthcare Extension Service
	CDC-funded Prevention Research Centers
	Bi-regional centers supported by SAMHSA Center for Mental Health: Dissemination, Implementation, and Sustainment
	Other training and technical assistance providers
	Community health centers
	Clearinghouses

continued

TABLE 1-1 Continued

Part of Ecosystem	Sample Relevant Entities
Knowledge sharers/ dissemination	SAMHSA National Mental Health and Substance Use Policy Laboratory, Society for Prevention Research
	Society for Research in Child Development and other research organizations
	National Prevention Science Coalition to Improve Lives
	National associations: National Association of State Alcohol and Drug Agency Directors, National Association of State Mental Health Program Directors, National Association of City and County Health Officials, National Association of County Behavioral Health and Disability Directors, CADCA, National Indian Health Board, National Council of Urban Indian Health, Association of State and Territorial Health Officials
Systems and settings	Human services (child welfare, aging services)
	Public health
	Education
	Criminal-legal
	Health care (including national associations)
	Tribal

NOTES: This table should not be considered an exhaustive description of the ecosystem. MEB = mental, behavioral, and emotional.

fault . . . then the psychiatrist must be willing to try to meet social needs and handle the wide range of psychiatric problems" (Erickson, 2021, p. 7).

Structuring governance for the field has also long been a key concern, as SAMHSA, National Institute of Mental Health, National Institute on Drug Abuse (NIDA), and National Institute on Alcohol Abuse and Alcoholism were once grouped together under the same agency, in a long-evolving effort to find the optimal forms of governance and funding for MEB health research, prevention, and treatment services (see Table 1-2). The history of the field reflects broader tensions between the biomedical and population health paradigms and between pathologizing approaches focused on the individual compared with a broad focus on social and environmental factors that shape risk for and protection from MEB disorders (Acolin and Fishman, 2023).

THE COMMITTEE'S APPROACH

The statement of task called on the committee to describe an infrastructure to deliver preventive interventions that target risk factors and enhance protective factors for behavioral disorders. In considering terminology for

TABLE 1-2 Timeline of Milestones in the History of MEB Health in the United States

Year	Event
1944	The Public Health Service Act enacted (Title V establishes Substance Abuse and Mental Health Services Administration [SAMHSA])
1946	National Mental Health Care Act, National Institute of Mental Health (NIMH), and National Advisory Mental Health Council
1949	NIMH opens
1952	First *Diagnostic and Statistical Manual of Mental Disorders (DSM-I)* published
1963	Community Mental Health Act enacted
1965	First Neighborhood Health Centers launched Medicare and Medicaid Act enacted
1966	National Center for Prevention and Control of Alcoholism, and Center for Studies of Narcotic Addiction and Drug Abuse launched
1968	NIMH reorganized, with a focus on service delivery
1970	National Institute on Alcohol Abuse and Alcoholism (NIAAA) established
1972	NIDA (National Institute on Drug Abuse) established (within NIMH)
1973	NIMH reorganized back to NIH
1974	Alcohol, Drug Abuse, and Mental Health Administration (ADAMHA) created, contained NIMH, NIDA, and NIAAA
1977	President's Commission on Mental Health created
1992	ADAMHA Reorganization Act—NIMH, NIDA, and NIAAA move back to NIH, while service components become part of SAMHSA (a Public Health Service agency); Act includes support for home visiting services (see Chapter 2)
1996	Health Centers Consolidation Act (under Section 330 of the Public Health Service Act, health centers serving communities, migrants, unhoused people, and public housing residents)
1996	Mental Health Parity Act enacted
1999	First U.S. Surgeon General's report on mental health released
2000	Children's Health Act of 2000 enacted
2002	President's New Freedom Commission on MH created
2004	Mentally Ill Offender Treatment and Crime Reduction Act signed into law to provide resources for alternatives to incarceration for youth and adults with mental disorders/SUD
2006	Sober Truth on Preventing Underage Drinking Act
2008	Mental Health Parity and Addiction Equity Act enacted
2009	American Recovery and Reinvestment Act (increased Supplemental Nutrition Assistance Program, expanded Earned Income Tax Credit) enacted
2010	Affordable Care Act enacted, creating the National Prevention, Health Promotion, and Public Health Council (NPC)

continued

TABLE 1-2 Continued

Year	Event
2010	Tribal Law and Order Act enacted, calling for "interagency coordination and collaboration between the Department of Justice, the Department of the Interior, and the Department of Health and Human Services (HHS)" to focus attention to "justice, safety, education, youth, and alcohol and substance abuse prevention and treatment issues relevant to Indian country"
2016	Comprehensive Addiction and Recovery Act enacted
2018	Support for Patients and Communities Act signed into law
2021	Protecting Youth Mental Health—Surgeon General's Advisory[9]
	Behavioral Health Coordinating Council established in HHS to coordinate "all federal government resources to address inequities and gaps within the mental health and substance use disorder system"
2021	HHS Overdose Prevention Strategy announced
2022	Roadmap to Behavioral Health Integration developed, and Behavioral Health Coordinating Council tasked with its implementation
	Restoring Hope for Mental Health and Wellbeing Act
	Surgeon general's framework Workplace Mental Health & Well-Being
2023	Surgeon General issues new advisory about effects of social media use on youth mental health
2024	National Strategy for Suicide Prevention announced, and federal action plan released
	Surgeon General: Why I'm Calling for a Warning Label on Social Media Platforms
	Surgeon General issues advisory on the public health crisis of firearm violence in the United States

NOTE: MEB = mental, emotional, and behavioral.
SOURCES: NIMH, n.d.; NIDA, 2025.

this report, particularly the use of "mental, emotional, and behavioral (MEB) disorders" or "MEB health," the committee noted the use of the phrase "behavioral health disorders" in the statement of task, sponsors' remarks to the committee at the first meeting, and context provided by related National Academies reports that provide detailed reviews of the evidence base of interventions (NASEM, 2019; NRC and IOM, 2009).

---

[9] From the Advisory: "A Surgeon General's Advisory is a public statement that calls the American people's attention to an urgent public health issue and provides recommendations for how it should be addressed. Advisories are reserved for significant public health challenges that need the nation's immediate awareness and action" https://www.hhs.gov/sites/default/files/surgeon-general-youth-mental-health-advisory.pdf (accessed February 28, 2025).

"Behavioral" or "mental" disorders include a variety of conditions defined in the *Diagnostic and Statistical Manual of Mental Disorders* and the *International Classification of Diseases* with clear diagnostic criteria, which can be diagnosed in clinical settings by health care providers. Federal and state agencies, advocacy groups, professional organizations, and other groups use broader terminology to avoid stigma and ensure relevance to a wider audience (see later for examples of some audiences of this report). Accordingly—and, as *Fostering Health Mental Emotional, and Behavioral Development in Children and Youth* did—this report primarily uses "mental, emotional, and behavioral" to describe "both disorders diagnosable using [DSM-V] criteria and the problem behaviors associated with them, such as violence, aggression, self-injury, suicide, and antisocial behavior" (NASEM, 2019, p. 16), thus encompassing mental illness, SUDs, and a broader range of concerns associated with problem behaviors and conditions. This is also reflected in the prevention science field, which largely targets risk and protective factors (which are the same for many conditions and disorders).

The committee offers a blueprint to implement and sustain prevention of MEB disorders in the United States. The infrastructure includes evidence-based programs and policies, funding, workforce, data, and governance and partnerships. The committee did not conduct a comprehensive review of programs, but rather focused on a sampling of different types of programs to illustrate the extant evidence base; the needs for the workforce, data systems, funding, and governance; and needs for future research and the dissemination of evidence. The committee briefly examined high-level economic and social policies that are interventions delivered by policy makers who allocate taxpayer funding to support them and are informed by high-level data, such as Census data and Congressional Budget Office cost calculations. Although the report primarily focuses on the infrastructure for delivering evidence-based programs, the committee interpreted its charge in the light of sponsor remarks at its first open information-gathering meeting in December 2023. In response to clarifying questions from the committee, NIDA director Nora Volkow and SAMHSA Center for Substance Abuse Prevention director Captain Christopher Jones shared reflections on the population-level and structural factors, such as poverty and exposure to adverse childhood experiences, that shape BH outcomes, and the interventions that operate upstream of the disease process.

Given the clarification and urging by the study's sponsors, the committee focused on primary, and, to a lesser extent, primordial and secondary prevention. In addition to describing and making recommendations about the infrastructure needed to support the delivery of preventive programs, the committee also made policy-related recommendations relevant to preventing risk factors and enhancing protective factors. The committee was informed by the socio-ecological model of health that shows the levels of influences on trajectories to certain kinds of outcomes at every level from intrapersonal (genetic and biological—not discussed in this report because they are not modifiable), to interpersonal (e.g., family), institutional, community, and ultimately, public policy. Sloboda (2009) provides an extensive discussion of socialization and related processes and mechanisms that influence behavior along the life course and identifies the points where interventions can be applied.

The committee asserts, echoing the sponsors' comments at the giving of the charge, that social, economic, and environmental policies constitute "upstream" or primordial prevention. Policies may be considered interventions because their enactment can lead to changed outcomes at a population level. But policies also shape the broader social and economic context within which programs are implemented, workers deliver services, and other components of the infrastructure operate. This explains why the report treats policies differently from programs. The report's closing chapter (7) recognizes policy as context for the infrastructure. An in-depth discussion of policy makers as "workforce," national data systems (with the U.S. Census as foundation), and funding needed for high-level policies seemed out of scope or at least unreasonably broad for the present report. Chapter 7 outlines policies that could enhance MEB health opportunities for all. These include evidence-based early-life investments such as home-visiting programs and quality early childhood care and education, and policies and investments that are impactful later in life such as Social Security and housing vouchers. The chapter discusses in more detail the broad categories (and specific examples) of policies shown to have direct effects on MEB outcomes.

The committee approached its task with a few guiding principles front and center in developing this report. The first two are perhaps the most important. First, the use of lessons learned from implementation science (IS) is crucial if the infrastructure and delivery systems it supports are to achieve their goals. IS, a "systematic, scientific approach to ask and answer questions about how we get 'what works' to people who need it, with greater speed, fidelity, efficiency, quality and relevant coverage" (UWDGH, 2024). IS provides not only key insights into implementing discrete interventions or policies but also strategies to sustain a successful infrastructure. IS offers frameworks and approaches that can be used to support sustaining delivery of the intervention as intended and adapting it intentionally and rigorously in response to community and population need. Second, achieving health equity—"the state in which everyone has a fair opportunity to attain full health potential and well-being, and no one is disadvantaged from doing so because of social position or any other socially defined circumstance"—is a key objective of the infrastructure to prevent MEB disorders and promote

MEB well-being (NASEM, 2023). Each chapter includes these guiding principles.

The statement of task asked the committee to "consider embedding prevention services within existing systems and settings, establishing an independent prevention delivery system to which existing systems and settings can refer individuals and families for the receipt of prevention services, and/or other possible approaches by which behavioral health prevention programs can be delivered and sustained." As shown in Figure 1-1, the committee's information gathering demonstrated that existing systems (e.g., education, human services) and settings provide a good foundation for the prevention infrastructure. The committee viewed creating an independent delivery system as inefficient and suboptimal. Taking workforce as an example, teachers and staff in education settings are well placed to implement interventions that are both promotive and protective.

Other principles reflected across and within each chapter: prevention is inherently multidisciplinary (NASEM, 2019; NRC and IOM, 2009); it cannot happen successfully without community-driven partnerships or considerations related to local and cultural contexts.

This report describes the components needed to successfully support the implementation of approaches to prevent MEB disorders and promote MEB health on a national scale. Boxes in each chapter highlight (1) needs and considerations for the successful implementation and sustainment of evidence-based interventions, and (2) specific interventions/approaches that are intended to be illustrative and may be useful to communities and their partners. The evidence-based programs mentioned in the report were selected for illustrative purposes only, for being evidence-based or promising, and for exemplifying strategies for a variety of settings and populations. The committee does not endorse these specific sample programs, but shares them to illustrate the types of interventions that are available, and to help explore implementation, workforce, and other dimensions.

The committee conducted four public information-gathering meetings, extensive reviews of the literature, public listening sessions and staff conversations with additional stakeholders or constituents, and closed working meetings to deliberate and write the report.

A Vision for the Prevention Infrastructure for MEB Disorders

A national MEB prevention infrastructure requires "systems, competencies, frameworks, relationships, and resources that enable [state and local governments and agencies, along with communities, community-based organizations, and their partners,] to perform core functions" central to preventing MEB disorder and promoting health and well-being (NACCHO, n.d.).

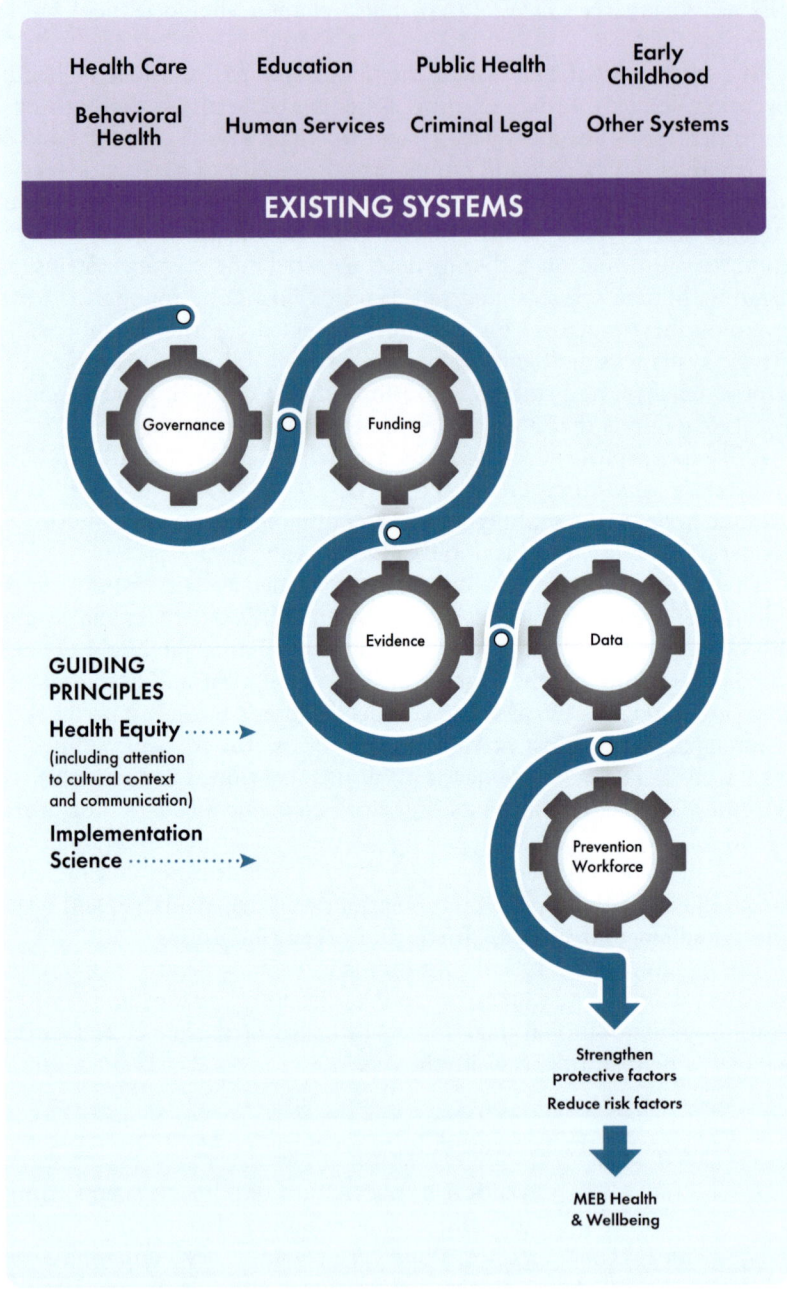

FIGURE 1-1 A depiction of the prevention infrastructure for MEB disorders.

FIGURE 1-1 Continued
NOTES: This graphic illustrates (1) the major components of the infrastructure that is embedded in existing systems and operates across varied settings, delivering interventions along the life course, and (2) the guiding principles that should permeate it. The interlocking gears represent how each element is complementary and critical to the others: governance and partnerships at federal, state, local, and tribal levels; sustained funding; supportive data systems; a constantly evolving evidence base; and a competent, supported workforce comprise a flexible and responsive infrastructure to prevent MEB disorders. The blueprint for such an infrastructure includes guidance on turning, engaging, and fine-tuning the "gears" to foster implementation of preventive strategies that is fully responsive to the communities that need them. The infrastructure operates in the context of policies (not included in the graphic) that shape the economic, social, and environmental conditions that enhance protective factors against or present risk factors for MEB disorders. MEB = mental, emotional, and behavioral.

This report proposes recommendations to support a well-functioning prevention infrastructure, which

- Is organized around delivering **evidence-based programs** that are effectively disseminated, continually evaluated, and well known, with easily accessed details about effectiveness and implementation, and feedback loops that add to the evidence base (a feature of a learning prevention infrastructure) (Chapter 2), and operate in a supportive policy environment (Chapter 7);
- Has a **workforce** that is appropriately trained to deliver those strategies, representative of the populations served, and able to provide linguistically and culturally appropriate services,[10] fairly paid, supported, and provided with career ladders (Chapter 3);
- Has **data systems** that draw on all existing resources to inform needs assessment and selection of strategies, and to support evaluation and accountability (Chapter 4);
- Has clear governance structures at the federal, state, tribal, and local levels, including shared governance through cross-sector and community partnerships (Chapter 5);
- Is adequately and sustainably **funded** (Chapter 6);

---

[10] The committee endorses the recommendation in the recent National Academies report that called on CMS and SAMHSA to "restructure current workforce and training mechanisms and their funding to better incentivize robust training environments that support career choices that will more directly impact care for Medicare and Medicaid beneficiaries" (NASEM, 2024, p. 241). The restructuring, the committee said, should "focus on the providers serving populations with highest need for greater access to behavioral health provision in Medicaid such as rural, child/adolescent, and racial/ethnic minoritized populations" and "focus on workforce demographic diversity."

- Exists in the context of **supportive evidence-based policies** that create and strengthen the social, economic, and environmental conditions necessary for MEB disorder prevention and undergird population health (Chapter 7); and
- Prioritizes **implementation with an emphasis on (communities and populations) at highest risk**—collaborating and co-creating with communities at each step, from pre-implementation (assessing readiness, defining the problem and goals) to implementation planning (e.g., training, resource distribution), to implementation (discussed throughout the report).

The committee identified a prevention infrastructure that is fragmented and better developed for substance use disorders (SUD) than for MH—and it is embedded in a broad ecosystem of public and private entities and networks. It can be nurtured, strengthened, and robustly funded to close gaps and provide the interventions and packages of interventions needed in every community and at every level of society, with a focus on greater support for areas of greatest need.

It includes parts of several other infrastructures, including public health, health care, social and human services, and education. The major infrastructure components are funding, governance, data, the workforce, and the evidence base; together, these allow for sustained delivery of interventions affecting both upstream and downstream factors related to MEB health. Expanding opportunities for all to reach their full health potential, local and cultural contexts, and community-driven partnerships are necessary throughout these components. For example, workers drawn from the community bring deep knowledge and earned trust. The evidence base must reflect the communities to whom interventions are being delivered and must determine whose voices, perspectives, and contributions shape or lead these decisions.

The charge to the committee underscores the lack of uptake of proven prevention interventions, and that, the committee shows, is fundamentally an implementation issue—having to do with adequate, sustained funding; reliable dissemination of the evidence base with feedback loops to update it and fill gaps; data access, collection, and use to inform decision making and implementation; a well-trained and fairly compensated workforce with opportunities for growth; and a structure of oversight and leadership—governance—that is well coordinated, integrates MH and SUD functions and organizations, and engages community voice and lived expertise.

HOW TO USE THIS REPORT

It is important to first identify partners in the prevention ecosystem who will implement and/or are affected by implementation (as discussed below in the "map constituents" step for supporting the infrastructure).

The ecosystem includes many of the constituents and audiences for the report. In addition to this report's sponsors, which include several institutes, centers, and offices across NIH, CDC, and SAMHSA, it may be of interest to other federal entities such as other HHS agencies, the Department of Agriculture, Department of Veterans Affairs, Department of Defense, Department of Education, and Department of Justice. This blueprint for the prevention infrastructure will also be useful to state leaders and decision makers, researchers, community coalitions, prevention research centers, academic and community partnerships, government and academic partnerships, and philanthropic and community organizations. It also could be useful to community leaders and members, and other implementers and partners who are not, strictly speaking, responsible for the infrastructure per se but interact with it in various ways.

As noted, this report emphasizes health equity ("the state in which everyone has a fair opportunity to attain their full potential for health and well-being and no one is disadvantaged from doing so because of social position or other socially defined circumstances" [NASEM, 2023]) and applying implementation science in the infrastructure and the interventions. Considerations related to these two points of emphasis appear throughout the report.

When thinking about supporting the prevention infrastructure or delivering interventions in communities, any constituents will benefit from referring to lessons from implementation processes. On multiple levels—the "meta," or the infrastructure; the "macro," or social policy; or the "meso" and "micro," as more discrete interventions implemented on a community level—the overarching steps are the same, but the steps are characterized here with some detail as it would apply to the meta level (e.g., the sustainers, funders, or builders of the infrastructure).

1. **Identify the gap or need:** Sustainers must gather data and establish priorities for the infrastructure itself, which this report in part helps to do. A key component for identifying needs or gaps is doing so in a way that is community driven.
2. **Select the intervention:** Sustainers will consider the major components of the infrastructure (chapter topics in this report) to address identified needs and may look to recommendations from this report and other expert advice or resources to inform selection as well. This step might include redirecting funds or issuing new funds for practice or research, developing methods or support for data collection, or identifying criteria for workforce development. Sustainment is also something to consider during this step, such as designing for dissemination and sustainability of updated or new evidence on preventive interventions (Kwan et al., 2022).
3. **Map the constituents:** Sustainers will likely have done some version of this already but will need to map the constituents invested in the

infrastructure (see Table 1-1 for examples) to identify partners and assets, increase buy-in, and ensure that the approaches to support the infrastructure are addressing the needs of its constituents.[11]

4. **Assess barriers and facilitators, and understand context:** Barriers and facilitators, or "determinants," enable or hinder adoption, implementation, and sustainment of approaches to support the infrastructure. As part of the process, sustainers must have rapid ways to measure their context and those determinants. There are many tools to help support this assessment, such as a pragmatic context assessment tool (see pCAT[12]).
5. **Create a logic model:** Once sustainers have identified determinants, they can create a logic model for implementation. Smith and colleagues offer one example, but the crucial component is intentionally and prospectively mapping out the whole approach based on the work already done so there is a clear path forward (Smith et al., 2020).
6. **Evaluate:** Sustainers will need consistent metrics to evaluate if their approaches to support the infrastructure are effective. They will also need to select and assess data in partnership with different constituents—this may include the data discussed in Chapter 4 and also data about research funding and outcomes, governance, and the workforce that are not specific to outcomes from specific interventions.
7. **Adapt:** As sustainers begin to collect data and other information about the outcomes of their approaches to support prevention research translation, dissemination, and sustainment, they will need to adapt to ensure maximum success and fit to context.
8. **Sustain:** Sustainment is a key consideration at both the end and the beginning of the process; it is important to plan for it from the start. Sustainers can use tools such as a program sustainability assessment tool to help with planning (e.g., PSAT) (PSAT, n.d.).

This list is semilinear, in that implementers will often be engaged in more than one step at one time. This type of process is a continuous cycle of engagement, supported by data and partnerships with groups that can help with interpretation, adaptation, and ongoing iteration to maintain the infrastructure's adaptability for new evidence and ways to support the delivery of interventions.

---

[11] See Potthoff and colleagues (2023) for one example of a constituent engagement model.
[12] See https://cfirguide.org/tools/tools-and-templates/ (accessed October 28, 2024). As of October 28, 2024, the tool is updated; in the interim, follow instructions in link to see the tool in "Additional File 2" from Robinson and Damschroder (2023).

REPORT OVERVIEW

The report contains seven chapters and six appendixes. Chapter 2 provides a brief overview of the evidence base for prevention programs and strategies, along with a discussion of IS and the guidance it offers to ensuring that implementation is robust and includes all keys to success and sustainment. Chapter 3 discusses the workforce for prevention, which is considerably different from the traditional, largely clinical, licensed professions in BH (psychiatrists, psychologists, social workers, etc.). Chapter 4 discusses the data infrastructure to support the delivery of interventions in a wide range of settings. Chapter 5 discusses the governance and partnerships that set the pace, motivate, and lead the way at different levels. Chapter 6 identifies the gaps in funding that need to be addressed, especially by Congressional and state-level attention, and generating additional resources and devoting them to this essential work. Finally, Chapter 7 offers a brief overview of the social, economic, and environmental policies that create the conditions for primordial prevention of MEB health and population well-being.

REFERENCES

Abramson, B., J. Boerma, and A. Tsyvinski. 2024. *Macroeconomics of mental health.* National Bureau of Economic Research. https://www.nber.org/system/files/working_papers/w32354/w32354.pdf (accessed December 30, 2024).

ACF (Administration for Children and Families). 2021. *Child care stabilization grants appropriated in the American Rescue Plan (ARP) Act (Public Law 117-2) signed into law on March 11, 2021.* https://www.acf.hhs.gov/sites/default/files/documents/occ/CCDF-ACF-IM-2021-02.pdf (accessed December 30, 2024).

Acolin, J., and P. Fishman. 2023. Beyond the biomedical, towards the agentic: A paradigm shift for population health science. *Social Science & Medicine* 326:115950. https://doi.org/10.1016/j.socscimed.2023.115950.

CDC (Centers for Disease Control and Prevention). 1992. A framework for assessing the effectiveness of disease and injury prevention. *MMWR Morbidity and Mortality Weekly Report* 41. https://www.cdc.gov/mmWR/preview/mmwrhtml/00016403.htm (accessed December 30, 2024).

CDC. 2024a. *Tribal suicide prevention.* https://www.cdc.gov/suicide/programs/tribal.html (accessed December 16, 2024).

CDC. 2024b. *Youth risk behavior survey data summary & trends report.* https://www.cdc.gov/yrbs/dstr/index.html (accessed December 30, 2024).

CDC. n.d.-a. *Provisional drug overdose death counts.* https://www.cdc.gov/nchs/nvss/vsrr/drug-overdose-data.htm (accessed October 28, 2024).

CDC. n.d.-b. *Suicide in rural America.* https://www.cdc.gov/rural-health/php/public-health-strategy/suicide-in-rural-america-prevention-strategies.html (accessed October 28, 2024).

CFIR (Consolidated Framework for Implementation Research). 2025. *Tools and templates.* https://cfirguide.org/tools/tools-and-templates/ (accessed January 2, 2025).

Dawes, D. E., J. Bhatt, N. J. Dunlap, C. Amador, K. Gebreyes, B. Rush, J. Westfall, M. Fendrich, A. Davis, M. Keita Fakeye, C. Philip, N. Wade, D. Hernandez, and A. Dhar. 2024. *Projected cost and economic impact of mental health inequities in the United States.* https://meharryglobal.org/research-scholarship/projected-cost-and-economic-impact-of-mental-health-inequities/ (accessed January 2, 2025).

Erickson, B. 2021. Deinstitutionalization through optimism: The Community Mental Health Act of 1963. *American Journal of Psychiatry Residents' Journal* 16(4):6–7. https://doi.org/10.1176/appi.ajp-rj.2021.160404.

Esser, M. B., A. Sherk, Y. Liu, and T. S. Naimi. 2024. Deaths from excessive alcohol use–United States, 2016–2021. *MMWR Morbidity and Mortality Weekly Report* 73(8):154–161. https://doi.org/10.15585/mmwr.mm7308a1.

Friedman, J., M. Godvin, C. L. Shover, J. P. Gone, H. Hansen, and D. L. Schriger. 2022. Trends in drug overdose deaths among US adolescents, January 2010 to June 2021. *JAMA* 327(14):1398–1400. https://doi.org/10.1001/jama.2022.2847.

Gunja, M. Z., E. D. Gumas, and R. D. Williams II. 2023. *U.S. health care from a global perspective, 2022: Accelerating spending, worsening outcomes*. The Commonwealth Fund. https://www.commonwealthfund.org/publications/issue-briefs/2023/jan/us-health-care-global-perspective-2022 (accessed December 30, 2024).

Gunja, M. Z., E. D. Gumas, and R. D. Williams II. 2024. *Mental health needs in the U.S. compared to nine other countries: Findings from the commonwealth fund 2023 international health policy survey*. https://www.commonwealthfund.org/publications/2024/may/mental-health-needs-us-compared-nine-other-countries (accessed December 16, 2024).

Harrington, A. 2023. Mental health's stalled (biological) revolution: Its origins, aftermath & future opportunities. *Daedalus*. 2023;152(4):166–185. https://doi.org/10.1162/daed_a_02037.

Helliwell, J. F., R. Layard, J. D. Sachs, J-E. De Neve, L. B. Aknin, & S. Wang. 2024. *World happiness report 2024*. University of Oxford: Wellbeing Research Centre.

Heymann, J., A. Raub, W. Waisath, M. McCormack, R. Weistroffer, G. Moreno, E. Wong, and A. Earle. 2020. Protecting health during Covid-19 and beyond: A global examination of paid sick leave design in 193 countries. *Global Public Health* 15(7):925–934. https://doi.org/10.1080/17441692.2020.1764076.

HHS (Department of Health and Human Services). n.d. *Mental and behavioral health–American Indians/Alaska Natives*. https://minorityhealth.hhs.gov/mental-and-behavioral-health-american-indiansalaska-natives (accessed December 16, 2024).

Hidalgo-Padilla, L., M. Toyama, J. H. Zafra-Tanaka, A. Vives, and F. Diez-Canseco. 2023. Association between maternity leave policies and postpartum depression: A systematic review. *Archives of Women's Mental Health* 26(5):571–580. https://doi.org/10.1007/s00737-023-01350-z.

Hostetter, M., and S. Klein. 2021. *Making it easy to get mental health care: Examples from abroad*. The Commonwealth Fund. https://www.commonwealthfund.org/publications/2021/feb/making-it-easy-get-mental-health-care-examples-abroad (accessed December 30, 2024).

IOM (Institute of Medicine). 1991. *Research and service programs in the PHS: Challenges in organization*. Washington, DC: National Academy Press. https://doi.org/10.17226/1871.

IOM. 1994. *Reducing risks for mental disorders: Frontiers for preventive intervention research*. Washington, DC: The National Academies Press. https://doi.org/10.17226/2139.

Ivey-Stephenson, A. Z., A. E. Crosby, S. P. D. Jack, T. Haileyesus, and M. J. Kresnow-Sedacca. 2017. Suicide trends among and within urbanization levels by sex, race/ethnicity, age group, and mechanism of death–United States, 2001–2015. *MMWR Surveillance Summaries* 66(18):1–16. https://doi.org/10.15585/mmwr.ss6618a1.

Jackson-Morris, A., C. L. Meyer, A. Morgan, R. Stelmach, L. Jamison, and C. Currie. 2024. An investment case analysis for the prevention and treatment of adolescent mental disorders and suicide in England. *European Journal of Public Health* 34(1):107–113. https://doi.org/10.1093/eurpub/ckad193.

Kobau, R., J. Sniezek, M. M. Zack, R. E. Lucas, and A. Burns. 2010. Well-being assessment: An evaluation of well-being scales for public health and population estimates of well-being among US adults. *Applied Psychology: Health and Well-Being* 2:272–297. https://doi.org/10.1111/j.1758-0854.2010.01035.x.

Kwan, B. M., R. C. Brownson, R. E. Glasgow, E. H. Morrato, and D. A. Luke. 2022. Designing for dissemination and sustainability to promote equitable impacts on health. *Annual Review of Public Health* 43(1):331–353. https://doi.org/10.1146/annurev-publhealth052220-112457.

Luo, F., M. Li, and C. Florence. 2021. State-level economic costs of opioid use disorder and fatal opioid overdose–United States, 2017. *MMWR Morbidity and Mortality Weekly Report* 70(15):541–546. https://doi.org/10.15585/mmwr.mm7015a1.

MHTTC (Mental Health Technology Transfer Center). 2024. *Mental Health Technology Transfer Center.* https://mhttcnetwork.org/ (accessed January 2, 2025).

Miller, M., C. Barber, R. A. White, and D. Azrael. 2013. Firearms and suicide in the United States: Is risk independent of underlying suicidal behavior? *American Journal of Epidemiology* 178(6):946–955. https://doi.org/10.1093/aje/kwt197.

Morales, D. A., C. L. Barksdale, and A. C. Beckel-Mitchener. 2020. A call to action to address rural mental health disparities. *Journal of Clinical and Translational Science* 4(5):463–467. https://doi.org/10.1017/cts.2020.42.

NACCHO (National Association of County and City Health Officials). n.d. *Public health infrastructure and systems.* https://www.naccho.org/programs/public-health-infrastructure (accessed November 22, 2024).

NASEM (National Academies of Sciences, Engineering, and Medicine). 2019. *Fostering healthy mental, emotional, and behavioral development in children and youth: A national agenda.* Washington, DC: The National Academies Press. https://doi.org/10.17226/25201.

NASEM. 2023. *Federal policy to advance racial, ethnic, and tribal health equity.* Washington, DC: National Academies Press. https://doi.org/10.17226/26834.

NASEM. 2024. *Expanding behavioral health care workforce participation in Medicare, Medicaid, and marketplace plans.* Washington, DC: The National Academies Press. https://doi.org/10.17226/27759.

NIDA (National Institute on Drug Abuse). 2024. *U.S. Overdose deaths by sex, 1999–2022.* https://nida.nih.gov/research-topics/trends-statistics/overdose-death-rates#Fig1 (accessed December 12, 2024.)

NIDA. 2025. NIDA has supported scientific research on drug use and addiction for 50 years, https://nida.nih.gov/about-nida/50th-anniversary (accessed January 3, 2025).

NIMH (National Institute of Mental Health). 2024. Celebrating 75 years: Transforming the understanding and treatment of mental illnesses. https://www.nimh.nih.gov/sites/default/files/documents/NIMH-Celebrating-75-Years-508_0.pdf (accessed January 2, 2025).

NIMH. n.d. *Suicide.* https://www.nimh.nih.gov/health/statistics/suicide (accessed October 22, 2024).

NRC (National Research Council) and IOM. 2009. *Preventing mental, emotional, and behavioral disorders among young people: Progress and possibilities.* Washington, DC: The National Academies Press. https://doi.org/10.17226/12480.

OMH (HHS Office of Minority Health). 2024. *Mental and behavioral health–Asian Americans.* https://minorityhealth.hhs.gov/mental-and-behavioral-health-asian-americans (accessed December 30, 2021).

OSG (Office of the Surgeon General). 2024. *Firearm violence: A public health crisis in America.* https://www.hhs.gov/sites/default/files/firearm-violence-advisory.pdf (accessed December 30, 2021).

Panchal, N. 2024. *Recent trends in mental health and substance use concerns among adolescents.* KFF. https://www.kff.org/mental-health/issue-brief/recent-trends-in-mental-health-and-substance-use-concerns-among-adolescents/ (accessed December 30, 2024).

Potthoff, S., T. Finch, L. Bührmann, A. Etzelmüller, C. R. van Genugten, M. Girling, C. R. May, N. Perkins, C. Vis, and T. Rapley. 2023. Towards an Implementation-Stakeholder Engagement Model (I-STEM) for improving health and social care services. *Health Expectations* 26(5):1997–2012. https://doi.org/10.1111/hex.13808.

Pronk, N., D. V. Kleinman, S. F. Goekler, E. Ochiai, C. Blakey, and K. H. Brewer. 2021. Promoting health and well-being in healthy people 2030. *Journal of Public Health Management and Practice* 27(Supplement 6):S242–S248. https://doi.org/10.1097/PHH.0000000000001254.

PSAT (Program Sustainability Assessment Tool). n.d. *Find planning resources.* https://www.sustaintool.org/psat/resources/ (accessed October 28, 2024).

Randi, O. 2021. *American rescue plan act presents opportunities for states to support school mental health systems.* NASHP. https://nashp.org/american-rescue-plan-act-presents-opportunities-for-states-to-support-school-mental-health-systems/ (accessed December 30, 2024).

Robinson, C. H., and L. J. Damschroder. 2023. A pragmatic context assessment tool (PCAT): Using a think aloud method to develop an assessment of contextual barriers to change. *Implementation Science Communications* 4(1):3. https://doi.org/10.1186/s43058-022-00380-5.

Rule, A., C. Abbey, H. Wang, S. Rozelle, and M. K. Singh. 2024. Measurement of flourishing: A scoping review. *Frontiers in Psychology* 15:1293943. https://doi.org/10.3389/fpsyg.2024.1293943.

SAMHSA (Substance Abuse and Mental Health Services Administration). 2019. *Risk and protective factors.* https://www.samhsa.gov/sites/default/files/20190718-samhsa-risk-protective-factors.pdf (accessed December 12, 2024).

Smith, J. D., D. H. Li, and M. R. Rafferty. 2020. The implementation research logic model: A method for planning, executing, reporting, and synthesizing implementation projects. *Implementation Science* 15:1–12. https://doi.org/10.1186/s13012-020-01041-8.

Spencer, M. R., A. M. Miniño, and M. Warner. 2022. *Drug overdose deaths in the United States, 2001–2021.* https://www.cdc.gov/nchs/data/databriefs/db457.pdf (accessed December 30, 2024).

Stelmach, R., E. L. Kocher, I. Kataria, A. M. Jackson-Morris, S. Saxena, and R. Nugent. 2022. The global return on investment from preventing and treating adolescent mental disorders and suicide: A modelling study. *BMJ Global Health* 7:e007759. https://doi.org/10.1093/eurpub/ckad193.

TFA (Trust for America's Health). 2008. *Prevention for a healthier America.* https://www.tfah.org/wp-content/uploads/archive/reports/prevention08/Prevention08Exec.pdf (accessed December 30, 2024).

TFA. 2009. *Prevention for a healthier america: Investments in disease prevention yield significant savings, stronger communities.*

UWDGH (University of Washington Department of Global Health). 2024. *Step 4: Select research methods.* https://impsciuw.org/implementation-science/research/select-research-methods/ (accessed October 29, 2024).

WHO (World Health Organization). 2024. *Constitution.* https://www.who.int/about/governance/constitution (accessed December 13, 2024).

Williams, R. 2024. International Comparisons & International Health, presented to the Committee on Blueprint for a National Prevention Infrastructure for Behavioral Health Disorders, Meeting 3. https://www.nationalacademies.org/event/42281_04-2024_blueprint-for-a-national-prevention-infrastructure-for-behavioral-health-disorders-meeting-3 (accessed December 16, 2024).

Zilkha, C., V. Agarwal, and R. G. Frank. 2024. Suicide rates are high and rising among older adults in the US. *Health Affairs Forefront.* https://doi.org/10.1377/forefront.20240228.27143.

2

The Evidence Base on Programs

This report is focused on the infrastructure needed to support the successful adoption and implementation of interventions to prevent mental, emotional, and behavioral (MEB) disorders and promote well-being. The breadth and quality of preventive interventions for MEB disorders are the focus of several National Academies of Sciences, Engineering, and Medicine (National Academies) reports (for example, NRC and IOM, 2009; NASEM, 2019a,b,c, 2020). As noted in these reports and elsewhere, the evidence base regarding the prevention of MEB disorders is robust in some crucial ways and lacking in others: there are a number of interventions with decades of high-quality research to support their effectiveness, particularly focused on children, youth, and families. However, there are related to gaps in the evidence and the mechanism through which high-quality evidence is disseminated to would-be adopters and implementers. This chapter begins with a brief discussion of the translation pipeline from pre-implementation to implementation studies, followed by discussion of approaches (used interchangeably with "interventions" and "package of interventions") across settings and stages of the life course and a discussion of the gaps in evidence and research needs related to both intervention research and dissemination and implementation research.

RESEARCH TO TRANSLATION PIPELINE

Figure 2-1 illustrates the pipeline from intervention research to implementation research (Brown et al., 2017). Intervention research here also encompasses more foundational questions related to disorder processes, such as pathophysiology, etiology, natural history, and comorbidities. It also encompasses research questions related to

- psychometric properties such as reliability, generalizability, and validity;
- risk assessment and health equity considerations, which includes a wide range of complex risk and protective factors, ranging from individual behaviors or individual biological (including genetic, metabolic, and physiological) risk factors to social drivers of health and lack of fair opportunities to attain one's full potential for MEB health; and
- intermediate and long-term outcomes, i.e., potential benefits or harms of interventions.

Implementation research encompasses questions about the dissemination and implementation of those interventions: how information about new

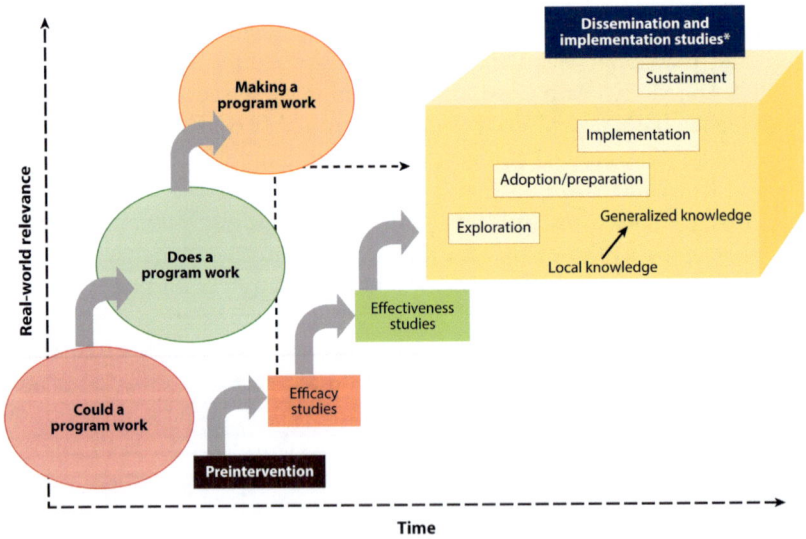

*These dissemination and implementation stages include systematic monitoring, evaluation, and adaptation as required.

FIGURE 2-1 Traditional translational pipeline from preintervention, efficacy, effectiveness, and dissemination and implementation studies.
SOURCE: Brown et al., 2017. Copyright © 2017 *Annual Reviews*. CC-BY-SA.

interventions is collected and shared and how interventions can be effectively implemented in real-world settings. This can include research related to the following:

- The effectiveness of evidence-based clearinghouses and improving them, along with other knowledge-sharing resources; and
- Strategies and resources needed to deliver interventions within communities with fidelity and sustainment, including access to and ability to use relevant data, a competent workforce to deliver interventions, and training and other technical support.

It is important to note that this research and practice pipeline is fundamentally a loop, requiring constant feedback to improve research, practice, and ultimately, MEB outcomes—see Smith and colleagues (2024) for another example of the research pipeline. As with a learning health care system, a learning infrastructure focused on prevention of MEB disorders may incorporate data-driven, embedded learning that feeds back into the infrastructure, continuous improvement, collaboration and transparency, and health equity and representativeness. This focus on learning and continuous improvement applies both to the research on interventions and each component of the infrastructure as discussed in each chapter (Abraham et al., 2016; IOM, 2013).

As is discussed in Chapter 1, the committee directed most of its attention to questions related to the infrastructure that would support primary (before MEB disorders occur) and universal (targeted at the entire population) prevention approaches. Primary prevention as used here includes health promotion and consists of approaches to reduce the incidence of MEB disorders and support MEB health (see Figure 2-2 for a visual representation of the spectrum of possible prevention approaches). Secondary and tertiary prevention are grouped together in this report—encompassing approaches to reduce the prevalence of MEB disorders or treatment modalities to prevent relapse. Examples include screenings for depression before clinical MEB symptoms become apparent; medication-assisted treatment for individuals diagnosed with clinical MEB disorders, such as schizophrenia; or lethal means counseling to reduce risk of suicide. Although the committee understood its charge largely to focus on primary prevention, the report touches briefly on secondary and selective interventions—targeted to people or groups with above-average risk, or tertiary and indicated preventive interventions—for people or groups already engaging in high-risk behaviors or experiencing an MEB disorder.

Many preventive interventions have targeted risk and protective factors. The former are characteristics that are associated with negative MEB outcomes. The latter are positive conditions that lower risk factors or prevent negative MEB outcomes. Both can occur in many domains, including

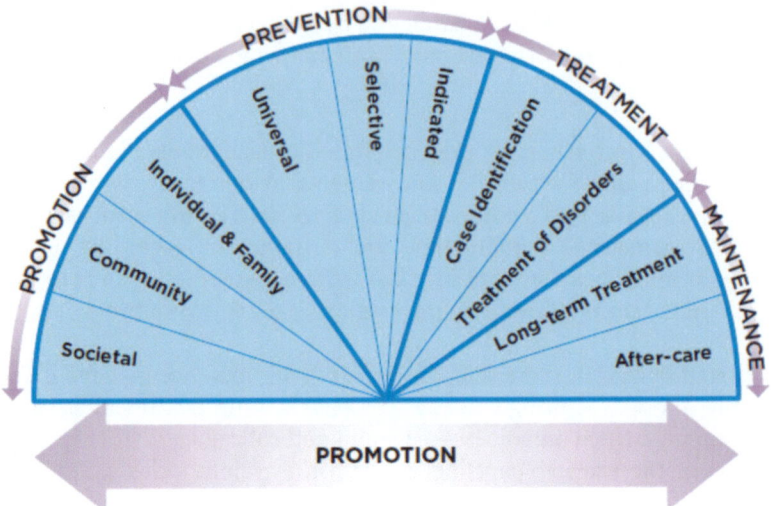

FIGURE 2-2 Prevention spectrum for mental, emotional, and behavioral disorders.
SOURCE: NASEM, 2019a.

individual, family, partner, peer, community, school, and workplace, and intersect in daily life across the entire life course. Risk factors for MEB disorders across the life course include adverse childhood experiences (ACEs), (see Box 2-1), trauma and stress, grief/bereavement, lack of a consistent caring adult during childhood, in utero exposure to maternal stress, racial discrimination, co-occurring psychiatric conditions, adult unemployment,

---

BOX 2-1
A Note About Adverse Childhood Experiences (ACEs)

One crosscutting and multifaceted risk factor for developing an MEB disorder is ACEs, which broadly refers to "childhood exposure to potentially traumatic experience including violence, abuse or neglect, witnessing violence in the home or community or having a family member attempt or die by suicide" (CDC, 2024a). Felitti and colleagues (1998) showed that children with high ACEs scores are far more likely than their peers to face poor health outcomes, including depression, violence, being a victim of violence, and suicide. Phillips and colleagues (2017) suggest that evidence-based home visiting could help prevent the intergenerational transmission of ACEs.

abrupt cessation of pain medication, and bullying. Protective factors include healthy social and emotional development; positive/benevolent childhood experiences; accessible and affordable mental health (MH) care services; building resilience to stress; social support, connectedness, and opportunities for positive socialization; and promotion of parental and family MH (Latimore, 2023; NASEM, 2019a). As illustrated by the socio-ecological framework, risk factors operate at the individual, family, and community levels, as do the social determinants of health (SDOH) that influence them, including economic stability, education access and quality, health care access and quality, neighborhood and built environment, and social and community context (see Chapter 7 for a discussion of broader social policies that relate to the SDOH at a more macro level).

Over the last 50 years, the field of prevention science has focused on how best to "promote health and well-being and prevent health conditions from starting or getting worse" (ODP, 2024), drawing from multiple disciplines, including public health, psychology, sociology, and neurobiology. Prevention research explores how biology, behavior, environments, physical and MEB health services and systems, and physical- and MEB-health–related policies can affect physical and MEB health and well-being by identifying risk factors and protective factors to target, developing and evaluating interventions, and developing best practices to disseminate and implement those interventions (NPSC, 2019; ODP, 2024; SPR, 2011).

Much of this research is focused on the beginning of the life course—preconception through young adulthood—and can be found in National Academies reports (see NASEM, 2019a,b,c, 2020) that provide details about healthy development in early life. However, the prevention of MEB disorders and promotion of MEB health can occur later in life as well, which is why this committee also briefly discusses approaches to prevent MEB disorders in adulthood.

PREVENTION APPROACHES

This section offers a brief overview of evidence-based and promising approaches that can prevent MEB disorders and promote MEB health across the life course; it is not a comprehensive review of all relevant interventions, nor does it attempt to assess their reach or impact. As discussed in the introduction, examples of different approaches are used to explore the characteristics of programs that may be delivered within the proposed prevention infrastructure, rather than an endorsement of any particular intervention. Most programs or approaches discussed as exemplars were named in multiple evidence clearinghouses (also referred to as "registries") for prevention science, healthy youth development, or MEB health promotion and substance use prevention. Some exemplars are newer and may not be found in any clearinghouses. For newer exemplars that show promise featured in the report, sources are noted.

While many types of approaches are cited in literature as "evidence based," this report also refers to "practice-based evidence." In this report, evidence-based programs (EBPs) comprise a rigorous evidence base (often including randomized controlled trials [RCTs]), include considerations for clinical judgment and patient context, and are often considered the "gold standard" for preventive interventions (APA, 2005; NIHB, 2009). Practice-based evidence encompasses interventions that are "derived from, and supportive of, the positive [culture] of the local society and traditions" (NIHB, 2009, p. 10). These categories offer something of a false dichotomy by indicating that interventions can *either* be rigorously evaluated *or* culturally appropriate and co-designed with people with lived expertise. However, these concepts need not be mutually exclusive (see "Healing of the Canoe" discussed below for one example). Some examples in this report also highlight what is often called "community-based evidence," which may lean more heavily on consensus from coalitions and community members (Bartgis, n.d.; Wolfson et al., 2017). Green and Allegrante (2020) outlined three sources of practice-based evidence: participatory research and Practice-Based Research Networks, systems science (helpful in addressing complex problems that affect an entire community), and systematic reviews (which analyze and assemble multiple studies, including practice-based experience).

National Academies reports have provided extensive descriptions of evidence-based interventions (IOM and NRC, 2009; NASEM, 2019a,b,c). In the section that follows, the committee provides a very brief, non-exhaustive overview of some interventions implemented across different settings and for different age groups, and in some cases, for specific groups of people, to underscore that they are one component of the infrastructure and illuminate the infrastructure considerations needed to support the delivery of such a wide range of interventions. This chapter also includes some examples of promising practices that may not have a well-developed evidence base but offer new ideas about preventive interventions among populations or in contexts that are historically lacking (for example, see Box 2-7, a brief review of web-based preventive interventions). The inclusion of a preventive intervention in this chapter is not an endorsement from the committee for its implementation, as this was well outside the committee's charge. The descriptions are intended to conceptually ground the later chapters on the workforce needed to deliver the interventions; the data needed to select, implement, and evaluate them; the funding needed to support the infrastructure; and the governance and partnerships needed to lead the way in MEB promotion. These examples highlight the considerations needed for a prevention infrastructure to support the delivery of interventions across a variety of settings and life stages, as illustrated by the "exemplar" boxes throughout the other chapters.

THE EVIDENCE BASE ON PROGRAMS 51

The illustrative approaches below are grouped both by settings and/or stage of the life course.

Approaches for Children, Adolescents, and Young Adults

Approaches in Family and Community Settings

Approaches for family and childhood settings include strategies that address parent, family, and other primary caregiver needs to support healthy parenting strategies and home environments, mitigating risk factors and promoting protective factors from conception through young adulthood. As noted in Box 2-2, the Nurse-Family Partnership program targets pre-birth outcomes by addressing risk factors that are associated with poor birth outcomes and continuing the support during the early days of parenting. Group-based parenting interventions can address mental health, particularly depression during pregnancy and postpartum, and prevent substance use disorders (SUDs) and child neglect and abuse. Programs focused particularly on supporting the development of positive parenting skills can also have indirect positive effects on reducing maternal depression and reducing substance and alcohol use (Barlow et al., 2002; Cioffi et al., 2021; Forgatch et al., 2009; Patterson et al., 2010; Shaw et al., 2009).

Overall, the evidence base connects positive MEB outcomes among children and adolescents with interventions that can be tailored to cultural and other community contexts, treat parents as knowledgeable and equal partners in childrearing, integrate services for families with multiple service needs, support peer networks for parents, address trauma among parents, and increase fathers' involvement in parenting (NASEM, 2019a).

BOX 2-2
Evidence-Based Program: Nurse-Family Partnership

The Nurse-Family Partnership is a home-visiting program that sends registered nurses to visit the families of low-income, first-time mothers from pregnancy through the child's second birthday. These nurses deliver a strengths-based and trauma-informed program and develop a therapeutic relationship with participants. Child abuse and neglect, arrests, behavioral impairments due to use of alcohol or other drugs, and child mortality are reduced. The results have been sustained over time.

SOURCE: CEBC, 2024.

Approaches in Education-Based Settings

Decades of research supports the use of preventive interventions in school settings, from preschool through college. The committee considered the large base of research of preventive interventions in education settings. For example, socio-emotional learning (SEL) programs have demonstrated effectiveness for improved social skills, MH, prosocial behavior, academic achievement, and the prevention of antisocial behavior and substance misuse. Early childhood education programs are associated with increased educational attainment, consistent employment, and improved self-control and self-esteem. All of these are protective factors to support MEB health and reduced the likelihood of receipt of public assistance, involvement in the criminal legal system, and substance misuse (Latimore, 2023; Reynolds et al., 2011). Many classroom-based programs (including those for adolescents) prevent and reduce disruptive behavior, depression, posttraumatic stress and trauma, substance misuse and SUD, and bullying (NASEM, 2019a). One such example, LifeSkills Training, is a classroom-based universal prevention program designed to address substance use initiation and violence for 12–14-year-olds (Blueprints for Healthy Youth Development, 2024b). Teaching three major skills (personal self-management, social skills, and information and resistance skills) over 3 years, the program has shown to significantly lower rates of polysubstance use at 6.5-year follow-up and violent behavior at posttest and significantly slower growth rates in cigarette initiation and alcohol use at 5.5 years after baseline. Similar types of skills training programs along with brief motivational interviewing programs focused on the risks of alcohol use can reduce problematic use in college students as well, particularly when introduced as a package of multiple interventions (environmental and individual) (NIAAA, 2019a). See Box 2-3 for a description of the Good Behavior Game, which is used in school settings and is part of the U.S. Department of Education evidence clearinghouse.

Out-of-school-time programs can provide similar opportunities as classroom-based programs for children and adolescents. In addition to supporting food security and nutrition education and providing avenues for healthy physical activity, they often offer SEL programs for youth (CDC, 2023; Sparr et al., 2020). Programs that focus on developing interpersonal skills are linked with positive social behavior, another protective factor to support MEB well-being (see Box 2-4 for a promising program) (CDC, 2023).

Healing of the Canoe is one example of PBE specifically developed for tribal youth—an intervention developed in partnership between the Suquamish Tribe, Port Gamble S'Klallam Tribe, and University of Washington Addictions, Drug & Alcohol Institute (ADAI) (Healing of the Canoe,

> **BOX 2-3**
> **Evidence-Based Program: Good Behavior Game**
>
> The Good Behavior Game (GBG) is an intervention designed for children grades Pre-K through 6th, delivered by teachers or other adults (parents or school staff). The GBG can be integrated into the school day and involves a set of self-management and self-regulation exercises that can promote healthy social behavior by having children predict good and bad behaviors during transitions between activities. Recipients of the GBG intervention showed reduced drug/alcohol use later in life, reduced conduct problems, and reduced mental health service need.
>
> Teachers can be trained in implementing GBG in the classroom through an initial two-day training, booster training sessions, and GBG coaches. GBG coaches undergo an extra day of training and are audited by the American Institutes for Research on the implementation of GBG in their schools. Coaches can become certified GBG trainers with an additional year of training.
>
> SOURCE: Blueprints for Healthy Youth Development, 2024a.

2024). Suquamish and Port Gamble S'Klallam leaders identified community needs to prevent substance use and develop a sense of cultural belonging among youth. They partnered with ADAI to develop a curriculum adapted from the traditional Canoe Journey, tailored specifically for their tribes, for youth to build healthy social and interpersonal skills and prevent the initiation of substance use (Donovan et al., 2015). See also Box 2-5 for details about Family Spirit, an EBP developed for Indigenous families to improve pregnancy and child development outcomes.

Approaches for Adults

Faith-Based and Community Settings

Faith-based settings, such as churches, mosques, synagogues, and other houses of worship, along with other community groups, are well positioned to provide universal preventive interventions and promote social norms that encourage help-seeking (HHS Partnership Center, 2023). Interventions can include support groups, SEL programs, and parenting courses. Leaders may serve as role models, changing social norms and reducing stigma around MEB disorders, by being open about MH or addiction issues, encouraging

> **BOX 2-4**
> **Boys and Girls Clubs of Washington State Association's Promising Out-of-School Program**
>
> Afterschool programs provide another setting for delivering prevention services to school-age children and adolescents. One example is the Boys & Girls Clubs of Washington State Association (BGCWA), which has developed and is implementing a 3-year pilot program in 14 of its club organizations to provide behavioral health staff support and trauma-informed training in partnership with the Washington State Office of Superintendent of Public Instruction, Paxis Institute, and Norcliffe Foundation.
>
> BGCWA deployed three implementation strategies. First, it hired 14 full-time behavioral support specialists, one for each of the 14 clubs (representing 169 different communities). They also led staff training, student socio-emotional learning programming, and family engagement. Second, guided by Paxis Institute, BGCWA trained 398 full-time staff and 674 part-time youth development professionals across Boys & Girls Clubs in the state in behavior management approaches that include trauma-informed care. As its third strategy, BGCWA implemented SEL programming using the SMART Moves Emotional Wellness program along with other efforts to provide environments responsive to a range of needs (i.e., "Quiet Corners and Sensory Tools") and engage teens in small group sessions and build relationships with families and the community through its Family Nights (reprioritized after COVID-19 pandemic disruption).
>
> The BGCWA initiative demonstrated that the workforce pipeline can be enhanced by community organizations participating in this work. The 14 clubs were asked to identify anyone on their staff who was on the continuum of psychology, counseling, or pursuing licensure or study, and if they were not licensed, the club arranged for supervision from a licensed professional in the community and paid for the supervisory contact. The program was viewed as a way to popularize the concepts related to MEB health, destigmatizing the topic, and normalizing the Boys & Girls Club as a place to go for help.
>
> SOURCE: Day, 2023, 2024.

community members to seek help if they are struggling, and providing referrals to MH care providers. A variety of programs supporting protective factors and reducing risk or screening for risk have demonstrated effectiveness in exercise clubs and community spaces, such as libraries, parks, hair salons, and barber shops. Community-partnered depression screenings were

> **BOX 2-5**
> **Evidence-Based Program: Family Spirit**
>
> Family Spirit is a home visiting program designed for Indigenous pregnant women and families. Family Spirit meets Department of Health and Human Services criteria for model effectiveness in tribal populations and can be used for non-Native populations with disparities in maternal and child behavioral health. Family Spirit sends paraprofessional home visitors to conduct visits starting during pregnancy and up until the child's third birthday to deliver a curriculum that incorporates problem-solving skills and traditional tribal teachings. This curriculum involves 63 lessons that cover prenatal care, infant care, child development, toddler care, life skills and healthy living. The model was shown to be effective in improving child development and school readiness, maternal health, and positive parenting practices.
>
> Family Spirit recommends that home visitors be members of the participating community and allows affiliates to make enhancements to meet needs at the local level. They also encourage paraprofessionals to have familiarity with local or tribal culture, traditions, and languages.
>
> SOURCE: HomVEE, 2022.

demonstrated to be more effective than resources for individual programs improving MH-related quality of life, "physical activity, and homelessness risk factors, and shifted [use] away from hospitalizations and specialty medication visits toward primary care and other sectors, offering an expanded health-home model to address multiple disparities for depressed safety-net clients" (Wells et al., 2013, p.1268).

Approaches for Older Adults

Because the social and MEB needs of older adults are linked, strategies to improve MEB health will ideally be delivered along with health and social services to meet the MEB needs of low-income and homebound older adults (Forsman et al., 2011; Heisel, 2006). Strategies include supporting people by securing low-income senior housing and Section 8 housing vouchers, addressing social isolation and loneliness by providing opportunities for social engagement and volunteering, and facilitating access to improved access to MEB health services (see Box 2-6 for a promising program for older adults).

> **BOX 2-6**
> **PEARLS: A Promising Preventive Intervention for Older Adults**
>
> PEARLS (Program to Encourage Active, Rewarding Lives) at University of Washington screens older adults for symptoms of depression and helps them build skills for more active and self-sufficient living. It is an evidence-based "program for all older adults, especially those who have limited access to depression care because of systemic racism, trauma, language barriers, low income, and/or where they live. This is because PEARLS was designed in collaboration with the organizations that deliver it, validated in partnership with the communities who use it, and adaptable to the people who need it" (UW, 2025).
> It is delivered in the older adult's home or "a community-based setting that is more accessible and comfortable for older adults who do not see other mental health programs as a good fit for them." Staff at community-based organizations are trained to deliver the program. No counseling training or higher education is required.
>
> SOURCE: Smith et al., 2023.

Workplace Settings

Workplaces can contribute to preventing MEB disorders and promote worker well-being through approaches that target the organization or target the individual worker. Individually targeted approaches are primarily employee assistance programs,[1] which have been proliferating despite a lack of evidence of effectiveness (Fleming, 2024). At the organizational level, however, a psychosocial safety climate can play a role in worker well-being and requires organizational change strategies and work redesign (Bouzikos et al., 2022; Zadow et al., 2019). Organizational and group-level interventions also have a universal prevention focus—to support all workers by changing work conditions—addressing workplace stressors by strengthening protective factors (e.g., flexwork and self-scheduling) that benefit even those who do not pursue workplace resources for well-being (Fox, 2021). A systematic review by Fox and colleagues (2021) found that "[i]nterventions that most reliably improved well-being incorporated multiple facets of

---

[1] EAPs are "voluntary, work-based program that offers free and confidential assessments, short-term counseling, referrals, and follow-up services to employees who have personal and/or work-related problems." See https://www.opm.gov/frequently-asked-questions/work-life-faq/employee-assistance-program-eap/what-is-an-employee-assistance-program-eap/ for more detail.

> **BOX 2-7**
> **Promising Approach: Web-Based Apps**
>
> Kaiser Permanente, Veterans Health Administration (VHA), and other U.S. health care systems have launched digital ecosystems for MEB wellness (Wakefield et al., 2024). Many programs have been adapted for web- or app-based delivery, and others are being digitized to promote scale-up, with VHA programming being a great example. MEB health programs include varying types of professional support, from face-to-face interaction in a teleconference setting to entirely digital interactions through a web-based app. Digital apps have proliferated in recent years, intensified by pandemic-era needs for virtual delivery. Estimates indicate as many as 20,000 MEB health apps focused on a wide range of outcomes, from mindfulness and medication to symptoms of anxiety and depression. There is evidence of effectiveness for some telehealth interventions. For example, the Pathways for African American Success was tested in a randomized controlled trial comparing a telehealth to control and group arms and found to be effective (Murry et al., 2019).

change within their overall intervention and provided many opportunities for employee engagement" (p. 46).

Approaches for Veterans

One of the Department of Veterans Affairs' (VA) many approaches to preventing suicide among veterans aims to increase safety planning and follow-up by caring contacts through emergency settings. When a veteran is "assessed as being at risk of suicide but still safe enough to be discharged home, VA deploys a suicide safety planning intervention, including lethal means safety counseling, while the person is still in the emergency department or urgent care center" (Carroll et al., 2020, p.3). This program was found to reduce "suicidal behaviors by almost half" (45 percent) "in the 6 months following emergency department visits" (Carroll et al., 2020, p.3). Box 2-7 discusses web-based apps.

IMPLEMENTATION SCIENCE

Although dissemination and implementation (D&I) science is a relatively new field—with the first conference by the National Institutes of Health (NIH) on the Science of Dissemination and Implementation in

Health 17 years ago—like prevention science, it has been a part of scientific inquiry since at least the early 20th century (Dearing et al., 2023; Estabrooks et al., 2018). Implementation science is the "systematic, scientific approach to ask and answer questions about how we get 'what works' to people who need it, with greater speed, fidelity, efficiency, quality and relevant coverage" (UWDGH, 2024). The uptake of EBPs can take decades, and implementation science has emerged to reduce this gap, to speed the translation of discovery into real-world impact for all people. It can be drawn upon, with established frameworks, methods, outcomes, and strategies, when considering how to implement a national infrastructure to prevent MEB disorders. Implementation occurs at multiple levels, with each being related and optimally collaborative but having differing roles and responsibilities of the constituents. The overall meta-process of setting up a prevention infrastructure for MEB disorders speaks to policy makers, funders, and decision makers, while the hyperlocal community level that will be charged with frontline implementation activities and processes will include providers, faith leaders, educators, activists, and community partners. The interactions between and across these levels of constituents will happen within each community related to implementation of the infrastructure needed for the prevention effort, in a nuanced contextually appropriate way.

Implementation Strategies and Considerations

These implementation strategies encompass a variety of resources, organizations, individuals, and practical and conceptual tools to support the successful sustained implementation of an intervention or group of interventions. In addition to numerous frameworks, there are also blended implementation strategies, in which multiple strategies that address multiple levels or barriers to change are blended as one package (Powell et al., 2012). These include the Communities That Care framework (CTC), Promoting School-community-university Partnerships to Enhance Resilience (PROSPER) or Getting to Outcomes (GTO). CTC is a program that uses a "blended implementation strategy aimed at developing community-based prevention systems that take advantage of multiple evidence-based programs" (NASEM, 2019a, p. 225). This approach aims to foster comprehensive and coordinated community-led prevention that meets the needs of all young people in the community. Trained CTC coaches provide training and technical support to build capacity in community coalitions to use data to assess strengths, needs, and prevention gaps; develop prevention priorities and select and implement appropriate programs; and monitor results. PROSPER is a system that links university researchers with communities to support the delivery of programs related to promoting youth and family MEB well-being—the focus is on maximizing existing education infrastructure to build capacity and allow for sustained program delivery in partnership with others who are attuned to local needs. The GTO toolkit offers support for community leaders to follow 10 steps: focus on problems; target goals, population, and outcomes; adopt programs; adapt programs; assess capacity and resources for implementation; plan to get started; monitor implementation; evaluate implementation; improve continuously; and sustain if successful. GTO is "intended to strengthen agencies' and organizations' use of prevention programs regardless of prior evidence of effectiveness"; it provides tools and supports to help communities identify the best EBP for their needs and context (see *Fostering Healthy MEB Development in Youth* [2019] for greater detail about blended implementation strategies) (NASEM, 2019a, p. 237). Federally funded implementation organizations include the Prevention Transfer Technology Centers and National Center for Mental Health: Dissemination, Implementation, and Sustainment.

Community Partnerships and Community-Led Work

A wealth of literature suggests that the most successful implementations are led by the community but supported by research and rigor to develop an infrastructure that can evaluate, realize, and sustain outcomes. Prevention requires a long-term lens, where outcomes might not be realized for years or until later in the life-span, and sustained implementation is critical.

Implementing preventive interventions must center the community, be led by it, and result in partnership between community members (see Box 2-8 for steps towards successful implementation of an intervention) (Gunn et al., 2022). Policy makers and funders must have relationships with the communities they represent to identify service gaps, new needs, and emerging prevention issues (NASEM, 2023). Researchers must have relationships with community partners to identify feasible methods and strategies to activate in real-world contexts and prioritize resources toward prevention that is meaningful to communities (NCDD, 2009). And community partners themselves must come together with a shared vision and motivation to enact change through adoption of EBP. While individual "go-it-alone" implementations help bring in innovation, community partnership is necessary to develop the infrastructure for sustained change.

Implementation research has identified that trust and respect are the most important facilitators of community partnerships, while time commitment is a potential barrier (Pellecchia et al., 2018). Implementation partnerships must consider the feasibility of time and resources necessary for success.

Funding Needs

Implementing evidence-based interventions requires adequate and sustained funding. There is some information about the costs of evidence-based

> **BOX 2-8**
> **Eight Steps for Implementation of Preventive Interventions in Communities**
>
> As noted in Chapter 1, these steps are not necessarily sequential, and many can and should be concurrent.
>
> 1. **Identify the Need:** To address a problem, communities will need to take steps to clearly identify it. This can be achieved through needs assessments, such as a community health assessment or improvement plan (CDC, 2024b).
> 2. **Select the Intervention:** Choosing an intervention or package of interventions can be daunting. To support this process, communities can use implementation strategies, such as the GTO toolkit, partner with a university (i.e., PROSPER), or consult the University of Washington's Center for Communities that Care. Communities can also independently refer to any number of clearinghouses, such as the ACF Title IV-E Prevention Services Clearinghouse (ACF, n.d.). Planning for sustainment should also be considered at this step, and tools such as A Designing for Dissemination & Sustainability Action Planner may be of use (D4DS, n.d.).
> 3. **Map the Constituents:** Mapping the constituents allows communities to determine key players for implementation to ensure that those who are affected by the problem are part of the problem-solving process. Constituent mapping and collaboration also increase buy-in and ensure the implementation addresses the need. I-STEM is one tool that can offer key considerations and activities for conducting constituent engagement activities during implementation (Potthoff et al., 2023).
> 4. **Assess Barriers and Facilitators and Understand Context:** Barriers and facilitators, or "determinants," are categories of enablers

programs (e.g., from evidence clearinghouses, such as Blueprints for Healthy Youth Development[2] and the National Center for Education Statistics). However, communities have different demographics, needs, and assets,

---

[2] In July 2024, external funding concluded for Blueprints for Healthy Youth Development. Blueprints' leadership opted to "put Blueprints into dormancy until it is possible to secure a sustainable, high-impact path forward. The dormancy process entails updating information on the existing programs listed on our website and ensuring that Blueprints will remain freely available and searchable while in dormancy. This process will be completed by June 2025" (Buckley, 2024).

or hindrances to intervention adoption, implementation, and sustainment and may include costs, workforce, and political or collective will in addressing the issue. Communities will need to be able to rapidly assess barriers and facilitators and develop strategies to address them. There are many tools to help support this assessment, such as a pragmatic context assessment tool (Robinson and Damschroder, 2023).

5. **Create a Logic Model:** Once Steps 1–4 are completed, communities can create a road map for the implementation. There is no one correct way to do this, and the important part is that the approach is mapped out intentionally and prospectively and documents the identified need or problem, proposed intervention, required resources, target outcomes, and data and evaluation. The Implementation Research Logic Model may be a helpful starting point (Smith et al., 2020).

6. **Evaluate:** As documented in the logic model, communities will need ongoing evaluation of the intervention to assess if it is effective or changes should be made.

7. **Adapt:** A possible outcome of early evaluations may indicate to a community that an intervention is on the right track but needs to be adapted to suit the community's needs. Adaptation is necessary to ensure maximum success and fit to context (Chambers, 2023) (Geng et al., 2023; Wiltsey Stirman et al., 2019).

8. **Sustain:** Sustainment is a throughline for the entire process, as noted. In addition to tools such as D4DS, emerging evidence of types of sustainment strategies may be helpful information for communities (Wolfenden et al., 2024).

NOTE: ACF = Administration for Children and Families; CTC = Communities That Care; GTO = Getting to Outcomes; PROSPER = Promoting School-Community-University Partnerships to Enhance Resilience.

and each community will require a package of evidence-based interventions that is best suited to the local context. Very little published research is available on the cost of scaling prevention programs and associated components of the infrastructure, such as data and resources (see Fagan and colleagues [2019] for one review on increasing scale-up in U.S. public systems to prevent MEB disorders). The following examples are provided to (1) illustrate potential ways to estimate costs of programs, and (2) to help answer the question "what does an investment in prevention infrastructure buy a community?"

TABLE 2-1 Examples of General Cost Estimates for Selected Interventions

Example of program	Cost
Delivering Parent Corps projected to cost $111,000 per school to each of more than 13,000 school districts in the nation (annually)	$1.45 billion
Delivering Nurse-Family Partnership (an evidence-based intervention) that costs $12,437 to each eligible family (465,000 eligible families in a year)	$5.78 billion
Delivering an evidence-based intervention (e.g., Good Behavior Game) to each elementary school student in birth cohort (approximately 3.6 million/year) at a per student cost of $160/individual	$576 million

SOURCES: Blueprints for Healthy Youth Development, 2024a,c,d; Zaid et al., 2022.

One could assume an average of five evidence-based programs per county, with programs ranging in cost from an early childhood intervention, such as Nurse-Family Partnership, at $12,437 per family given the intense one-to-one nature of the intervention, to $10,000 to $12,000 per school for school-based interventions that involve training teachers and staff, and delivery to students and/or parents/guardians (Blueprints for Healthy Child Development, 2024b,c). Table 2-1 gives a general idea—for illustration purposes only—of the resources needed by states and localities to ensure that every community has the necessary support for MEB prevention programs.

Another way to think about program costs is to consider the full cost of planning and implementing an evidence-based program in a community (e.g., staffing, technology, office and space). A micro costing study estimated that first year cost of a community-based mental health prevention program in a population of 272,000 across 10 ZIP codes would cost $1,382,669 for the first year in 2022 dollars (Roy et al., 2024). Multiplying by 3,142 U.S. counties (acknowledging the vast range in population across counties), the cost of year 1 of a similar program being implemented in every county in the United States would be $4.3 billion. Note that counties vary widely in size, need, and local resources of all kinds, that the number of counties does not cover some tribal places and communities, and the 574 federally recognized tribal nations would need comparable levels of investment.

RESEARCH NEEDS TO IMPROVE THE EVIDENCE BASE ON INTERVENTIONS AND THEIR IMPLEMENTATION

Developing, testing, and establishing numerous evidence-based preventive interventions for MEB health is a notable achievement within the field of prevention science. However, there are evidence gaps and research needs related to the existing body of knowledge and the D&I of the interventions. Although many interventions have been developed and demonstrated to show positive outcomes in rigorous trials, EBPs continue to be plagued with low rates of adoption in real-world community settings and even lower rates of sustainment (Wong et al., 2022).

Improving and Maintaining the Evidence Base on Existing Interventions

NIH and other research funders have invested significantly in rigorous research to establish dozens of demonstrated effective programs, policies, and practices that improve MEB outcomes (Murray et al., 2021). As noted, much of the evidence for prevention comes from studies of interventions targeting the early stages of life, among infants, children, adolescents, or their parents and caregivers. Other stages of life are less frequently represented, meaning the prevention and health promotion needs of middle-aged and older adults do not yet have the same volume of evidence-based strategies (Epstein et al., 2023).

Although the fields of prevention and implementation science have steadily increased their focus on developing interventions that reduce health disparities and can be used in any community and cultural context, the longest-established interventions in the evidence base to prevent MEBs predate this shift (Shelton and Brownson, 2023). There is a long history of research that does not include Black and Latino subpopulations, people with disabilities and LGBTQ people, and that was almost exclusively reliant on White male participants (NASEM, 2022; NIMHD, 2024). As such, some interventions with the longest history of RCTs or other research may not be applicable in diverse communities for a number of reasons. Therefore:

- Well-tested interventions may still not apply to groups that were excluded from any of the original studies.
- The interventions may not be well received or applicable in all communities (NIHB, 2009).
- The interventions were not developed to and are not equipped to reduce MEB health disparities (Sanchez et al., 2023).

The first and third points above do not mean that existing EBPs cannot be useful in populations in which they were not included when programs were tested but careful attention must be given to needs and cultural contexts of every community where an EBP is being implemented (Sanchez et al., 2023). These considerations can be developed by focusing on research that assesses generalizability of interventions not only to different groups of people but across different real-life settings.

RECOMMENDATION 2-1: The National Institutes of Health, Centers for Disease Control and Prevention, and philanthropic organizations should fund more research on the prevention of mental, emotional, and behavioral (MEB) disorders that addresses research gaps related to intervention development (to identify what works and the certainty and magnitude of outcomes) and implementation (to identify how to deliver and sustain interventions with fidelity). This research should prioritize interventions that target MEB health inequities, are needed for different age groups, and are co-created with the populations they are intended to serve.

A few process options may be helpful for funders to practically identify research needs, further health equity, and focus on community cocreation in research going forward. Funders can use existing taxonomies,[3] develop new ones, or a combination thereof to systematically and consistently identify further evidence gaps and research needs and set priorities so appropriate proposals are funded and the research needs are addressed. Additionally, funders could request that study sections, scientific review officers, and others in similar roles familiarize themselves with theoretical frameworks for expanding fair opportunities for all people to attain their full health potential to be used during the proposal review process. Funders also can set aside sufficient resources for community–academic partnerships specifically for evaluation to support communities that have or are developing practice-based evidence to partner with scientists.

When developing requests for proposals, funders can emphasize the need for

- Interventions that can be tailored for different contexts, settings, and age ranges, using data that has been disaggregated by race and ethnicity, and for an array of participants, from those who are easily engaged to those who have been historically excluded or underrepresented or who experience language access barriers;
- Co-design, co-production, or co-creation of intervention and implementation approaches between investigators, community members, and/or future participants in research proposals and projects; and
- Implementation plans for interventions that prove successful including adequate attention to pre-implementation timelines and resource allocation, understanding that pre-implementation requires different timelines under different community contexts.

---

[3] See, for example, the clinical prevention foundational issues, analytic framework, and dissemination and implementation taxonomies for identifying research gaps at https://nap.nationalacademies.org/resource/26351/ or the Reconnecting Youth Evidence Gap Map at https://youth.gov/youth-topics/opportunity-youth/reconnecting-youth?q=egm.

Improving Knowledge Dissemination

I get bombarded, as a school district director, from calls all over the country trying to sell me programs as evidence-based practices, and you look at the effect sizes, if they have any, and they're only observable in laboratory settings. Our school leadership doesn't know how to discern that.

—Joe Neigel, Monroe School District Director of Prevention Services, Washington

NIH and other research funders have invested significantly in rigorous research to establish dozens of demonstrated effective programs, policies, and practices that improve MEB health outcomes (Murray et al., 2021). Two major ways new research is disseminated and eventually implemented are public health campaigns and evidence-based clearinghouses. The former tend to focus more on shifting social norms and behaviors toward promoting health and well-being and reducing disease (ODP, 2023) but can include concrete tips and strategies for communities or leaders to adopt. For example, CollegeAIM is an implementation guide that can be found on NIH's Office of Disease Prevention's public health campaigns webpage; it not only evaluates 60 different interventions designed to prevent harmful drinking among college students but provides detailed preimplementation considerations (how administrators can evaluate needs, assess which blend of strategies to use, and assess cost and other resources needed) (NIAAA, 2019b). Evidence-based clearinghouses[4] are web-based collections of programs and practices often centered around a particular topic or age group (Lee et al., 2022). Their landscape is dotted with multiple sets of standards, multiple sources, and a range of proprietary or trademarked interventions (see Appendix B for a sample of some of the evidence-based clearinghouses available that share information about preventive interventions for MEB disorders, although most of them do not exclusively cover these).

Barriers to adopting interventions include implementers not being aware of existing interventions or knowing which are applicable to their population or setting needs. Implementers may not be aware of evidence clearinghouses that list and, in some cases, evaluate and rate interventions. In addition, implementers may not understand these rating systems. Many of these issues are compounded by a related challenge: at least three dozen prevention-related evidence clearinghouses exist (Burkhardt et al., 2015; Lee-Easton and Magura, 2023; Lee et al., 2022). The evidence base of interventions is not disseminated or implemented well across communities for a variety of reasons, and developing interventions with validity for

---

[4] Also called "registries," although this report uses "clearinghouses" whenever possible.

diverse groups of people and settings is needed, as is continued research and development for existing interventions.

Some clearinghouses only include interventions for child and adolescent populations, and some are broad, spanning prevention *and* treatment interventions to support physical and MEB health. Clearinghouses can collate and rank prevention programs to support decision makers considering which interventions to implement to promote MEB health. However, the landscape is not able to support these decision makers, because clearinghouses are created, overhauled, and closed without harmonized goals and standards. Reinforcing the overlapping and sometimes confusing aspect of this is a kind of cross-referencing by clearinghouses. For example, Blueprints for Healthy Youth Development included "Endorsements" where applicable in each intervention it reviews, noting which other clearinghouses also recommend the program, presumably to strengthen its credibility. Another example is Youth.gov, which has a webpage titled "The Federal Understanding of the Evidence Base," linking to clearinghouses managed by AmeriCorps (two), U.S. Agency for International Development (one), U.S. Department of Agriculture (USDA, one); Department of Defense and USDA-collaboration (one), Department of Education (two); Department of Health and Human Services (HHS, 16); Department of Justice (three); and Department of Labor (one) (Youth.gov, n.d.). These clearinghouses cover topics mostly related to youth but have vast range among what part of the prevention-treatment continuum they address, settings, types of programs, and intended outcomes (some are focused on risk and protective factors, while others focus on reducing specific discrete outcomes, such as teen pregnancy).

The proprietary nature of programs poses barriers as well. These include challenges to transparency and collaboration, and potential conflicts of interest or biases in how those interventions are evaluated (Supplee et al., 2022). Clearinghouses typically include limited information about implementation factors that affect whether impacts from efficacy trials are achieved in real-world delivery. The patchwork nature of the landscape is exacerbated by inconsistent evaluation of programs: many clearinghouses lack transparency about inclusion criteria, and those that offer grades (e.g., "highly recommended" or "strong evidence for. . .") do not use standardized evaluation measures (Lee-Easton and Magura, 2023). Between the standard for which evidence is assessed and the potentially differing criteria (e.g., one clearinghouse highly prioritizes a criterion, such as health equity, while another does not explicitly consider it at all), high grades may mean vastly different things. One study by Zheng, Wadhwa, and Cook (2022) reviewed 13 clearinghouses and found that 82 percent of 2,525 programs were rated by a single clearinghouse, and of those rated by more than one, agreement of effectiveness was reached about half the time. Similarly, a 2024 study reviewed 1,359 programs over 10 clearinghouses and found "83% of them were assessed by a single clearinghouse and, of those rated by more than one, similar ratings were achieved for only about 30% of the programs" (Wadhwa et al., 2024). This analysis reveals that the majority of programs are only included in one clearinghouse, limiting replication opportunities for evaluation, and when they are evaluated by multiple clearinghouses, they receive dissimilar ratings more often than not. This inconsistency in inclusion and grading renders clearinghouses less useful to communities trying to determine which programs would be most effective. As an example, one of the programs identified in this report was not endorsed and another was considered "promising" by one clearinghouse. In both cases, another clearinghouse had fully endorsed both programs. For example, Familias Unidas (see Box 3-3) is rated as a Promising Program on Blueprints for Healthy Child Development but given the highest endorsement for the strength of evidence by the California Evidence-Based Clearinghouse for Child Welfare (Pantin et al., 2009). Again, reference in this report to a specific program should not be considered an endorsement by this committee, but illustrative of the needs of the prevention infrastructure.

Perhaps the most well-known clearinghouse of preventive interventions for MEB disorders was the Substance Abuse and Mental Health Services Administration (SAMHSA) National Registry of Effective Prevention Programs (NREPP), which was launched in 1997. SAMHSA renamed this the National Registry of Evidence-based Programs and Practices and added treatment interventions. In late 2017, NREPP was suspended, and in early 2018 funding for the work of evaluating and rating the evidence for programs listed was terminated (Dodge Foundation, 2018). An effort to standardize and preserve the data in the original evidence clearinghouse was undertaken by the Pew-MacArthur Results First Initiative, which archived 80 percent of the NREPP links (Bryant-Comstock, 2019). In 2018, SAMHSA launched the Evidence-Based Practices Resource Center (EBPRC) which is extant and is simply a collection of resources that are not rated or evaluated. This has left the field of MEB disorder prevention with incomplete, outdated, and discordant resources to navigate the evidence base.

Despite these challenges, evidence based clearinghouses have significant potential to improve MEB outcomes for all communities, particularly those that are disproportionately affected, by supporting the dissemination of interventions that promote MEB health and being transparent about the process used to evaluate the intervention (Hirsch et al., 2023). The committee learned from a Federal Register notice and SAMHSA outreach to the field that the agency has been seeking input on the importance and organization of a potentially relaunched centralized clearinghouse of evidence-based prevention programs. The Federal Register notice stated that the EBPRC does not meet the 21st Century Cures Act vision to "make the metrics used to evaluate applications . . . and any resulting ratings of such applications, publicly available,"[5] emphasizing a transparent rating and review system for EBPs (Mayo-Wilson et al., 2022). SAMHSA's actions are good steps forward. To support SAMHSA's work, the committee underscores key components of an evaluation system that are necessary to fill the gap of a "decision support tool," as NREPP was designed to be:

1. A set of criteria for both including and evaluating programs that considers both EBP and PBE, implementation, dissemination, fit to population, and generalizability.
2. A clear focus on including programs that are diverse and already are/can be tailored to meet the needs of underserved and excluded subpopulations, which should include groups across the life course and settings outside of school.
3. A system that can clearly sort programs between levels of prevention and, in particular, includes community-level universal primary/primordial interventions.
4. A system that accounts for the proprietary nature of many programs, protects against bias in the evidence submitted and review process, and does not include programs that have not been evaluated. For example, in 2017, one review of 112 programs newly added to NREPP found that 78 percent had some conflict of interest. In the majority of those cases, the point of contact for the program also authored at least one document reviewed as evidence for inclusion (Gorman, 2017); and
5. Clear cost/funding information for each program, which should include up-front and reoccurring costs to run programs once they have been implemented in a community and the potential cost of hiring workforce as applicable.

Many clearinghouses have no dedicated and sustained funding source, making it hard to maintain quality or respond dynamically as the evidence base changes. Sustained, non-grant-dependent resourcing is needed. Ideally, support for select clearinghouses would be built into SAMHSA's budget as a permanent component. In addition to procedures for regularly updating and maintaining the clearinghouse, a feedback loop is needed to outline data collection needs as a program is implemented, so that evaluation can take place during implementation and adjustments made—and learnings (such as tailoring of an intervention for a specific cultural or language contexts) integrated in the clearinghouse.

---

[5] 21st Century Cures Act, Public Law 114-255, §7002, 114th Cong., 1st sess. (December 13, 2016).

Prevention leaders, such as coordinators and directors, in partnership with implementers, are making decisions with significant resource constraints. Opacity and fragmentation of the evidence of effective MEB disorder prevention programs for their communities should not be one of them. With the resources they are able to dedicate to prevention, the committee believes these prevention leaders should be able to explore existing programs that may work for them and use that information to consider which innovative new programs would be promising for the community if there is a gap. A centralized decision support tool is needed to navigate the evidence base, and the committee believes that SAMHSA's efforts on this point are laudable and important to continue and ultimately lead to the re-establishment of NREPP or something like it.

An evidence base exists of tested and effective MEB disorder preventive and health promotive interventions particularly targeted for children, youth, and families, which address a variety of BH outcomes, and many are cost effective. The evidence base for other stages of the life course is not as robust. Also, the reach and impact of these interventions is limited for several reasons:

- Barriers to successful adoption (knowledge of interventions at all, or difficulty accessing them because of clearinghouse lack of usefulness or cost barriers);
- Other barriers to implementation: lack of tools/knowledge to implement them successfully (no preimplementation plan for sustainability), necessary funding levels not met in the real world and inadequate funding mechanisms, failure to consider implementation factors that moderate impact; and
- Generalizability and external validity: limitations include narrow age range and study demographics and lack of ecological validity (e.g., inadequate research with underrepresented racial, ethnic, and tribal populations, lack of cultural or language appropriateness, or lack of consideration for cultural or other ecological contexts that shape effectiveness of interventions).

CONCLUSION 2-1: *Existing prevention strategies and evidence clearinghouses—as critical aspects of the prevention and health promotion infrastructure—are necessary but not sufficient for meeting population mental, emotional, and behavioral (MEB) health needs and reducing disparities in MEB outcomes that originate during preconception and early life and can increase along the life course.*

RECOMMENDATION 2-2: The Substance Abuse and Mental Health Services Administration (SAMHSA) should manage and maintain a

centralized and dynamic evidence clearinghouse for mental, emotional, and behavioral health that promotes standardization of criteria for inclusion and evaluation. The clearinghouse should include information about intervention effectiveness, guidance for implementation, and a focus on prevention strategies that address the needs of diverse communities.

To support uptake of effective interventions and integrate practice-based evidence, SAMHSA should also

a. Develop clearinghouse navigation tools to help implementers find relevant strategies, ensure implementation quality, and increase the likelihood of impact; and
b. Work with state and other grantees to develop a mechanism to integrate evaluation of implementation, new knowledge, and community experience.

Possible criteria for inclusion within this centralized and dynamic clearinghouse could include:

1. Quality of the evidence: reliability and internal validity;
2. Generalizability of results to specific and new subpopulations, settings, and geographic locations (external validity); and
3. Preimplementation, implementation, and cost considerations.

Clearinghouse usability considerations include having straightforward search functions and being tailorable for different needs, concise, and jargon free. To operationalize a focus on health equity, SAMHSA could include a transparent and consistent section on health equity considerations, e.g., whether there are differential impacts across populations and if an intervention worsens, sustains, or reduces MEB health disparities (Hirsch et al., 2023). Managing this resource may fall under the role of the Evidence-Based Practices Innovation and Dissemination Team under SAMHSA's National Mental Health and Substance Use Policy Laboratory, as they currently disseminate information about programs through SAMHSA's EBPRC, along with training and technical assistance providers, listservs, and social media (GAO, 2024). SAMHSA could also provide technical assistance to communities to select appropriate, contextually relevant, and culturally responsive EBPs to meet their needs and active implementation support to ensure success. It could be a function of the HHS Behavioral Health Coordinating Council (or similar cross-departmental structure) to work with SAMHSA in accomplishing working with state grantees to develop a mechanism to further integrate evaluation along with dissemination of new research.

REFERENCES

Abraham, E., C. Blanco, C. Castillo Lee, J. B. Christian, N. Kass, E. B. Larson, M. Mazumdar, S. Morain, K. M. Newton, A. Ommaya, B. Patrick-Lake, R. Platt, J. Steiner, M. Zirkle, and M. Hamilton Lopez. 2016. Generating knowledge from best care: Advancing the continuously learning health system. *NAM Perspectives*. Discussion paper, National Academy of Medicine, Washington, DC. https://doi.org/10.31478/201609b.

ACF (Administration for Children and Families). n.d. *Title IV-E Prevention Services Clearinghouse.* https://preventionservices.acf.hhs.gov/ (accessed December 16, 2024).

APA (American Psychological Association). 2005. Policy Statement on Evidence-Based-Practice in Psychology. http://www2.apa.org/practice/ebpstatement.pdf. (accessed January 7, 2025).

Barlow, J., E. Coren, and S. Stewart-Brown. 2002. Meta-analysis of the effectiveness of parenting programmes in improving maternal psychosocial health. *British Journal of General Practice* 52(476):223–233. https://www.ncbi.nlm.nih.gov/pubmed/12030667 (accessed December 31, 2024).

Bartgis, D., and D. Bigfoot. n.d. *Evidence-based practices and practice-based evidence.* https://ncuih.org/ebp-pbe/ (accessed October 26, 2024).

Blueprints for Healthy Youth Development. 2024a. *Good behavior game.* https://www.blueprintsprograms.org/programs/20999999/good-behavior-game/ (accessed September 9, 2024).

Blueprints for Healthy Youth Development. 2024b. *Lifeskills training.* https://www.blueprintsprograms.org/programs/5999999/lifeskills-training-lst/ (accessed October 9, 2024).

Blueprints for Healthy Youth Development. 2024c. *Nurse-family partnership.* https://www.blueprintsprograms.org/programs/35999999/nurse-family-partnership/ (accessed December 11, 2024).

Blueprints for Healthy Youth Development. 2024d. *Parentcorps.* https://www.blueprintsprograms.org/programs/1291999999/parentcorps/ (accessed December 11, 2024).

Bouzikos, S., A. Afsharian, M. Dollard, and O. Brecht. 2022. Contextualising the effectiveness of an employee assistance program intervention on psychological health: The role of corporate climate. *International Journal of Environmental Research and Public Health* 19(9). https://doi.org/10.3390/ijerph19095067.

Brown, C. H., G. Curran, L. A. Palinkas, G. A. Aarons, K. B. Wells, L. Jones, L. M. Collins, N. Duan, B. S. Mittman, A. Wallace, R. G. Tabak, L. Ducharme, D. A. Chambers, C. Neta, T. Wiley, J. Landsverk, K. Cheung, and G. Cruden. 2017. An overview of research and evaluation designs for dissemination and implementation. *Annual Review of Public Health* 20(38):1–22. https://doi.org/10.1146/annurev-publhealth-031816-044215.

Bryant-Comstock, S. 2019. *Results first initiative saves NREPP from obscurity.* https://www.cmhnetwork.org/news/results-first-initiative-saves-nrepp-from-obscurity/ (accessed December 31, 2024).

Buckley, P. 2024. *The blueprints bulletin.* Issue 29, October 2024. https://www.blueprintsprograms.org/issue-no-29/ (accessed December 16, 2024).

Burkhardt, J. T., D. C. Schröter, S. Magura, S. N. Means, and C. L. Coryn. 2015. An overview of evidence-based program registers (EBPRS) for behavioral health. *Evaluation and Program Planning* 48:92–99. https://doi.org/10.1016/j.evalprogplan.2014.09.006.

Carroll, D., L. K. Kearney, and M. A. Miller. 2020. Addressing suicide in the veteran population: Engaging a public health approach. *Frontiers in Psychiatry* 11:569069. https://doi.org/10.3389/fpsyt.2020.569069.

CDC (Centers for Disease Control and Prevention). 2023. *Out-of-school time.* https://www.cdc.gov/healthyschools/ost.htm (accessed September 11, 2024).

CDC. 2024a. *About adverse childhood experiences.* https://www.cdc.gov/aces/about/index.html (accessed November 11, 2024).

CDC. 2024b. *Community planning for health assessment: CHA & CHIP*. https://www.cdc.gov/public-health-gateway/php/public-health-strategy/public-health-strategies-for-community-health-assessment-health-improvement-planning.html (accessed November 11, 2024).

CEBC (The California Evidence-Based Clearinghouse for Child Welfare). 2024. *Nurse-family partnership*. https://www.cebc4cw.org/program/nurse-family-partnership/detailed (accessed December 16, 2024).

Chambers, D. A. 2023. Advancing adaptation of evidence-based interventions through implementation science: Progress and opportunities. *Frontiers in Health Services* 3:1204138. https://doi.org/10.3389/frhs.2023.1204138.

Cioffi, C. C., D. S. DeGarmo, and J. A. Jones. 2021. Participation in the fathering through change intervention reduces substance use among divorced and separated fathers. *Journal of Substance Use and Addiction Treatment* 120:108142. https://doi.org/10.1016/j.jsat.2020.108142.

Day, L. 2023. *Mental health promotion pilot: Year 1 report*. http://www.washingtonclubs.org/wp-content/uploads/2023/09/BGCWA_Mental-Health-Promotion-Pilot_Year-1-report.pdf (accessed January 10, 2025).

Day, L. 2024. *Mental health promotion pilot: Year 2 report*. http://www.washingtonclubs.org/wp-content/uploads/2023/08/BGCWA_Mental-Health-Pilot-Report_Year-2.pdf (accessed January 10, 2025).

Dodge Foundation. 2018. SAMHSA's Registry of Evidence-Based Programs (NREPP) Suspended. News Release. https://pgdf.org/samhsas-registry-of-evidence-based-programs-nrepp-suspended/ (accessed January 2, 2025).

D4DS. n.d. *D4DS planner*. https://d4dsplanner.com/ (accessed October 25, 2024).

Dearing, W. J., F. K. Kee, and T.-Q. Peng. 2023. Historical roots of dissemination and implementation science. In *Dissemination and implementation research in health*, edited by D. Chambers: Oxford University Press. Pp. 69–85.

Donovan, D. M., L. R. Thomas, R. L. Sigo, L. Price, H. Lonczak, N. Lawrence, K. Ahvakana, L. Austin, A. Lawrence, J. Price, A. Purser, and L. Bagley. 2015. Healing of the canoe: Preliminary results of a culturally tailored intervention to prevent substance abuse and promote tribal identity for Native youth in two Pacific Northwest tribes. *American Indian and Alaska Native Mental Health Research Journal* 22(1):42–76. https://doi.org/10.5820/aian.2201.2015.42.

Epstein, M., R. Kosterman, and R. F. Catalano. 2023. The potential for prevention science in middle and late adulthood: A commentary on the special issue of prevention science. *Prevention Science* 24(5):808–816. https://doi.org/10.1007/s11121-023-01544-y.

Estabrooks, P. A., R. C. Brownson, and N. P. Pronk. 2018. Dissemination and implementation science for public health professionals: An overview and call to action. *Preventing Chronic Disease* 15:E162. https://doi.org/10.5888/pcd15.180525.

Fagan, A. A., B. K. Bumbarger, R. P. Barth, C. P. Bradshaw, B. Rhoades Cooper, L. H. Supplee, and D. K. Walker. 2019. Scaling up evidence-based interventions in US public systems to prevent behavioral health problems: Challenges and opportunities. *Prevention Science* 20:1147–1168. https://doi.org/10.1007/s11121-019-01048-8.

Felitti, V. J., R. F. Anda, D. Nordenberg, D. F. Williamson, A. M. Spitz, V. Edwards, and J. S. Marks. 1998. Relationship of childhood abuse and household dysfunction to many of the leading causes of death in adults: The adverse childhood experiences (ACE) study. *American Journal of Preventive Medicine* 14(4):245–258. https://doi.org/10.1016/s0749-3797(98)00017-8.

Fleming, W. J. 2024. Employee well-being outcomes from individual-level mental health interventions: Cross-sectional evidence from the United Kingdom. *Industrial Relations Journal* 55(2):162–182. https://doi.org/10.1111/irj.12418.

Forgatch, M. S., G. R. Patterson, D. S. Degarmo, and Z. G. Beldavs. 2009. Testing the Oregon delinquency model with 9-year follow-up of the Oregon divorce study. *Development and Psychopathology* 21(2):637–660. https://doi.org/10.1017/S0954579409000340.

Forsman, A. K., J. Nordmyr, and K. Wahlbeck. 2011. Psychosocial interventions for the promotion of mental health and the prevention of depression among older adults. *Health Promotion International* 26(suppl_1):i85–i107. https://doi.org/10.1093/heapro/dar074.

Fox, K. E., S. T. Johnson, L. F. Berkman, M. Sianoja, Y. Soh, L. D. Kubzansky, and E. L. Kelly. 2021. Organisational- and group-level workplace interventions and their effect on multiple domains of worker well-being: A systematic review. *Work & Stress* 36 (1):30–59. https://doi.org/10.1080/02678373.2021.1969476.

GAO (U.S. Government Accountability Office). 2024. Behavioral health: Activities of the National Mental Health and Substance Use Policy Laboratory. GAO-24-106760. https://www.gao.gov/assets/gao-24-106760.pdf (accessed December 31, 2024).

Geng, E. H., A. Mody, and B. J. Powell. 2023. On-the-go adaptation of implementation approaches and strategies in health: Emerging perspectives and research opportunities. *Annual Review of Public Health* 44(1):21–36. https://doi.org/10.1146/annurev-publhealth051920-124515.

Gorman, D. M. 2017. Has the national registry of evidence-based programs and practices (NREPP) lost its way? *International Journal of Drug Policy* 45:40–41. https://doi.org/10.1016/j.drugpo.2017.05.010.

Green, L. W., and J. P. Allegrante. 2020. Practice-based evidence and the need for more diverse methods and sources in epidemiology, public health and health promotion. SAGE Publications.

Gunn C. M., L. S. Sprague Martinez, T. A. Battaglia, R. Lobb, D. Chassler, D. Hakim, M. L. Drainoni. 2022. Integrating community engagement with implementation science to advance the measurement of translational science. *J Clin Transl Sci* 1;6(1):e107. https://doi.org/10.1017/cts.2022.433.

Healing of the Canoe. 2024. *About us.* https://healingofthecanoe.org/about/ (accessed September 11, 2024).

Heisel, M. J. 2006. Suicide and its prevention among older adults. *The Canadian Journal of Psychiatry* 51(3):143–154. https://doi.org/10.1177/070674370605100304.

HHS Partnership Center. 2023. *Youth mental health and well-being in faith and community settings: Practicing connectedness a toolkit of the HHS partnership center.* https://www.hhs.gov/sites/default/files/youth-mental-health-and-well-being-in-faith-and-community-settings.pdf (accessed September 11, 2024).

Hirsch, B. K., M. C. Stevenson, and M. L. Givens. Evidence clearinghouses as tools to advance health equity: What we know from a systematic scan. *Prevention Science* 24:613–624 (2023). https://doi.org/10.1007/s11121-023-01511-7.

HomVEE (Home Visiting Evidence of Effectiveness). 2022. *Family spirit.* https://homvee.acf.hhs.gov/models/family-spiritr (accessed December 11, 2024).

IOM (Institute of Medicine). 2013. *Best care at lower cost: The path to continuously learning health care in America.* Washington, DC: The National Academies Press. https://doi.org/10.17226/13444.

Latimore, A. D., E. Salisbury-Afshar, N. Duff, E. Freiling, B. Kellett, R. D. Sullenger, and A. Salman. 2023. Primary, secondary, and tertiary prevention of substance use disorders through socioecological strategies. NAM Perspectives 9(6). https://doi.org/10.31478/202309b.

Lee, M. J., M. J. Maranda, S. Magura, and G. Greenman. 2022. References to evidence-based program registry (EBPR) websites for behavioral health in U.S. state government statutes and regulations. *Journal of Applied Social Science* 16(2):442–458. https://doi.org/10.1177/19367244221078278.

Lee-Easton, M. J., and S. Magura. 2023. Discrepancies in ratings of behavioral healthcare interventions among evidence-based program resources websites. *Inquiry* 60:469580231186836. https://doi.org/10.1177/00469580231186836.

Mayo-Wilson E., S. Grant, and L. H. Supplee. July 2022. Clearinghouse standards of evidence on the transparency, openness, and reproducibility of intervention evaluations. *Prevention Science* 23(5):774–86. https://doi.org/10.1007/s11121-021-01284-x.

Murray, D. M., L. F. Ganoza, A. J. Vargas, E. M. Ellis, N. K. Oyedele, S. D. Schully, and C. A. Liggins. 2021. New NIH primary and secondary prevention research during 2012–2019. *American Journal of Preventive Medicine* 60(6):e261–e268. https://doi.org/10.1016/j.amepre.2021.01.006.

Murry, V. M., C. Berkel, M. N. Inniss-Thompson, and M. L. Debreaux. 2019. Pathways for African American success: Results of three-arm randomized trial to test the effects of technology-based delivery for rural African American families. *Journal of Pediatric Psychology* 44(3):375–387. https://doi.org/10.1093/jpepsy/jsz001.

NASEM (National Academies of Sciences, Engineering, and Medicine). 2019a. *Fostering healthy mental, emotional, and behavioral development in children and youth: A national agenda.* Washington, DC: The National Academies Press. https://doi.org/10.17226/25201.

NASEM. 2019b. *Vibrant and healthy kids: Aligning science, practice, and policy to advance health equity.* Washington, DC: The National Academies Press. https://doi.org/10.17226/25466.

NASEM. 2019c. *The promise of adolescence: Realizing opportunity for all youth.* Washington, DC: The National Academies Press. https://doi.org/10.17226/25388.

NASEM. 2020. *Promoting positive adolescent health behaviors and outcomes: Thriving in the 21st century.* Washington, DC: The National Academies Press. https://doi.org/10.17226/25552.

NASEM. 2022. Improving Representation in Clinical Trials and Research: Building Research Equity for Women and Underrepresented Groups. Washington, DC: The National Academies Press. https://doi.org/10.17226/26479.

NASEM. 2023. Federal Policy to Advance Racial, Ethnic, and Tribal Health Equity. Washington, DC: National Academies Press. https://doi.org/10.17226/26834.

NCDD (National Coalition for Dialogue & Deliberation), International Association for Public Participation, and the Co-Intelligence Institute. 2009. Core Principles for Public Engagement. https://www.ncdd.org/uploads/1/3/5/5/135559674/pepfinal-expanded.pdf (accessed February 25, 2025).

NIAAA (National Institute on Alcohal Abuse and Alcoholism). 2019a. *Individual-level strategies.* https://www.collegedrinkingprevention.gov/collegeaim/individual-strategies (accessed October 13, 2024).

NIAAA. 2019b. *Planning alcohol interventions using NIAAA's collegeaim alcohol intervention matirx.* https://www.collegedrinkingprevention.gov/sites/cdp/files/documents/NIAAA_College_Matrix_Booklet.pdf (accessed December 31, 2024).

NIHB (National Indian Health Board). 2009. *Healthy Indian country initiative promising prevention practices resource guide: Promoting innovative tribal prevention programs.* https://www.nihb.org/docs/04072010/2398_NIHB%20HICI%20Book_web.pdf (accessed September 9, 2024).

NIMHD (National Institute on Minority Health and Health Disparities). 2024. *Diversity and inclusion in clinical trials.* https://www.nimhd.nih.gov/resources/understanding-health-disparities/diversity-and-inclusion-in-clinical-trials.html (accessed September 11, 2024).

NPSC (National Prevention Science Coalition to Improve Lives). 2019. *What is prevention science?* https://www.npscoalition.org/prevention-science (accessed September 9, 2024).

NRC (National Research Council) and IOM (Institute of Medicine). 2009. *Preventing mental, emotional, and behavioral disorders among young people: Progress and possibilities.* Washington, DC: The National Academies Press.

ODP (Office of Disease Prevention). 2023. *Public health campaigns.* https://prevention.nih.gov/research-priorities/dissemination-implementation/nih-public-health-campaigns (accessed October 8, 2024).

ODP. 2024. *What is prevention research?* https://prevention.nih.gov/about-odp/prevention-research-defined (accessed September 9, 2024).

OPM (U.S. Office of Personnel Management). n.d. *What is an Employee Assistance Program (EAP).* https://www.opm.gov/frequently-asked-questions/work-life-faq/employee-assistance-program-eap/what-is-an-employee-assistance-program-eap/ (accessed January 2, 2025).

Patterson, G. R., M. S. Forgatch, and D. S. Degarmo. 2010. Cascading effects following intervention. *Devopment and Psychopathology* 22(4):949–970. https://doi.org/10.1017/S0954579410000568.

Pellecchia, M., D. S. Mandell, H. J. Nuske, G. Azad, C. B. Wolk, B. B. Maddox, E. M. Reisinger, L. C. Skriner, D. R. Adams, R. Stewart, T. Hadley, and R. S. Beidas. 2018. Community–academic partnerships in implementation research. *Journal of Community Psychology* 46(7):941–952. https://doi.org/10.1002/jcop.21981.

Phillips, M. A., T. W. McDonald, and D. I. Kishbaugh. 2017. Using evidence based home visiting for preventing intergenerational adverse childhood experiences. *Psychology* 8(14):2516. https://doi.org/10.4236/psych.2017.814159.

Potthoff, S., T. Finch, L. Bührmann, A. Etzelmüller, C. R. van Genugten, M. Girling, C. R. May, N. Perkins, C. Vis, and T. Rapley. 2023. Towards an Implementation-STakeholder Engagement Model (I-STEM) for improving health and social care services. *Health Expectations* 26(5):1997–2012. https://doi.org/10.1111/hex.13808.

Powell, B. J., J. C. McMillen, E. K. Proctor, C. R. Carpenter, R. T. Griffey, A. C. Bunger, J. E. Glass, and J. L. York. 2012. A compilation of strategies for implementing clinical innovations in health and mental health. *Medical Care Research and Review* 69(2):123–57. https://doi.org/10.1177/1077558711430690.

Reynolds, A. J., J. A. Temple, S.-R. Ou, I. A. Arteaga, and B. A. B. White. 2011. School-based early childhood education and age-28 well-being: Effects by timing, dosage, and subgroups. *Science* 333(6040):360–364. https://doi.org/10.1126/science.1203618.

Robinson, C. H., and L. J. Damschroder. 2023. A Pragmatic Context Assessment Tool (PCAT): Using a think aloud method to develop an assessment of contextual barriers to change. *Implementation Science Communications* 4(1):3. https://doi.org/10.1186/s43058-022-00380-5.

Roy, S., H. S. Brown III, L. S. Blinn, S. C. Narendorf, and J. E. Hamilton. 2024. A microcosting approach for planning and implementing community-based mental health prevention program: What does it cost? *Health Economics Review* 14(1):35. https://doi.org/10.1186/s13561-024-00510-w.

Sanchez, A. L., L. P. Cliggitt, N. L. Dallard, D. Irby, M. Harper, E. Schaffer, M. Lane-Fall, and R. S. Beidas. 2023. Power redistribution and upending white supremacy in implementation research and practice in community mental health. *Psychiatric Services* 74(9):987–990. https://doi.org/10.1176/appi.ps.20220209.

Shaw, D. S., A. Connell, T. J. Dishion, M. N. Wilson, and F. Gardner. 2009. Improvements in maternal depression as a mediator of intervention effects on early childhood problem behavior. *Development and Psychopathology* 21(2):417–439. https://doi.org/10.1017/S0954579409000236.

Shelton, R. C., and R. C. Brownson. 2023. Enhancing impact: A call to action for equitable implementation science. *Prevention Science.* 25:174–189. https://doi.org/10.1007/s11121-023-01589-z.

Smith, J. D., D. H. Li, and M. R. Rafferty. 2020. The implementation research logic model: A method for planning, executing, reporting, and synthesizing implementation projects. *Implementation Science* 15:1–12. https://doi.org/10.1186/s13012-020-01041-8.

Smith, J. D., S. F. Naoom, L. Saldana, S. Shantharam, T. A. Smith, J. M. Kohr. 2024. Preventing and managing chronic disease through implementation science: Editor's introduction to the supplemental issue. *Prevention Science.* 25(Suppl 1):1–9. https://doi.org/10.1007/s11121-023-01617-y.

Smith, M. L., L. E. Steinman, C. N. Montoya, N. Thompson, L. Zhong, A. L. Merianos. 2023. Effectiveness of the Program to Encourage Active, Rewarding Lives (PEARLS) to reduce depression: A multi-state evaluation. *Frontiers in Public Health* 11:1169257. https://doi.org/10.3389/fpubh.2023.1169257.

Sparr, M., S. Frazier, C. Morrison, K. Miller, and W. T. Bartko. 2020. *Afterschool programs help to improve socio-emotional, behavioral, and physical health in middle childhood: A targeted review of the literature.* https://aspe.hhs.gov/sites/default/files/private/pdf/265236/4_MCASP_LiteratureReview.pdf (accessed December 16, 2024).

SPR (Society for Prevention Research). 2011. *Standards of knowledge for the science of prevention.* https://preventionresearch.org/Society%20for%20Prevention%20Research%20Standards%20of%20Knowledge.pdf (accessed December 31, 2024).

Supplee, L. H., R. T. Ammerman, A. K. Duggan, J. A. List, and D. Suskind. 2022. The role of open science practices in scaling evidence-based prevention programs. *Prevention Science* 23(5):799–808. https://doi.org/10.1007/s11121-021-01322-8.

UW (University of Washington). 2025. *Program to Encourage Active, Rewarding Lives (PEARLS)* https://depts.washington.edu/hprc/programs-tools/pearls/?returnurl=%2FTraining%2FSchedule.aspx (accessed January 15, 2025).

UWDGH (University of Washington Department of Global Health). 2024. *Step 4: Select research methods.* https://impsciuw.org/implementation-science/research/select-research-methods/ (accessed October 29, 2024).

Wadhwa, M., J. Zheng, and T. D. Cook. 2024. How consistent are meanings of "evidence-based"? A comparative review of 12 clearinghouses that rate the effectiveness of educational programs. *Review of Educational Research* 94(1):3–32. https://doi.org/10.3102/00346543231152262.

Wakefield, M., J. Sankaranarayanan, J. M. Conroy, S. McLafferty, R. Moser, V. M. Murry, and R. Slifkin. 2024. National Institutes of Health pathways to prevention workshop: Improving rural health through telehealth-guided provider-to-provider communication. *Journal of Telemedicine and Telecare* 30(8):1320–1326. https://doi.org/10.1177/1357633x221139630.

Wells, K. B., L. Jones, B. Chung, E. L. Dixon, L. Tang, J. Gilmore, C. Sherbourne, V. K. Ngo, M. K. Ong, S. Stockdale, E. Ramos, T. R. Belin, and J. Miranda. 2013. Community-partnered cluster-randomized comparative effectiveness trial of community engagement and planning or resources for services to address depression disparities. *Journal of General Internal Medicine* 28(10):1268–1278. https://doi.org/10.1007/s11606-013-2484-3.

Wiltsey Stirman, S., A. A. Baumann, and C. J. Miller. 2019. The frame: An expanded framework for reporting adaptations and modifications to evidence-based interventions. *Implementation Science* 14:1–10. https://doi.org/10.1186/s13012-019-0898-y.

Wolfenden, L., A. Shoesmith, A. Hall, A. Bauman, and N. Nathan. 2024. An initial typology of approaches used by policy and practice agencies to achieve sustained implementation of interventions to improve health. *Implementation Science Communications* 5(1):21. https://doi.org/10.1186/s43058-024-00555-2.

Wolfson, M., K. G. Wagoner, S. D. Rhodes, K. L. Egan, M. Sparks, D. Ellerbee, E. Y. Song, B. Debinski, A. Terrillion, and J. Vining. 2017. Coproduction of research questions and research evidence in public health: The study to prevent teen drinking parties. *BioMed Research International* 2017(1):3639596. https://doi.org/10.1155/2017/3639596.

Wong, D. R., H. Schaper, and L. Saldana. 2022. Rates of sustainment in the universal stages of implementation completion. *Implementation Science Communications* 3(1):2. https://doi.org/10.1186/s43058-021-00250-6.

Youth.gov. n.d. *Federal understanding of the evidence base.* https://youth.gov/evidence-innovation/evidence-based-program-directories (accessed October 8, 2024).

Youth.gov. n.d. *Reconnecting youth evidence gap map.* https://youth.gov/youth-topics/opportunity-youth/reconnecting-youth?q=egm (accessed January 2, 2025).

Zadow, A., M. F. Dollard, L. Parker, and K. Storey. 2019. Psychosocial safety climate: A review of the evidence. In *Psychosocial safety climate: A new work stress theory*, edited by M. F. Dollard, C. Dormann and M. Awang Idris. Cham: Springer International Publishing. Pp. 31–75.

Zaid, S., McCombs-Thornton, K., Faucetta, K., Childress, L., Cachat, P., & Filene, J. (2022). Family Level Assessment and State of Home Visiting outreach and recruitment study report (OPRE Report No. 2022-110). Office of Planning, Research, and Evaluation; Administration for Children and Families; U.S. Department of Health and Human Services.

Zheng, J., M. Wadhwa, and T. D. Cook. 2022. How consistently do 13 clearinghouses identify social and behavioral development programs as "evidence-based"? *Prevention Science* 23(8):1343–1358. https://doi.org/10.1007/s11121-022-01407-y.

3

Workforce, Training, and Technical Assistance

In this chapter, the committee describes the workforce that must be cultivated to effectively select, implement, and sustain prevention programs and practices in all communities, across all settings, and along the life course. The workforce must reflect the local community to best facilitate adoption of evidence-based preventive interventions. This is especially important in populations experiencing the disproportionate burden of mental health (MH) and substance use–related challenges, including communities that are rural, have faced and continue to confront racial discrimination, that experience profound economic hardship, or face language barriers in receiving services.

The U.S. workforce in health care and public health is struggling to keep up with the demand for substance use (SU) and MH treatment. Most primary prevention activities take place outside of clinical settings, and the prevention workforce typically relies on a different set of skills than the behavioral health (BH) treatment workforce. The prevention workforce is widely distributed across multiple systems, including public health, behavioral health, child welfare, juvenile criminal-legal system, and the education system. Many prevention workers—for example, teachers, case managers, and nurses working as home visitors—may not view themselves as such, and may need additional support and resources (e.g., training and technical assistance) to enable them to integrate evidence-based programs as part of their roles.

This chapter describes the need for a prevention workforce; discusses the competencies, certification, training, and technical assistance needs of practitioners who can deliver the interventions discussed in Chapter 2; and presents the rationale for recommendations to develop and sustain this workforce.

THE WORKFORCE AND CURRENT CHALLENGES

In 2016, the Behavioral Health Workforce Research Center defined the BH workforce as "all workers involved in treatment or prevention of mental health conditions or substance use disorders or both" (Beck et al., 2018, p. 194). The definition includes "licensed and non-licensed workers, peer support workers, and volunteers" and "primary care workers who may be providing behavioral health services" but excludes professionals in other systems (e.g., education, law enforcement) who may provide relevant services (Beck et al., 2018, p. 194).

The committee adopts the broader definition; this report describes several categories of workers in the prevention workforce. The 2019 National Academies report *Fostering Healthy MEB Development in Children and Youth* outlines five categories of roles relevant to prevention work: (1) community members and partners, (2) funders and policy makers, (3) purveyors and intermediary organizations, (4) intervention developers and researchers, and (5) service providers. Service providers "are leaders, managers, supervisors, and practitioners who have a stake in the adoption, implementation, and outcomes of a program." (NASEM, 2019, p. 258). This chapter discusses primarily the first, third, and fifth types of roles—that is, the organizations and people that provide training, technical assistance, coaching, and other types of support and the people who deliver or oversee delivery of the interventions. The second and fourth categories refer to the role and organizations relevant to the chapters on governance and partnerships (5), funding (6), evidence for policy (7), and evidence for programs (2).

Prevention workers include a variety of generally non-licensed workers, such as community health workers, aides, and peer workers. Prevention workers also include those responsible for coordination and implementation of prevention programs. In a robust prevention workforce, expertise in prevention and implementation science is essential for selecting, adopting, implementing, evaluating, and sustaining interventions.

Poorly Characterized or Defined Workforce

Both Health Resources and Services Administration (HRSA) workforce projections and a Substance Abuse and Mental Health Services Administration (SAMHSA) workforce report characterize the BH workforce primarily as those in licensed, graduate degree–trained, and clinical BH professions

(HRSA and SAMHSA, 2016).[1] The prevention workforce is not reflected in a comprehensive manner in workforce reports. SAMHSA's 2021 Behavioral Health Workforce Report largely discusses the occupations and roles concerned with treatment and refers to nonclinical and non-licensed personnel only once—in relation to BH aides in schools (SAMHSA, 2021b). As noted, prevention services may be delivered by a wide variety of workers, but these have not been comprehensively described or enumerated.

Another key issue that shapes the workforce is that governance and funding of prevention efforts are siloed, even though most risk and protective factors for substance use disorder and mental disorders overlap. These silos are evident at federal, state, and local levels. SAMHSA has separate centers for mental health services, and for substance abuse prevention and substance abuse treatment, respectively. At the state level, mental health and substance use prevention are frequently funded by separate agencies and managed by different units in a public health agency (SAMHSA, 2017). Federal funding flows through separate channels to states—from the substance use or the mental health centers in SAMHSA and also from different parts of the Centers for Disease Control and Prevention.

Workforce Shortages and Related Issues

In many settings, such as schools, the prevention workforce is absent or insufficient and there is substantial variation in the non-licensed roles, occupational standards, training and competencies, and state-level certification. Most prevention workforce roles are not listed in the Bureau of Labor Statistics Standard Occupational Classifications (SOC),[2] which make categories of labor and their role in the economy visible (U.S. Census Bureau, 2019; BLS, 2024). That has implications for the ability to count and track these roles and efforts to professionalize and certify them and develop pathways to career advancement.

Pay and Other Workforce Issues

Some categories of prevention workers, like others in BH, are underpaid, may lack labor protections, and do not receive adequate training or pathways to advance their careers. Community health workers and similar

---

[1] Including adult psychiatrists, addiction counselors, child and adolescent psychiatrists, "child, family, and school social workers," health care "social workers, marriage and family therapists, mental health and substance abuse social workers, mental health counselors, psychiatric aides, psychiatric nurse practitioners, psychiatric physician assistants, psychiatric technicians, psychologists, and school counselors" (HRSA and SAMHSA, 2016).

[2] See https://data.bls.gov/search/query/results?q=prevention and https://data.bls.gov/search/query/results?q=behavioral (accessed December 30, 2024).

roles experience the same social and economic circumstances as their communities and thus also need additional support and resources (Schriger et al., 2024). Competitive remuneration will help recruit and build career ladders for the full spectrum of prevention workers (Last and Crable, 2024; Schriger et al., 2024).

It is important to acknowledge that because of the nature of many primary prevention interventions, some of the individuals working to deliver them have traditionally been volunteers or had responsibilities added to their job descriptions without additional compensation. This is not a sustainable model. Proper implementation requires a dedicated workforce in addition to task shifting (i.e., delegating specific tasks to less specialized workers) (Kanzler et al., 2024).

A Real-Life Model for Building the Workforce

The United Kingdom has implemented a broad effort to build up the BH workforce to deliver services to its people. Although this workforce is not prevention-focused, the effort illustrates that it is possible to gain and sustain broad-based policy maker support, including investment, for a transformative approach that demonstrated a return on investment (see Box 3-1).

PREVENTION WORKFORCE NEEDS

The prevention infrastructure needs three kinds of workers to move evidence-based prevention interventions for MEB disorders into routine practice. These categories are somewhat fluid, with differences by setting or community and a variety of titles for closely related roles. The workforce includes the following:

(1) Community/prevention coordinators, prevention specialists, implementation facilitators, implementation leads

These individuals can support the selection, adoption, implementation, evaluation, and sustainment of evidence-based interventions. The title may vary across settings. The prevention specialist title is most formalized in substance use prevention settings; the analog for mental health may be mental health promotion leads. These are individuals who may have public health, behavioral health, or related expertise and can help communities and their partners assess needs and assets, identify appropriate interventions, and build capacity toward implementation. Examples include someone who directs prevention programs at the local health department, a prevention coalition coordinator, or a director of a school-based health center. These

> **BOX 3-1**
> **A United Kingdom (U.K.) Model for Building an Infrastructure**
>
> The U.K. Improving Access to Psychological Therapies, now Talking Therapies for Anxiety and Depression, is largely a treatment program, but some of its dimensions of it hold lessons for implementing a broad-based prevention infrastructure.
>
> In 2007, 5 percent of people in the U.K. with depression or anxiety received an evidence based psychological therapy, wait times were often longer than one year, and research showed that these conditions depressed the nation's gross domestic product by 4 percent (presenteeism and absenteeism). The program trained a large workforce of 10,800 psychological therapists using an evidence-based curriculum and competency standards; deployed them in new and additional "stepped care" services; provided clinical supervision and continuing education; and measured and reported clinical outcomes for all patients to facilitate learning and demonstrate transparency. The program was launched with two pilot sites in 2005 and between 2005 and 2024 it has continued to expand with the support of six different governments. The program also integrated economic arguments in its rationale and ultimately demonstrated cost effectiveness and savings (exceeding the cost of delivering an average of 10 therapy sessions), with substantial economic return on investment to the National Health Service and Treasury.
>
> The program provides several useful lessons for the U.S. context about identifying a public health problem, building the workforce to address the problem with an evidence-based intervention, providing the necessary training and supports, earning and sustaining policy maker support through transparency, accountability, and results.
>
> SOURCE: Clark, 2024.

individuals have training in selecting evidence-based interventions, identifying best practices for prevention, and assessing the needs of the community in which they work. They also have established relationships with the community partners who will implement the preventive interventions.

Some communities may have *implementation leads*. These are individuals with specialized training to oversee implementing and delivering one or more evidence-based interventions, such as a specialized worker in a county agency supervised by the prevention specialist or a school-based health center director who oversees implementing evidence-based interventions across multiple schools. They ensure everyone receives training in the selected intervention(s), secure technical assistance, oversee evaluation and monitoring, and use the findings to inform ongoing program development and implementation. They could be the same person as the prevention specialist in places with fewer resources, but in places with larger populations, specific interventions require people to oversee implementation (see Table 3, Individuals domain, Roles subdomain in Damschroder et al., 2022). The need for different roles and the number of people in them will vary within a community based on population size, social vulnerability, and subgroups within communities (e.g., different ethnic groups, rural communities, refugees, unhoused individuals and families, or different languages spoken).

(2) Trainers

These individuals teach/train how to implement the intervention. They may be managers, coordinators, and other individuals with specific training in the intervention(s) and best practices for training others to use them; they also have training in monitoring adoption, and in consultation strategies to improve uptake and fidelity. Trainers may be associated with academic institutions, Prevention Technology Transfer Centers (PTTCs), other organizations that provide training and technical assistance, such as Centers for Disease Control and Prevention (CDC) Prevention Research Centers, and entities that developed the intervention. They may provide individual, group, or place-based training, in addition to policy-related training (e.g., for advocacy to change environmental policies for alcohol). Intervention developers include training, coaching, and technical assistance in the cost of program materials.

To be effective, the prevention team needs the following:

- A needs assessment that maps the problem areas, strengths, and risk and protective factors on which interventions would focus (this would require gathering or identifying necessary data and measures, as discussed in Chapter 5);
- A strategic plan that identifies prevention and health-promoting priorities and goals; the interventions that will be used to address them; an approach to monitoring, evaluating, and engaging in continuous quality improvement; and training and technical assistance that will be enlisted as support; and
- Ability to support fidelity of implementation and sustainment.

Because this work can be complex—requiring, for example, multisectoral collaboration and engaging diverse community members with different perspectives and agendas—prevention teams may find it beneficial to receive technical assistance from experts in external planning, implementation, and evaluation frameworks, such as Mobilizing for Action through Planning and Partnerships, Promoting School-Community-University Partnerships to Enhance Resilience (PROSPER), or Communities That Care (CTC). These frameworks can support local prevention teams in selecting, implementing, monitoring, and evaluating one or more interventions aligned with their priorities, strengths, needs, and values (RHIH, 2024b).

Implementing an evidence-based intervention (or a package of interventions) requires partnership with community members and oversight of different teams, each of which may be responsible for a different intervention, population or setting. The team member(s) leading this work are accountable for (and in turn, hold their team members accountable for) deliverables, such as selecting and implementing evidence-based programs (EBPs), getting buy-in and partnership from different community constituents, organizing and conducting training, and addressing other issues related to implementation.

(3) Implementers:

  (a) Frontline workers in other sectors/systems trained to deliver evidence-based programs (e.g., teachers, clergy, law enforcement);
  (b) Direct service practitioners (e.g., community health workers, BH support specialists, promotora/es); community health representatives (tribal); and
  (c) Volunteers.

Frontline workers in other systems or sectors (e.g., education, law enforcement, child welfare, agricultural extension, librarians, barbers, clergy) could integrate a BH promotion program or approach into their practice. They could be trained to deliver specific evidence-based prevention interventions to individuals, families, and various community groups (see Box 3-1 for some examples). For early childhood and K–12 settings, this could also include the classroom (NASEM, 2019).

Workers drawn from the community may have less than a bachelor's-level education but relevant life experience and can be trained to deliver EBPs in a variety of community settings. In their present roles, they may be titled BH support specialists, community health workers, peer counselors, family support specialists, etc. Two types of non-clinician BH workers in the federal government who deliver some preventive interventions are the BH technicians[3] in the Defense Health Agency and peer specialists in the Veterans Health Administration (Kanzler et al., 2024).

---

[3] For example, Combat and Operational Stress Control training (Health.mil, 2022).

Unpaid lay prevention workers include trained members of religious congregations. This category of worker requires careful consideration of workforce equity issues. The volunteer work of older adults serving as reading tutors to children (e.g., the AARP Experience Corps program) provides benefits to both. In other circumstances, however, unpaid services may be exploitative and perpetuate economic insecurity.

The workforce equity considerations for all prevention workers include the need for fair wages, career advancement ladders and opportunities, and continuing education (Barnett et al., 2018; Fernando et al., 2021; NACHW, 2022; Smithwick et al., 2023).

State and local government agencies require prevention specialists similar to the community-specific roles described above.

Prevention specialists or coordinators who support communities in selecting interventions require the knowledge and skills to convene community leaders and members, assess community needs, identify strategies to address the needs by building on community culture and strengths (e.g., social validity, acceptability, appropriateness), and undertake ongoing

---

BOX 3-2
Training Frontline Workers from Other Sectors: Sample Strategies

Rhode Island's 11 Health Equity Zones implement a variety of locally developed solutions for public health issues and include several sites providing prevention programming, ranging from cigarette and vaping bans to trauma-informed services, and tackling health-related social needs and social determinants of health, such as affordable housing and healthy built and natural environments. "The Washington County Health Equity Zone has provided evidence-based mental health (MH) first aid and suicide prevention training to more than 1,000 police officers, clergy, teachers, parents, and staff of youth-serving organizations and received federal funding to partner with local hospitals, community health centers, and residents to screen all patients for depression and support health care staff to provide high-quality, timely, and evidence-based care to patients at risk for suicide" (PFNYC, 2020, p.39). The West Warwick Health Equity Zone "partnered with the local high school to equip educators and staff to better address childhood traumatic stress" (in addition to the treatment-oriented action of embedding a behavioral health clinician in the local police department "to divert patients with substance misuse from the criminal justice system and into treatment") (RIDH, 2022).

Healing City Baltimore is a trauma-informed initiative co-led by young people (RWJF, 2024). Students advocated for their local government and

evaluation and process improvement. The workforce may not exist in a given setting or community. As efforts are undertaken to develop it, care is needed to ensure that workers are representative of the population they are serving and provide linguistically and culturally appropriate care.

There are many examples of state efforts to build the prevention workforce in a way that reflects the community and provides points of entry for people with varying educational backgrounds. Washington State, for example, offers prevention internship and fellowship programs for people with high school, college, and master's degrees. It also requires online completion of the Certified Prevention Professional training for the Health Care Authority staff and local providers (Mariani, 2024). Healing City Baltimore, an initiative described in Box 3-2, along with examples from Rhode Island's Equity Zones, illustrate in broad terms how the different types of prevention workers with varied backgrounds may function in one setting. Alaska developed the Community Health Aide Program in the 1960s to meet Alaska Native community needs in remote villages of the state. The program includes both community health aides and behavioral

---

schools to acknowledge and address the trauma affecting many city residents and the adverse childhood experiences of young Black people in the city. The initiative has been training thousands of public employees, including librarians, along with community healers, leaders, barbers, and beauticians to provide trauma-responsive care. (A public–private partnership, with funding from a health care insurer, also trained paid peer recovery coaches/navigators to work in the libraries [EPFL, 2024].) Implementation was launched by legislation enacted by the city's mayor—illustrating a community's journey through information gathering and needs assessment, organizing and advocacy, leading to the Elijah Cummings Healing City Act, which has put in place multiple components informed by community leaders, decision makers, and many people with lived expertise.

These examples illustrate how frontline workers from other sectors can be trained to implement evidence-based or promising preventive interventions. Rhode Island's efforts are described as implementing evidence-based interventions. Baltimore's efforts included restorative practices, a set of interventions with some evidence of effectiveness but also what has been called a "practice-to-research" gap (Darling-Hammond, 2023; Zakszeski and Rutherford, 2021).

Similarly, the Confess Project trains barbers to be MH advocates and mentors who help to combat MH stigma and provide social support to Black men and boys. The Beyond the Shop program has trained over 1,400 barbers across 47 cities (Stand Together, 2024).

health aides, and the latter role includes prevention of behavioral disorders (CHAP Alaska, 2024).

BUILDING THE PREVENTION WORKFORCE PIPELINE

There are multiple strategies for building the pipeline of prevention workers, including expanding training opportunities and resources for frontline workers from other sectors and systems. The first category of workers (prevention specialists and/or implementation leads) is composed of professionals, who lead the implementation of prevention programs. Their educational backgrounds will vary. The presence of the second category, trainers, will depend on context (setting and community) and institutional or system resources. Trainers may be licensed BH or public health professionals, but other types of individuals with relevant training and expertise can train frontline workers (or volunteers) in delivering preventive interventions. Trainers can include university faculty, those who have been trained in prevention science and its application to practice and trainers who train on specific programs. There are graduate and certification programs in prevention science. Some prevention professionals are trained in prevention science, others are not trained specifically in prevention science but have education or training in related fields.

The third group of workers, those who implement interventions, will vary with the setting and population. That is why strategies are needed to build a flexible workforce that can be adapted to a community's specific range of prevention needs (e.g., rural geography, demographics). Building that workforce would benefit from a convening of stakeholders to discuss assets and gaps, involving the public health agency, behavioral or mental health agency, community mental health centers or behavioral health centers, first responders, hospitals, community health centers, nonprofit organizations, school districts, and other relevant entities to, for example,

(1) Inventory existing capabilities, such as the following:
    - What kinds of workers already deliver prevention interventions for MEB disorders or could have prevention-related tasks added to their work,
    - Where/in what settings workers exist who already include prevention in their daily work,
    - What state resources (e.g., prevention technology transfer center, regional prevention resource center, academic institution with relevant departments, extension offices [Brown et al., 2023]) exist to support the effort, and
    - What resources exist to build community capacity (i.e., investment in standardized and experiential training to support knowledge of overarching best practices).

(2) Discuss what pathways can be built to better support training of frontline workers in other systems and train community workers.
(3) Identify constituents and partners for training and technical assistance to the workforce (including academic institutions, especially community colleges that may offer associate degree programs that lend themselves to community health worker or peer educator or related training and including high schools—perhaps the earliest opportunity to introduce young people to a potential career).

Workforce development programs could include collaboration across federal departments, including Labor, Treasury, and Commerce that focus on training, workforce, and community revitalization as they relate to building the human capital for prevention.

Linkages are needed between school districts that train peer counselors and area community and four-year college and other academic training programs to create pathways to careers in prevention (CSBHA, 2024; Dodd et al., 2022). Minority-serving institutions could also be a key partner in growing the prevention workforce at all levels, including, for example, tribal colleges that can train future prevention professionals in American Indian and Alaska Native communities and at historically Black colleges and universities (HBCUs) (see for example SAMHSA's HBCU Center for Excellence in Behavioral Health) (AIHEC, 2022; SAMHSA, 2024). SAMHSA's Voices of Youth program is designed to orient young people to the field, and the federal resource Youth Engaged 4 Change provides information about internship, training, and other opportunities (Youth Engaged 4 Change, n.d.; SAMHSA, 2023). In addition to the need to characterize and enumerate the prevention workforce, institutions of higher education and relevant associations could create pathways to entry-level professions/jobs (e.g., for college students who are already serving as peer counselors) with ladders for continuing education and advancement. Previously incarcerated individuals who are in recovery could also receive training and work as peer workers. For example, in North Carolina's Formerly Incarcerated Transition program (and 24 clinics across 10 states), formerly incarcerated individuals are trained as peer navigators to work with recently returned individuals, an approach that shows promise (NCCHCA, n.d.; Ray et al., 2021). Many recently returned individuals face an extremely high risk of overdose in the weeks post-release, and navigators play an essential role in supporting their well-being (NCCHCA, 2020).

Many prevention providers are employed by state and tribal[4] agencies to deliver MH and SUD prevention services, and those agencies or units

---

[4] The Indian Health Service's four branches that focus on mental health, alcohol and substance abuse, behavioral health initiatives, and tele-behavioral health center of excellence, respectively, refer to I/T/U providers, denoting ("I") Indian Health Service, ("T") Tribally operated facility/program, and ("U") Urban Indian clinics.

within agencies are generally separate. Due to the governance and funding silos discussed in Chapters 5 and 6 respectively, the functions associated with delivering prevention services for MH disorders and SUDs are separate. Prevention workers are also employed by local government, school districts or boards, and nonprofits, such as Boys and Girls Clubs and YMCA organizations, and by other organizations providing preventive services (YMCA of San Diego County, 2024).

Even in places with training programs, the number of prevention workers is often insufficient to meet the need. For example, the director of New York State's Office of Addiction Services and Supports, Chinazo Cunningham, stated at a public meeting of the committee that her office funds 175 credentialed prevention professionals (at least bachelor's level plus 4,000 hours supervised work experience) and 15 credentialed prevention specialists (at least high school diploma or GED plus 2,000 hours supervised work experience) for a state of over 18 million people. They deliver services through 306 state-contracted programs at private nonprofit organizations, schools and boards of cooperative educational services,[5] local prevention councils, and local governments. Cunningham shared that "the workforce is really struggling; 175 people for the state of New York, which is 18 million people, is nothing . . . [W]e really need to continue to expand and support the workforce. . . But we're decades behind in investing in the workforce in this field" (Cunningham, 2024).

The lack of data about workers who deliver prevention interventions for MEB disorders makes it difficult to ascertain adequacy, but given the shortages of related or overlapping workforces—direct care, public health, and BH—it is likely that the supply of trained workers is inadequate (Lyons and O'Malley Watts, 2024; NCHWA, 2024; NCSL, 2024; Yeager and Krasna, 2024).

Burnout is a related consideration that reflects both an input challenge and an outcome challenge related to the workforce, along with general retention, turnover, and attrition (NCHWA, 2023). Burnout manifests as sustained feelings of exhaustion, professional inefficiency, and depersonalization, evident in a sense of cynicism, withdrawal, and related behaviors (SAMHSA, 2022). Workforce development strategies should involve supporting worker well-being and resilience. Improving the mental health/resilience of existing behavioral health professionals can likely be facilitated by creating a more efficient system of early detection and support that is less dependent on higher levels of education/degrees. Building a stronger prevention workforce could include approaches to stepped care, with different levels of workers delivering different types of interventions or overseeing frontline workers, and the building of a larger workforce that ensures better worker-to-community ratios.

---

[5] NY state arrangement that allows schools to share the costs of certain educational and administrative services.

Coalitions

Coalitions are community-based, multisector collaborations that play an important role as grantees, conveners, planning entities and accountability mechanisms, and prevention champions. Coalitions may be led by community coordinators who can effectively lead and support the selection, adoption, implementation, evaluation, and sustainment of preventive interventions. Thousands of community-based coalitions across the United States work to improve health, reduce youth risk factors, and address social issues that affect community health, from community violence to homelessness. In the domain of MEB disorder prevention, the coalitions represented by CADCA (formerly the Community Anti-Drug Coalitions of America) can serve as hubs of prevention delivery systems. Many of the coalitions receive ONDCP Drug Free Communities funding.

With adequate financial and technical supports (and as informed by community needs), many of these coalitions could expand their focus on prevention to include mental disorders, which share many risk and protective factors with SUDs. Their potential to play a broader role in prevention will be enhanced by CDC funding to CADCA, which announced in October 2024 that it was awarded a 5-year grant under CDC's National Partners Cooperative Agreement Funding to Strengthen Public Health Infrastructure that would help it "enhance public health infrastructure, improve workforce capacity, and address equity-based public health priorities" (CADCA, 2024).

Research comparing multisector community coalition models to individual program technical assistance in the delivery of MH interventions found that the coalition approach was more effective in "reducing the probability of having poor mental health-related quality of life, behavioral health hospitalization, and homelessness risk factors" (Arevian et al., 2019, p. S206).

It is essential that primary prevention of MEB disorders be the central focus of community-based, multisector coalitions. Despite coalitions often working to address issues along the MEB disorder prevention-treatment spectrum, it is important to recognize that prevention requires devoted attention to ensure the delivery of effective interventions.

The coalition workforce—people leading and supporting coalitions to strengthen protective factors and mitigate risk factors for MEB disorders—needs the following key ingredients:

- Adequate financial resources to support coalition providers who are credentialed in the prevention field with adequate pay and benefits to encourage longer tenure and avoid the knowledge and relational loss of frequent turnover associated with prevention professionals;

- Trained people on the ground doing the work of primary prevention, providing information that is easy to understand so that it can facilitate the work; and
- Monitoring of data systems to assess delivery of evidence-based interventions with fidelity.

Coalitions also engage community members who have lived expertise with MEB disorders in themselves or their family members. Proposals for funding, and funding programs of government, health care, or philanthropic organizations need to include consideration of compensation needs for community members (Spencer and Scannelli Jacobs, 2023).

Getting a Complete Picture of the Workforce Status and Needs

Developing a complete picture of the state of the prevention workforce and ascertaining the gaps will require federal leadership, especially from HRSA, the agency that has historically led the characterization and enumeration of workforces in the health sector. It will be necessary to understand the full range of prevention roles, variety of job titles used across communities and states, responsibilities and duties of the various prevention jobs that exist, and range of state approaches to recognizing and supporting these categories of workers. Gathering this baseline information will inform efforts to build up the workforce, align standards, and facilitate sustainable payment mechanisms for programs in all communities and across all settings.

HRSA descriptions of the BH workforce are not expansive enough to include the prevention-focused occupations and roles noted in this report and outlined by Beck et al. (2018) in their description of the Minimum Data Set needed to fully describe the workforce. These roles include the following elements: enumeration (total count of provider type), demographics, education, training, licensure, certification, occupational category, area of practice, and employment setting. One challenge for non-licensed BH and prevention occupations is that few have SOCs. As a result, these occupations are "largely unidentifiable in BLS Occupation Employment Statistics, American Community Survey, and similar national databases" (Beck et al., 2018. p. 193). This makes it difficult to establish the legitimacy of a newer role for reimbursement, for example, and identify staffing needs, gaps in services, and risks for cessation of services.

RECOMMENDATION 3-1: In consultation with Substance Abuse and Mental Health Services Administration (SAMHSA), the Health Resources and Services Administration should describe and enumerate the workforce for mental, emotional, and behavioral (MEB) health promotion and prevention of MEB disorders. SAMHSA should add

the newly defined roles to its behavioral health workforce estimates and reports.

> RECOMMENDATION 3-2: The Department of Labor should use the most up-to-date description of the prevention workforce for mental, emotional, and behavioral disorders as the basis for updates to the Standard Occupational Classifications for behavioral and public health jobs.

For example, prevention specialists would be listed as a Department of Labor occupation, which will help inform the certification process and pathway from education to careers. In Chapter 5, focused on Governance and Partnership, the committee makes a recommendation on the founding of a new SAMHSA Center for Mental Health Promotion or a joint Center for Prevention of Behavioral Disorders that combines MH and SUD-related prevention activities, which will have bearing on what the committee recommends to further support the development of the workforce for MEB prevention.

In addition to counting and defining the workforce, there is an opportunity for federal agencies to estimate the relative need and forecast the supply. Part of this could also involve analyzing current wages and what wages (and thus reimbursement and funding) would be needed for adequate workforce supply.

COMPETENCIES AND TRAINING

The categories of workers who support the delivery of preventive programs are referred to as "coaches, improvement advisors, technical assistance providers, facilitators, consultants, mentors, and implementation specialists" (Metz et al., 2021, p. 239). This range in terminology reflects the fragmented literature base describing individuals who provide implementation support. Identifying and operationalizing the competencies needed for this broad category in the prevention workforce for MEB disorders will be necessary for effective implementation that will benefit individuals and communities (Metz et al., 2021).

States have varied requirements regarding competencies needed for certifying prevention specialists. SAMHSA's *Prevention Core Competencies* were developed based on its Prevention Strategy and integrate information from state requirements for certification: (1) crosscutting competencies: interdisciplinary foundations, multiple systems, family dynamics, ethical practice, basic knowledge, and communication; and (2) competencies in five domains (SAMHSA, 2021a):

  a. Assessment (data gathering, needs and resource identification, problem definition, analysis),

b. Capacity building (collaboration, organizational advocacy, organizational cultural proficiency),
   c. Planning (collaborative planning, cultural inclusion, systematic thinking, evidence-informed approaches, facilitation, strategic planning),
   d. Implementation (cultural responsiveness, collaboration, change management), and
   e. Evaluation (evaluation methods, data interpretation and use).

All of these are competency-based skills. The International Certification & Reciprocity Consortium Prevention Candidate Guide (IC&RC, 2022) provides a similar list of performance domains that has some overlap with the competencies above, and comprises:

   a. Planning and evaluation
   b. Prevention education and service delivery
   c. Communication
   d. Community organization
   e. Public policy and environmental change
   f. Professional growth and responsibility

Training and Pathways to Competency Attainment

People in adjacent professions already have these competencies and could start working in this area with minimal training. Further developing the workforce involves recruiting or identifying potential candidates who need competencies built, including investing in youth/young adults.

Community Health Workers are increasingly well studied and extensively discussed in the literature. A community health worker is a "frontline public health worker who is a trusted member of and/or has an unusually close understanding of the community served" (APHA, 2024). There have been many new developments in this workforce, which, according to the Bureau of Labor Statistics, was estimated at approximately 60,000 around the country (ASTHO, 2024a). The National Community Health Worker Core Consensus Project identified 10 core roles and competencies for the role—all of which apply to the MEB health context and most of which may apply to BH support specialists and other non-licensed or non-postsecondary-degree-trained occupations:

   1. Cultural mediation among individuals, communities, and service systems;
   2. Providing culturally appropriate health education and information;
   3. Care coordination, case management, and system navigation;

4. Providing coaching and social support;
5. Advocating for individuals and communities;
6. Building individual and community capacity;
7. Providing direct service;
8. Implementing individual and community assessments;
9. Conducting outreach; and
10. Participating in evaluation and research

This list of competencies seems sufficiently broad and comprehensive to apply to or at least warrant serious consideration for other community-based prevention worker roles.

Training and Technical Assistance

Training and technical assistance for the prevention workforce requires integrating knowledge about evidence-based programs (St. George, 2023). Education and training ranges from graduate degrees in BH, public health prevention science, or related fields (e.g., public administration, public policy) to program-specific training given to non-licensed prevention workers, also known as "direct service practitioners," who may deliver preventive interventions in a variety of community settings (see Box 3-3 for an example). The training paths for the former are already well developed, although a graduate of a Master of Public Health program will still need additional training to be able to identify prevention best practices and implementation supports needed to move those into practice. For teachers, resources include Classroom WISE (n.d.), a free 3-part training package for K–12 educators and other school staff, developed by the Mental Health Technology Transfer Centers (MHTTC) Network[6] and National Center for School Mental Health. The PTTC Network catalog offers 714 resources for educators on substance use prevention, along with free training courses on core competencies and prevention ethics that are key to supporting the prevention workforce. Educators can also use resources from the National Center on Safe Supportive Learning Environments from the U.S. Department of Education (NCSSLE, 2025).

The National Implementation Research Network at the University of North Carolina at Chapel Hill and the National Council for Mental Well-Being both offer training on how to effectively strengthen protective factors (MHFA, 2024). Other sources of training and resources for educators, community coalitions, and a variety of prevention workers include the National Associations of State Mental Health Program Directors, National

---

[6] As noted, the MHTTC Network was ended in September 2024, but its resources remain available on the webpage.

> **BOX 3-3**
> **Evidence-Based Program Case Example: Familias Unidas**
>
> Familias Unidas is a multilevel family-based program that targets risk and protective factors in Hispanic immigrant families. The program was designed with culturally specific models and uses culturally relevant parent training, parent support networks, facilitator visits to homes, parent–school meetings, and family-supervised activities with peers to prevent substance use in adolescents in middle and high school. Facilitators have a bachelor's degree and speak Spanish and must complete a 32-hour training program. After delivering the intervention six times, facilitators are eligible to take another 32-hour training and become a trainer to other facilitators (ACF, 2021).
>
> "Familias Unidas was efficacious in reducing past 90-day substance use, illicit drug use, and in reducing the proportion of youth with an alcohol dependence diagnosis, relative to Community Practice" (CEBC, 2024a).

Association of State Alcohol and Drug Abuse Directors, CADCA, and academic–community partnerships.

For early childhood care and education providers, child care health consultants are an important potential training resource. Their competencies are described by the Head Start Early Childhood Learning and Knowledge Center in the Administration for Children and Families, and resources include a toolkit to governors developed by the Departments of Education and Health and Human Services on the use of federal resources to improve child health and well-being (HSS, 2022).

Other opportunities exist to train staff of community-serving organizations in mental, emotional, and behavioral health promotion. For area agencies on aging and nonprofit organizations working with older adults, training (e.g., developed by SAMHSA) could be included as a condition for receiving Older Americans Act funding. To support faith communities, relevant programs could be packaged for integration into their congregations (ideally) with others in the community. SAMHSA could work with the Department of Agriculture to package and disseminate programs to extension offices. Coordination about disseminating EBPs could be one priority for the interagency taskforce to promote MEB health that could be convened by a White House advisor on prevention as proposed in Chapter 5.

For frontline workers from other sectors and systems, training on delivering prevention interventions could be integrated into pre-service training or through professional development and continuing education requirements.

Recruiting direct service practitioners (e.g., CHWs) from the community can solve multiple problems concurrently. It can serve as an effective preventive intervention in itself, providing employment, harnessing workers' knowledge of and commitment to their community (and earned trust), and contributing to community economic stability.[7] Established and ongoing research demonstrates that professionals without a formal degree can effectively support change with the appropriate training (Smithwick et al., 2023).

Community health worker training varies greatly nationwide, and varied delivery models have been catalogued by the National Association of Community Health Workers. In addition to training in core skills/competencies described, specific modules could be developed. Training could also include a basic orientation to prevention and implementation sciences. Training direct service practitioners in prevention needs to include at least the following broad domains or standards:

1. Community-based participatory action and other community-engaged approaches;
2. Prevention science and how it is applied in evaluating evidence-based interventions;
3. Implementation science and implementation facilitation—including evaluation strategies and process frameworks, such as a two- or three-part course on frameworks, models, and theories and evaluation with a practice-based component;
4. Delivery of evidence-based interventions through a community implementation process (e.g., CTC, PROSPER, Getting to Outcomes, the Icelandic model, CDC frameworks); and
5. Data best practices (e.g., brief primer on locally available data, use of other data sources, such as state surveys, and strategies for collecting and analyzing data relevant to the program being implemented).

These training standards and competencies can form the basis for building knowledge and skills that can be delivered in a variety of settings, whether associated with a hiring entity or an education setting in an institution that may or may not partner with a hiring entity.

Informal opportunities to promote well-being in the community can be a powerful way to address social isolation and support social connection

---

[7] See, for example, https://www.newyorkfed.org/newsevents/events/regional_outreach/2023/0623-2023 (accessed October 2, 2024).

across the life course. Volunteers play an important role in prevention and related work (Namkung, 2024; Benson, 2024), and in some settings there may be an overreliance on them (Cohen, 2024). There are concerns about community or peer workers being expected to provide services on a volunteer basis, without pay. This can be exploitative in many contexts. There may be circumstances where the financial and occupational/professional incentive of a paid, formalized role working in the community does not apply, such as when members of a religious congregation provide some services as a part of a desire to serve as volunteers (English, 2024; Neigel, 2024) or communities where individuals volunteer to help older members (Ormel et al., 2019). For example, the Public Health AmeriCorps program, launched in 2023, is a volunteer opportunity (with a modest "living allowance") to work in communities to improve public health, and also connect with pathways to community health worker certification (AmeriCorps, n.d.).[8]

Technical Assistance

Providing technical assistance for prevention workers is generally not a function appropriate for local-level government agencies or entities for reasons of capacity, efficiency, and effectiveness. Well-established resources and technical assistance are available from several sources, including SAMHSA, in collaboration with state agencies, and academic institutions, including those with SAMHSA-supported technology transfer centers. Technical assistance may also be part of the purchase cost for a specific evidence-based intervention, so intervention developers provide technical assistance to organizations and entities.

Like other aspects of the landscape, technical assistance itself is siloed, with state substance use agencies providing it on prevention of substance use and state MH agencies providing it primarily on treatment of mental illness and related issues (most prevention efforts appear focused on suicide prevention). On the SUD side, New York State's Office of Addiction Services and Supports, for example, has several prevention resource centers that work with community coalitions and schools to implement evidence-based prevention strategies.

The PTTC Network provides technical assistance to the "substance misuse prevention field" (PTTC Network, 2024). Its services include providing learning resources and technical assistance on prevention science and implementation and training to emerging prevention professionals.

---

[8] AmeriCorps and CDC provided $76 million to 89 Public Health AmeriCorps grant recipients to support more than 4,000 AmeriCorps members across most states, Washington, DC, Guam, and Puerto Rico (AmeriCorps, n.d.).

The PTTC Network comprises 10 regional centers and a coordinating office that serve all 50 states, the District of Columbia, and the U.S. territories.

The MHTTC Network was closed in September 2024, but its focus, like that of the National Association of State Mental Health Program Directors, had been largely on the treatment of mental illness and suicide prevention. Some recent research findings from the MHTTCs have broader relevance, however. Gotham and colleagues surveyed the MH workforce and learned their top technical assistance needs were "equitable and culturally responsive services," "co-occurring mental and substance use disorders," and "mental health awareness and literacy" (Gotham et al., 2024, p. 1). Regarding the top technical assistance need, the authors observed that "this finding reflects continued inequities in mental health services, particularly for communities of color that face long-standing disparities in health care, racism, and stressors" (Gotham et al., 2024 p. 3).

CDC's Prevention Research Centers can also play a role in delivering training and technical assistance, in addition to conducting applied research in collaboration with community-based organizations and community residents. Of the 26 PRCs operating during the 2019–2024 funding cycle, nearly a dozen performed research that addressed one or more dimensions of preventing MEB disorders. Their 2019–2024 work focused on partnerships in varied settings and with a range of collaborators, including schools, afterschool providers, aging services providers, and the criminal-legal system (CDC, 2024).

Other academic centers, such as the EPIS Center at Pennsylvania State University, can provide technical assistance to community-based coalitions and other groups working in prevention of MEB disorders (J. Welsh, personal communication, June 18, 2024). The EPIS Center works closely with the Pennsylvania state agencies and receives funding from the state's Commission on Crime and Delinquency Office of Children, Youth, and Services. Academic providers of technical assistance are crucial because they are knowledgeable about the state, value community-engaged research and community partnerships, and play a key role as part of a triad of crucial relationships: academic entity, state agency, and community organization(s) or coalition(s). EPIS oversees the Prevention Learning Portal at Penn State, a key resource to everyone working in substance use prevention (PSU, 2024).

The U.S. Department of Health and Human Services Administration for Children and Families provides technical assistance from its National Center on Substance Abuse and Child Welfare, which is funded by SAMHSA, ACF, and the Children's Bureau. The center's resources are focused on "strategies for working with families affected by substance use and involved in the child welfare and family courts systems" (NCSACW, n.d.).

The significance of technical assistance in achieving gains in MEB health cannot be understated. Multiple studies have shown, for example, that when communities received technical assistance through PROSPER or CTC, more young people and families were reached with preventive interventions, and better and enduring MEB outcomes were attained. These improvements have been demonstrated in both rural and urban communities (Chilenski et al., 2019; Crowley et al., 2024; Gorman-Smith et al., 2024) and underscore the importance of good implementation practice, particularly pre-implementation processes, or "taking the time to get it right" (see Box 3-4). The last decade has provided evidence in support of the critical role of pre-implementation. Without such support, less than one third of implementation efforts succeed (Wong et al., 2022). Multiple studies have found a significant positive association between pre-implementation completion and program competency (Alley et al., 2023). Thus, it is critical to engage in appropriate training and technical assistance and implementation support to maximize the likelihood of success. That period before implementation can be a huge contributor to whether the eventual effort is successful. Blended implementation organizations and other kinds of technical support can help the workforce, and their community partners identify needs, make decisions about next steps, and plan for sustained implementation, also supporting monitoring and evaluation (or de-implementation, if appropriate).

Certification

Certification has implications for both funding and legitimizing and professionalizing newer roles in the prevention workforce. For community health workers, or community health representatives in tribal communities, certification is linked with payment because Medicaid reimbursement also requires certification, and not all states certify them (APHA, 2014; ASTHO, 2024b; NASHP, 2019). As one example, New Mexico offers both state generalist certification and three kinds of certifications with specialized training: community health representative, BH/MH specialty track, and peer support workers (in collaboration with the state's Department of Human Services) (Jones et al., 2021; Kelly, 2024). The state has reported that developing paths to certification is allowing more community health workers and representatives to bill Medicaid (Kelly et al., 2024).

For prevention specialists, most states provide certification and have a heterogeneous but overlapping list of requirements (PTTCN, 2024). In general, that includes passing the International Certification & Reciprocity Consortium (IC&RC) Prevention Specialist exam. Some states only require IC&RC certification, but most require certification by a state board (Jones et al., 2021). IC&RC certification has specific education and training and experience and supervision requirements (Jones et al., 2021).

> **BOX 3-4**
> **Implementation Considerations for the Workforce**
>
> **Expanding Opportunities for Health**
>
> - Some prevention workers need to be drawn from the community, have lived experience, and have the community's trust, especially for the role of community health worker or equivalent.
> - Living wage: workers with a lower level of education and training need fair remuneration, benefits, and protections.
> - Promise for promotion: entry-level prevention workers need pathways to advance their careers.
> - No uncompensated volunteers except for specific and clearly defined circumstances (e.g., generational programs where an older community member tutors a child in reading).
> - Addressing issues specific to rural communities (e.g., "lower population densities for program economies of scale coverage" (RHIH, 2024a).
> - Addressing issues of language access for all relevant populations.
>
> **Implementation Science**
>
> - Create coalitions, build capacity, and hire a coordinator.
> - Coordinator oversees prevention teams, brings pieces together.
> - Learn from aligned and parallel disciplines (including community-based participatory research practices, cocreation with community).
> - Engage and equip different levels of the workforce in assisting with implementation.
> - Assess level of workforce needed for different aspects of implementation.
> - Provide the prevention workforce with education, training, and technical assistance on implementation science.

Building an effective workforce will require review of competencies, training and certification needs, strategies for developing a pipeline and pathways to professional development, opportunities to expand and support the prevention workforce to implement EBPs in a variety of settings, and fair pay and labor protections. To begin, several changes are needed to better characterize and enumerate the prevention workforce, and a SAMHSA office devoted to the prevention workforce could provide a point of coordination and support for all workforce matters, including better integration of prevention related to mental health and to substance use (NASEM, 2024).

RECOMMENDATION 3-3: The Substance Abuse and Mental Health Services Administration should establish a Coordinating Office on the Mental, Emotional, and Behavioral Prevention Workforce or designate a lead office to coordinate prevention to delineate core competencies, develop a strategic plan, review agency programs and grants for workforce linkages, coordinate with the Centers for Disease Control and Prevention and accrediting and licensure bodies, and strengthen academic–community partnerships.

Specifically, the new or designated office would

- Delineate, with input from local community that centers lived experience, how the prevention core competencies described in SAMHSA's 2021 Prevention Core Competencies report apply to each set of prevention workforce roles, especially those that help communities select evidence-based programs and train implementers to deliver them (SAMHSA, 2021a).
- Develop a strategic plan for the prevention workforce, with a focus on fair treatment of different types of workers and nurturing workforce pathways for community members.
- Review SAMHSA prevention programs and grants to ensure they support and enable a distinct workforce for prevention of MEB disorders in communities.
- Collaborate with CDC and relevant accrediting and licensure bodies (e.g., Council for Education in Public Health, Society for Public Health Education, IC&RC) to ensure that academic institutions and training programs equip prevention workers with the knowledge, skills, and competencies needed to implement evidence-based preventive interventions in a variety of settings and age groups.
- Strengthen academic–community partnerships that provide technical assistance to communities and community-based prevention workers to support implementation of preventive interventions for MEB disorders (i.e., MH and SUD together).

The office will ideally be a collaboration of the Center for Substance Abuse Prevention and a new, parallel Center for Mental Health Promotion or a joint Center for Prevention of Behavioral Disorders, options suggested in Chapter 5. If creating a new office is not feasible, SAMHSA could conduct an analysis of its current capacity and resources, and of the additional resources, needed to support the building of a prevention workforce for MEB disorders.

RECOMMENDATION 3-4: The Substance Abuse and Mental Health Services Administration and Centers for Disease Control and Prevention should work with the Administration for Community Living, Administration for Children and Families, U.S. Department of Education, and Department of Justice to incorporate strategies for training on prevention of mental, emotional, and behavioral disorders for frontline personnel in those settings.

Options for training include collaboration with colleges and universities to build or expand prevention programming in their curriculum.

The recommended Coordinating Office on the MEB Prevention Workforce could build on existing competencies, such as SAMHSA's own prevention competencies, to

- Define and adopt a common set of national competencies for prevention-focused community coordinators, with aligned national training and supportive infrastructure;
- Develop a tracking system to understand the achievement of competencies for community coordinators who have the responsibility for facilitating community decision making to carry out steps in the implementation process; and
- Work with relevant entities, such as the Association of State and Territorial Health Officials, to provide guidelines for certification of non-licensed workers.

Brief Overview of Workers in Different Settings

This section provides several examples of how, with the appropriate training, practitioners working in different systems, community workers, or lay or peer workers can deliver evidence-based preventive interventions. For family-focused and parenting interventions, the workforce may include trained community workers in addition to specially licensed workers; additional consultation or support may be needed for the former (CEBC, 2024b). A program in Wisconsin trained both home visitors and community MH providers to deliver the evidence-based Mother-Infant Therapy Group screening and treatment for postpartum depression (IMI, 2023; UW-Madison PRC, 2024). Program implementers and community liaisons in the Strong African American Families and Pathways to African American Success programs were originally required to have a college degree in a related field, but that requirement was removed to acknowledge that it was not necessary for implementer effectiveness (Murry and Brody, 2004; Kogan et al., 2012).

Nonprofit organizations (e.g., Boys and Girls Clubs) that provide after-school programming may have a variety of staff who can be trained to deliver preventive interventions. Box 2-4 in Chapter 2 provides an example where one staff member for each club received specific training in delivering evidence-based interventions. In community and 4-year college settings, campus prevention professionals, counselors, teaching assistants, and other personnel can be trained to deliver Question, Persuade, Refer (QPR) Suicide Prevention Gatekeeper Training, and other evidence-based interventions, but additional training may be needed for cultural competence (Harris et al., 2022).

Non-degreed workers in community-based organizations that work with older adults can be trained to deliver evidence-based interventions, such as the Program to Encourage Active, Rewarding Lives (PEARLS) (see Box 2-6), which has been shown to be effective when delivered by these staff (UW PRC, 2025). Older adults themselves can be trained to be peer interventionists with dual benefit (Benson, 2024). Professionals in some types of workforce settings could be trained to deliver preventive interventions. For example, agricultural extension agents in rural Georgia were trained to deliver MH first aid to agricultural workers (who experience higher rates of risk factors for suicide) and to train additional extension agents.

Clergy and congregation members can deliver evidence-based prevention interventions, as has long been demonstrated around the country. In one region of Pennsylvania, INTERSECT trainers provide evidence-based MH and prevention training to clergy, social services providers, and community members, including MH first aid, Applied Suicide Intervention Skills Training, and QPR, while in San Antonio, a multisector (faith community, public health, health care, and nonprofit organization) partnership trains congregation members to deliver evidence-based interventions and certifies congregations as "Behavioral Friendly" (Access Services, 2024; NAMI, 2024). As faith community partnerships that deliver mental health intervention are becoming more common, so are evaluation and research to ascertain their effectiveness (Perez et al., 2024). Although more research is needed, there are promising findings of improved outcomes, as well as insights about facilitators and barriers in implementing such partnerships (Perez et al., 2024).

Exploring funding needs for the workforce

A well-trained and competent workforce requires funding, although given the lack of a workforce description and enumeration, there is limited information about workforce costs.

The 2017 SAMHSA profile of single state agencies (SSAs, focused on substance use) and mental health agencies (SMHAs) highlighted several workforce needs:

- Out of 47 SMHAs 96 percent rated "provider readiness to deliver an evidence-based program" as a barrier "sometimes to always" and 91 percent rated "shortage of an appropriately trained

workforce" as a barrier "sometimes to always" (SAMHSA, 2017, p. 67).
- Approximately 30 SSAs reported that they do not have "sufficient workforce to meet current SUD demands." It is unclear what proportion of the workforce provides SUD-related prevention services, but the workforce shortage is notable nonetheless (SAMHSA, 2017, p. B-2 – B-125).
- According to the SAMHSA report, 2,450 primary prevention providers were funded with the 20 percent set-aside from the Substance Use Prevention, Treatment, and Recovery Services Block Grant (SUBG) (then called the Substance Abuse Prevention and Treatment Block Grant) funds through the SSAs. In 2024, the 20 percent set-aside amounted to approximately $400 million (from the $2 billion SUBG; see Appendix C).

The following examples of potential workforce costs are provided solely for illustration as to what prevention dollars could pay for.

Prevention coordinators are one important role in the prevention workforce, and the cost for a coordinator will range depending on qualifications and setting (e.g., local vs. state government, college or graduate degree required or not, local cost of living). Taking as an example a county-level position in the Midwest requiring a bachelor's degree, the pay (roughly $65,000) plus benefits could reach $90,000. Having each county in the United States have a prevention coordinator would result in annual costs of approximately $280 million ($90,000 × 3,142 counties) (Wisconsin Counties, 2023).

The salary and benefits for a community health worker or equivalent are estimated at approximately $65,000 (median CHW pay of $48,200 plus approximately 30 percent of salary spent on benefits) (Mayer, 2023; BLS, 2024). Direct service practitioners such as community health workers may work in a variety of community settings but will also require supervision—such as from prevention coordinators. If every county had a community health worker promoting MEB health, that would cost approximately $205 million (Gurley-Calvez and Williams, 2020; U.S. Census Bureau, 2023).

REFERENCES

Access Services. 2024. *Intersect faith and mental health.* https://www.accessservices.org/intersect/#whatwedo (accessed October 22, 2024).

ACF (Administration for Children and Families). 2021. Familias unidas. https://preventionservices.acf.hhs.gov/programs/641/show (accessed December 15, 2024).

ACL (Administration for Community Living). n.d. *Program to Encourage Active, Rewarding Lives for Seniors (PEARLS).* https://acl.gov/sites/default/files/programs/2017-03/PEARLS_InterventionSummary.pdf (accessed October 28, 2024).

AIHEC (American Indian Higher Education Consortium). 2022. *American Indian Higher Education Consortium*. https://www.aihec.org/ (accessed January 2, 2025).

Alley, Z. M., J. E. Chapman, H. Schaper, and L. Saldana. 2023. The relative value of pre-implementation stages for successful implementation of evidence-informed programs. *Implementation Science* 18(1):30. https://doi.org/10.1186/s13012-023-01285-0.

ASTHO (Association of State and Territorial Health Officials). 2024a. *Opportunities for public health agencies to advance sustainable financing of community health worker programs*. https://www.astho.org/globalassets/report/advancing-sustainable-financing-of-community-health-workers.pdf (accessed December 30, 2024).

ASTHO. 2024b. *State approaches to community health worker certification*. https://www.astho.org/topic/brief/state-approaches-to-community-health-worker-certification/ (accessed December 30, 2024).

AmeriCorps. n.d. *2024 public health AmeriCorps*. https://americorps.gov/funded-grants/public-health-americorps#grants (accessed September 11, 2024).

APHA (American Public Health Association). 2014. *Support for community health worker leadership in determining workforce standards for training and credentialing*. https://www.apha.org/policies-and-advocacy/public-health-policy-statements/policy-database/2015/01/28/14/15/support-for-community-health-worker-leadership (accessed December 30, 2024).

APHA. 2024. *Community health workers*. https://www.apha.org/apha-communities/member-sections/community-health-workers (accessed December 30, 2024).

Arevian, A. C., F. Jones, L. Tang, C. D. Sherbourne, L. Jones, and J. Miranda. 2019. Community partners in care writing. Depression remission from community coalitions versus individual program support for services: Findings from community partners in care, Los Angeles, California, 2010–2016. *American Journal of Public Health* 109(S3):S205–S213. https://doi.org/10.2105/AJPH.2019.305082.

Barnett, M. L., A. Gonzalez, J. Miranda, D. A. Chavira, and A. S. Lau. 2018. Mobilizing community health workers to address mental health disparities for underserved populations: A systematic review. *Administration and Policy in Mental Health and Mental Health Services Research* 45(2):195–211. https://doi.org/10.1007/s10488-017-0815-0.

Beck, A. J., P. M. Singer, J. Buche, R. W. Manderscheid, and P. Buerhaus. 2018. Improving data for behavioral health workforce planning: Development of a minimum data set. *American Journal of Preventive Medicine* 54(6 Suppl 3):S192–S198.

Benson, K. 2024. Infrastructure supporting prevention among older adults, presented to the Committee on Blueprint for a National Prevention Infrastructure for Behavioral Health Disorders, Meeting 3. https://www.nationalacademies.org/event/42281_04-2024_blueprint-for-a-national-prevention-infrastructure-for-behavioral-health-disorders-meeting-3 (accessed December 16, 2024).

BLS (Bureau of Labor Statistics). 2024. *Community Health Workers*. https://www.bls.gov/ooh/community-and-social-service/community-health-workers.htm (accessed January 2, 2025).

BLS. n.d. *Search results: Behavioral*. https://data.bls.gov/search/query/results?q=behavioral (accessed December 30, 2024).

Brown, V., M. Bowie, D. Bales, A. Scheyett, R. Thomas, and G. Cook. 2023. Cooperative extension offices as mental health hubs: A social ecological case study in rural Georgia, United States. *SSM—Mental Health* 3:100191. https://doi.org/10.1016/j.ssmmh.2023.100191.

CADCA. 2024. *CADCA awarded National Partners Cooperative Agreement funding to strengthen public health infrastructure*. https://www.cadca.org/news-release/cadca-awarded-national-partners-cooperative-agreement-funding-to-strengthen-public-health-infrastructure/ (accessed October 28, 2024).

CDC (Centers for Disease Control and Prevention). 2024. *Prevention research centers 2019–2024*. https://www.cdc.gov/prevention-research-centers/php/funded-prcs-2019-2024/index.html (accessed October 24, 2024).

CEBC (The California Evidence-Based Clearinghouse for Child Welfare). 2024a. *Familias unidas*. https://www.cebc4cw.org/program/familias-unidas/ (accessed March 11, 2025).
CEBC. 2024b. *Family Check-Up (FCU)*. https://www.cebc4cw.org/program/family-check-up/detailed (accessed October 22, 2024).
CHAP (Community Health Aide Program) Alaska. 2024. *Health Aides of Alaska*. https://www.akchap.org/ (accessed December 31, 2024).
Chilenski, S. M., J. Frank, N. Summers, and D. Lew. 2019. Public health benefits 16 years after a statewide policy change: Communities That Care in Pennsylvania. *Prevention Science* 20:947–958. https://doi.org/10.1007/s11121-019-01028-y.
Clark, D. M. 2024. Large scale roll-out of evidence-based psychological therapies through the UK Talking Therapies Program (formerly known as IAPT): Clinical & economic benefits, presented to the Committee on Blueprint for a National Prevention Infrastructure for Behavioral Health Disorders, Meeting 2. https://www.nationalacademies.org/event/41980_02-2024_blueprint-for-a-national-prevention-infrastructure-for-behavioral-health-disorders-meeting-2 (accessed December 16, 2024).
Classroom WISE. n.d. *Introducing Classroom WISE*. https://www.classroomwise.org/ (accessed October 28, 2024).
Crowley, D. M., J. Welsh, S. Chilenski-Meyer, J. Gayles, E. Long, D. Jones, M. McCauley, M. Donovan, and T. Scott. 2024. Integrated prevention infrastructure: A framework for addressing social determinants of health in substance use policy making. *Focus* 22(4):483-491.
CSBHA (California School-Based Health Alliance). 2024. *Peer-to-peer mental health support: Students helping students*. https://www.schoolhealthcenters.org/resources/student-impact/peer-support/ (accessed October 13, 2024).
Cunningham, C. 2024. State-level infrastructure to support prevention, presented to the Committee on Blueprint for a National Prevention Infrastructure for Behavioral Health Disorders, Meeting 3. https://www.nationalacademies.org/event/42281_04-2024_blueprint-for-a-national-prevention-infrastructure-for-behavioral-health-disorders-meeting-3 (accessed December 16, 2024).
Damschroder, L. J., C. M. Reardon, M. A. Opra Widerquist, and J. Lowery. 2022. The updated Consolidated Framework for Implementation Research based on user feedback. *Implementation Science* 17(1):75. https://doi.org/10.1186/s13012-022-01245-0.
Darling-Hammond, S. 2023. *Fostering belonging, transforming schools: The impact of restorative practices*. Learning Policy Institute. https://doi.org/10.54300/169.703 (accessed December 30, 2024).
Dodd, S., E. Widnall, A. E. Russell, E. L. Curtin, R. Simmonds, M. Limmer, and J. Kidger. 2022. School-based peer education interventions to improve health: A global systematic review of effectiveness. *BMC Public Health* 22(1):2247. https://doi.org/10.1186/s12889-022-14688-3.
EPFL (Enoch Pratt Free Library). 2024. *Peer Navigators*. https://www.prattlibrary.org/services/peer-navigators (accessed October 2, 2024).
Federal Reserve Bank of New York. 2023. *The economic case for community health workers*. https://www.newyorkfed.org/newsevents/events/regional_outreach/2023/0623-2023 (accessed October 2, 2024).
Fernando, S., T. Brown, K. Datta, D. Chidhanguro, N. V. Tavengwa, J. Chandna, E. Munetsi, L. Dzapasi, C. Nyachowe, B. Mutasa, B. Chasekwa, R. Ntozin, D. Chibanda, and A. J. Prendergast. 2021. The Friendship Bench as a brief psychological intervention with peer support in rural Zimbabwean women: A mixed methods pilot evaluation. *Global Mental Health* 8:e31. https://doi.org/10.1017/gmh.2021.32.
Gorman-Smith, D., R. C. Garthe, M. E. Schoeny, F. N. Cosey-Gay, C. Harris Sr., C. H. Brown, and J. A. Villamar. 2024. The impact of the Communities That Care approach in reducing violence and crime within an urban, high-burden community. *Prevention Science* 25(6):863–877. https://doi.org/10.1007/s11121-024-01707-5.

Gotham, H. J., F. Benson, R. Canelo, E. R. Walker, M. Navarro, C. N. Clayton, D. Orobitg-Brenes, I. Carrión-González, K. Tomlin, and J. R. Olson. 2024. A national snapshot of training and technical assistance needs within the mental health workforce. *Psychiatric Services.* https://doi.org/10.1176/appi.ps.202306.

Gurley-Calvez, T., and J. A. R. Williams. 2020. *Cost Analysis of KC Care Community Health Worker Program: Using National Estimates of Avoided Care.* University of Kansas Medical Center. https://nachw.org/wp-content/uploads/2020/07/NACDD/MO49_CHW_Cost_final.pdf (accessed December 11, 2024).

Harris, B. R., B. M. Maher, and L. Wentworth. 2022. Optimizing efforts to promote mental health on college and university campuses: Recommendations to facilitate usage of services, resources, and supports. *Journal of Behavioral Health Services & Research* 49(2):252–258. https://doi.org/10.1007/s11414-021-09780-2.

Health.mil. 2022. Combat and operational stress control (COSC). https://www.health.mil/Military-Health-Topics/Centers-of-Excellence/Psychological-Health-Center-of-Excellence/Psychological-Health-Readiness/Combat-and-Operational-Stress-Control (accessed December 31, 2024).

HHS (Department of Health and Human Services). 2022. School-based health services—HHS resources: March 2022. https://www.hhs.gov/sites/default/files/school-based-health-services-resources.pdf (accessed December 30, 2024).

HRSA and SAMHSA (Health Resources and Services Administration/National Center for Health Workforce Analysis, and Substance Abuse and Mental Health Services Administration/Office of Policy, Planning, and Innovation, Planning, and Innovation). 2016. *National projections of supply and demand for selected behavioral health practitioners: 2013-2025.* Rockville, MD. https://www.modernhealthcare.com/assets/pdf/CH10852216.PDF 9 (accessed December 30, 2024).

IC&RC (International Certification & Reciprocity Consortium). 2022. *Candidate guide for the IC&RC prevention specialist examination.* https://internationalcredentialing.org/wp-content/uploads/2024/08/Prevention_Candidate_Guide_Final_06.28.24.pdf (accessed January 2, 2025).

IMI (Institute for Medicaid Innovation). 2023. *Innovation in Perinatal And Child Health In Medicaid.* https://medicaidinnovation.org/wp-content/uploads/2023/04/IMI-2023-Innovation-in-Perinatal-and-Child-Health-in-Medicaid-FINAL.pdf (accessed December 30, 2024).

Jones, T. M., A. Schulte, S. Ramanathan, M. Assefa, S. Rebala, and P. J. Maddox. 2021. Evaluating the association of state regulation of community health workers on adoption of standard roles, skills, and qualities by employers in select states: A mixed methods study. *Human Resources for Health* 19:1–12.

Kanzler, K. E., M. E. Kunik, and C. A. Aycock. 2024. Increasing access to behavioral health care: Examples of task shifting in two U.S. government health care systems. *Fam Syst Health* 42(4):626-636. https://doi.org/10.1037/fsh0000886.

Kelly, L., A. Bartels, and A. Cram. 2024. *Opportunities for public health agencies to advance sustainable financing of community health worker programs.* ASTHO and Center for Health Care Strategies. https://www.chcs.org/resource/opportunities-for-public-health-agencies-to-advance-sustainable-financing-of-community-health-worker-programs/ (accessed December 30, 2024).

Kogan, S. M., G. H. Brody, V. K. Molgaard, C. M. Grange, D. A. Oliver, T. N. Anderson, R. J. DiClemente, G. M. Wingood, Y. F. Chen, and M. C. Sperr. 2012. The Strong African American Families-teen trial: Rationale, design, engagement processes, and family-specific effects. *Prevention Science* Apr;13(2):206–217. https://doi.org/10.1007/s11121-011-0257-y.

Last, B. S., and E. L. Crable. 2024. Policy recommendations for coordinated and sustainable growth of the behavioral health workforce. *Milbank Quarterly* 102(3):0723. https://doi.org/10.1111/1468-0009.12711.

Lyons, B., and M. O'Malley Watts. 2024. Addressing the shortage of direct care workers: Insights from seven states. The Commonwealth Fund. https://www.commonwealthfund.org/publications/issue-briefs/2024/mar/addressing-shortage-direct-care-workers-insights-seven-states (accessed December 30, 2024).

Mariani, S. 2024. State-level infrastructure to support prevention, presented to the Committee on Blueprint for a National Prevention Infrastructure for Behavioral Health Disorders, Meeting 3. https://www.nationalacademies.org/event/42281_04-2024_blueprint-for-a-national-prevention-infrastructure-for-behavioral-health-disorders-meeting-3 (accessed October 28, 2024).

Mayer, K. 2023. Growth in Total Compensation Cost Slows for Employers. Society for Human Resources Management. https://www.shrm.org/topics-tools/news/benefits-compensation/growth-total-compensation-cost-slows-employers (accessed January 2, 2025).

Metz, A., B. Albers, K. Burke, L. Bartley, L. Louison, C. Ward, and A. Farley. 2021. Implementation practice in human service systems: Understanding the principles and competencies of professionals who support implementation. *Human Service Organizations: Management, Leadership & Governance* 45(3):238–259. https://doi.org/10.1080/23303131.2021.1895401.

MHFA (Mental Health First Aid). 2024. *Mental health first aid for youth.* https://www.mentalhealthfirstaid.org/population-focused-modules/youth/ (accessed August 5, 2024).

Murry, V. M., and G. H. Brody. 2004. Partnering with community stakeholders: Engaging rural African American families in basic research and the Strong African American Families preventive intervention program. *Journal of Marital and Family Therapy* 30(3):271–283. https://doi.org/10.1111/j.1752-0606.2004.tb01240.x.

NACHW (National Association of Community Health Workers). 2022. Community health worker pay equity. https://nachw.org/wp-content/uploads/2022/12/CHW_pay_equity.pdf (accessed July 9, 2024).

NAMI (National Alliance on Mental Illness). 2024. *NAMI Bridges to Care—Greater San Antonio: June 2024 Course Calendar.* https://nami-sat.org/wp-content/uploads/sites/370/2024/06/June-2024-Bridges-to-Care-Course-Calendar.pdf (accessed October 22, 2024).

NASEM (National Academies of Sciences, Engineering, and Medicine). 2019. *Fostering healthy mental, emotional, and behavioral development in children and youth: A national agenda.* Washington, DC: The National Academies Press. https://doi.org/10.17226/25201.

NASEM. 2024. *Addressing workforce challenges across the behavioral health continuum of care: Proceedings of a workshop.* Washington, DC: The National Academies Press, https://doi.org/10.17226/28583.

NASHP (National Academy for State Health Policy). 2019. *50-state scan: How medicaid agencies leverage their non-licensed substance use disorder workforce.* https://nashp.org/50-state-scan-how-medicaid-agencies-leverage-their-non-licensed-substance-use-disorder-workforce/ (accessed October 16, 2024).

NCCHCA (North Carolina Community Health Center Association). 2020. *Formerly incarcerated transitions: NC health care for returning inmates.* https://www.ncchca.org/community-resources/programs-services/formerly-incarcerated-transitions/#:~:text=Only%20prisoners%20with%20HIV%2FAIDS,first%202%20weeks%20post%2Drelease (accessed October 4, 2024).

NCCHCA. n.d. *Formerly incarcerated transitions.* https://www.ncchca.org/community-resources/programs-services/formerly-incarcerated-transitions/ (accessed January 14, 2025).

NCHWA (National Center for Health Workforce Analysis). 2023. *Behavioral health workforce, 2023.* https://bhw.hrsa.gov/sites/default/files/bureau-health-workforce/Behavioral-Health-Workforce-Brief-2023.pdf (accessed December 13, 2024).

NCSACW (National Center on Substance Abuse and Child Welfare). n.d. *Technical assistance.* https://ncsacw-stage.acf.hhs.gov/technical/ (accessed October 24, 2024).

NCSL (National Conference of State Legislatures). 2024. *Behavioral health workforce shortages and state resource systems.* https://www.ncsl.org/labor-and-employment/behavioral-health-workforce-shortages-and-state-resource-systems (accessed October 24, 2024).

NCSSLE (National Center on Safe Supportive Learning Environments). 2025. *Mental health.* https://safesupportivelearning.ed.gov/topic-research/environment/mental-health (accessed October 28, 2024).

Ormel, H., M. Kok, S. Kane, R. Ahmed, K. Chikaphupha, S. F. Rashid, D. Gemechu, L. Otiso, M. Sidat, and S. Theobald. 2019. Salaried and voluntary community health workers: Exploring how incentives and expectation gaps influence motivation. *Human Resources for Health* 17(59):1–12. https://doi.org/10.1186/s12960-019-0387-z.

Pantin, H., G. Prado, B. Lopez, S. Huang, M. I. Tapia, S. J. Schwartz, E. Sabillon, C. H. Brown, and J. Branchini. 2009. A randomized controlled trial of Familias Unidas for Hispanic adolescents with behavior problems. *Psychosomatic Medicine* 71(9):987–995. https://doi.org/10.1097/PSY.0b013e3181bb2913.

Perez, L. G., C. Cardenas, T. Blagg, and E. C. Wong. 2024. Partnerships between faith communities and the mental health sector: A scoping review. *Psychiatric Services*: appi-ps. https://doi.org/10.1176/appi.ps.20240077.

PFNYC (Partnership for New York City). 2020. *Lessons from COVID-19: Toward a resilient system of health.* https://pfnyc.org/wp-content/uploads/2020/10/Lessons%20from%20COVID-19%20Toward%20a%20Resilent%20System%20of%20Health%20-%20PFNYC.pdf (accessed January 15, 2025).

PSU (Penn State University). 2024. *Prevention learning portal.* https://plp.psu.edu/ (accessed October 24, 2024).

PTTC Network (Prevention Technology Transfer Center Network). 2024. *Prevention specialist certification states.* https://pttcnetwork.org/prevention-specialist-certification-states/ (accessed September 11, 2024).

Ray, B., D. P. Watson, H. Xu, M. P. Salyers, G. Victor, E. Sightes, K. Bailey, L. R. Taylor, and N. Bo. 2021. Peer recovery services for persons returning from prison: Pilot randomized clinical trial investigation of support. *Journal of Substance Abuse Treatment* 126:108339. https://doi.org/10.1016/j.jsat.2021.108339.

RHIH (Rural Health Information Hub). 2024a. *Barriers to Health Promotion and Disease Prevention in Rural Areas.* https://www.ruralhealthinfo.org/toolkits/health-promotion/1/barriers (accessed October 24, 2024).

RHIH. 2024b. *Community Coalitions Prevention Models.* https://www.ruralhealthinfo.org/toolkits/substance-abuse/2/prevention/community-coalition (accessed September 5, 2024).

RIDH (Rhode Island Department of Health). 2022. *Health equity zones: Building healthy and resilient communities across Rhode Island.* https://health.ri.gov/publications/brochures/HealthEquityZones.pdf (accessed August 7, 2024).

RWJF (Robert Wood Johnson Foundation). 2024. *Healing City Baltimore and its many partners show that lived experience is expertise.* https://www.rwjf.org/en/grants/grantee-stories/2023/2023-winner-baltimore-md.html (accessed October 2, 2024).

SAMHSA (Substance Abuse and Mental Health Services Administration). 2017. *Funding and Characteristics of Single State Agencies for Substance Abuse Services and State Mental Health Agencies, 2015.* HHS Pub. No. (SMA) SMA-17-5029. Rockville, MD.

SAMHSA. 2021a. Prevention core competencies. https://store.samhsa.gov/sites/default/files/pep20-03-08-001.pdf (accessed September 11, 2024).

SAMHSA. 2021b. *Behavioral health workforce report.* https://annapoliscoalition.org/wp-content/uploads/2021/03/behavioral-health-workforce-report-SAMHSA-2.pdf (accessed December 12, 2024).

SAMHSA. 2022. *Addressing burnout in the behavioral health workforce through organizational strategies.* https://store.samhsa.gov/sites/default/files/pep22-06-02-005.pdf (accessed January 2, 2025).

SAMHSA. 2023. *Voices of youth.* https://www.samhsa.gov/prevention-week/voices-of-youth (accessed October 13, 2024).

SAMHSA. 2024. *Historically Black Colleges and Universities Center for Excellence in Behavioral Health (HBCU-CFE).* https://www.samhsa.gov/resource/tta/historically-black-colleges-universities-center-excellence-behavioral-health-hbcu-cfe (accessed January 2, 2025).

Saunders, H., M. Guth, and G. Eckart. 2023. *A look at strategies to address behavioral health workforce shortages: Findings from a survey of state Medicaid programs.* https://www.kff.org/mental-health/issue-brief/a-look-at-strategies-to-address-behavioral-health-workforce-shortages-findings-from-a-survey-of-state-medicaid-programs/ (accessed May 22, 2024).

Schriger, S. H., M. Knowles, T. Daglieri, S. Kangovi, and R. S. Beidas. 2024. Barriers and facilitators to implementing an evidence-based community health worker model. *JAMA Health Forum* 5(3):e240034. https://doi.org/10.1001/jamahealthforum.2024.0034.

Smithwick, J., J. Nance, S. Covington-Kolb, A. Rodriguez, and M. Young. 2023. "Community health workers bring value and deserve to be valued too:" Key considerations in improving CHW career advancement opportunities. *Frontiers in Public Health* 11:1036481. https://doi.org/10.3389/fpubh.2023.1036481.

Spencer, A., and L. Scannelli Jacobs. 2023. Engaging community members: A guide to equitable compensation. https://www.chcs.org/resource/engaging-community-members-a-guide-to-equitable-compensation/ (accessed December 31, 2024).

St. George, D. 2023. In a crisis, schools are 100,000 mental health staff short. *The Washington Post*, August 31. https://www.washingtonpost.com/education/2023/08/31/mental-health-crisis-students-have-third-therapists-they-need/ (accessed December 30, 2024).

SU (Stanford University). 2024. National Center for Mental Health: Dissemination, Implementation, and Sustainment. https://med.stanford.edu/cdi/mhdis (accessed December 31, 2024).

Stand Together. 2024. The Confess Project: Starting a mental-health movement in Black barbershops. https://standtogether.org/stories/health-care/the-confess-project-mental-health-movement-in-black-owned-barbershops (accessed December 31, 2024).

TTC (Technology Transfer Centers). n.d. Technology transfer centers funded by Substance Abuse and Mental Health Services Administration. https://techtransfercenters.org/ (accessed December 31, 2024).

U.S. Census Bureau. 2019. *Implementing the 2018 standard occupational classification system into Census surveys.* https://www.census.gov/library/working-papers/2019/demo/SEHSD-WP2019-19.html (accessed October 22, 2024).

U.S. Census Bureau. 2023. Counties with large colleges and universities experience population gains once again. https://www.census.gov/newsroom/press-releases/2023/population-estimates-counties.html (accessed December 30, 2024).

UW HPRC (University of Washington Health Promotion Research Center). 2025. Prevention Research Centers Promoting Healthy Aging: Addressing chronic conditions and cognitive health. https://depts.washington.edu/hprc/wp-content/uploads/2024/12/Older-Adults-Issue-Brief_Final_508-1-compressed.pdf (accessed October 28, 2024).

UW-Madison PRC (University of Wisconsin-Madison Prevention Research Center). 2024. *Adaptation of staying health after childbirth (stac) to prevent and reduce racial disparities in postpartum morbidity and mortality.* https://prc.wisc.edu/research/core-research-project/ (accessed October, 17 2024).

Wisconsin Counties. 2023. Job Opening: Prevention Coordinator. https://www.wicounties.org/job/prevention-coordinator/ (accessed January 2, 2025).

Yeager, V. A., and H. Krasna. 2024. When money is not enough: Reimagining public health requires systematic solutions to hiring barriers. *Health Affairs (Millwood)* 43(6):840–845.

YMCA of San Diego County. 2024. *Behavioral & Mental Health Services in San Diego, CA.* https://www.ymcasd.org/community-support/ymca-youth-and-family-services/behavioral-and-mental-health-services (accessed October 6, 2024).

Youth Engaged 4 Change. n.d. *Opportunities.* https://engage.youth.gov/opportunities (accessed October 13, 2024).

Zakszeski, B., and L. Rutherford. 2021. Mind the gap: A systematic review of research on restorative practices in schools. *School Psychology Review* 50(2–3):371–387. https://doi.org/10.1080/2372966X.2020.1852056.

4

Data and Data Systems to Support the Infrastructure

Data are a core infrastructure component—important at every step of implementing evidence-based programs (EBPs) and informative to other components of the infrastructure, from enumerating the workforce and identifying shortages to demonstrating the value of prevention to funders. The prevention infrastructure needs both surveillance and monitoring data systems that are regularly updated to determine not only the prevalence and incidence of mental, emotional, and behavioral (MEB) disorders but also any changes in trends (e.g., new and emerging substances, new routes of administration, change in demographics of those affected). Communities and their partners need data about the MEB outcomes they are trying to enhance and the drivers of those outcomes, as the latter are the focus of prevention and health promotion interventions. Those drivers include structural (e.g., discrimination), environmental (e.g., high retail availability of substances), and social-interpersonal (e.g., family conflict, community violence) factors. These data can be used at federal, state, tribal, regional, and local levels to identify strengths and areas of concern; point to factors to intervene on for the purpose of improving outcomes; and monitor and evaluate results of policy, program, and practice interventions.

At the federal level, the implementation of the Foundations for Evidence-Based Policymaking Act of 2018 included guidance from the Office of Management and Budget (Vought, 2020) "to be used to continually improve the capacity of Federal agencies to generate evidence about effectiveness and implementation, identify areas for improvement of programs, policies, or organizations, and inform mission-critical decisions and policies." This memo and related efforts provide a starting point for considering a whole-of-government data infrastructure for evaluating prevention, which could be replicated at, or at least inform, program evaluation efforts at the state and local level.

At the local level, data need to be available at sufficient levels of granularity to serve the needs of local communities. They also need to be available by subgroup, particularly those that continue to be marginalized and experience persistent MEB health disparities. As with other aspects of the infrastructure, data to meet these needs may be incomplete or not easily accessible to communities, including due to funding constraints.

This chapter describes the purposes of data collection and systems to support prevention initiatives, along with key questions and principles for developing and using data. It provides a brief overview of the data sources that inform the promotion of MEB health and well-being and related gaps; outlines federal/national, state, and local models; and discusses key issues related to extant data and their use. It also identifies some sources of technical assistance and promising approaches for developing and using data systems, especially by and for the communities in which these prevention activities and associated data collection and analysis would take place.

The Centers for Disease Control and Prevention (CDC) Public Health Approach provides a simple framework (slightly updated in Figure 4-1) for discussing how data are used at different points when implementing preventive interventions. First, decision makers at the state or community level define and monitor the problem. What are the rates of substance use disorder (SUD) or mental illness in the community or in a specific setting, such as a school district? What are the trends, and how do they compare to similar communities and to the state as a whole?

Identifying risk and protective factors requires asking what increases the likelihood a person or a group will experience poor outcomes, such as developing an SUD or mental illness. These factors include structural

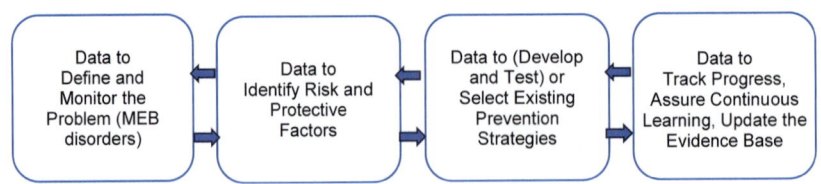

FIGURE 4-1 Adapted depiction of the public health approach to inform local data systems.
NOTE: MEB = mental, emotional, behavioral
SOURCE: CDC, 2024a.

drivers of MEB outcomes (e.g., health care access, poverty) and other aspects of the social-ecological context (see Chapter 2), such as adverse childhood experiences (ACEs). Sources of data to inform efforts to address ACEs or community and individual trauma may include population-level data available from the Behavioral Risk Factor Surveillance System (BRFSS) and data on physical or emotional trauma, including exposure to community violence (data such as homicide rates from the National Violent Death Reporting System) (CDC, 2024d; Swedo et al., 2023). Developing and testing prevention strategies generally takes place through research, but communities can also gather important data about implementation of programs in novel settings or populations or collect data that constitutes practice-based evidence. As a prevention strategy (program, communication campaign, etc.) is implemented, the implementation team and collaborators evaluate its effectiveness and the data collected from it (e.g., pre/post or other) can inform developers of the intervention, funders, and other communities considering the approach. A strong data system—as a key characteristic of a learning prevention infrastructure—is also important to feeding back into the evidence base about an intervention's effectiveness or lack thereof in preventing MEB disorders.

Finally, data are crucial to ensure widespread adoption of a preventive intervention if the following and similar questions are answered affirmatively: Did the strategy achieve the desired effect? Did outcomes improve as a result of the intervention?

TYPES OF DATA SOURCES

There are five sources of data relevant to MEB health and related prevention efforts. These data sources and systems already exist. There are some limitations, such as a gap in local data, or difficulty accessing and using available data sources, but there are efforts to facilitate access to more locally relevant data that can be used, or built on, to support the data needs for delivering preventive interventions and to help communities work with data (PTTC Network, 2024).

1. Administrative data from a range of public systems, including health care, education, criminal-legal, employment, housing, and human services;
2. Electronic health records (EHRs), distinguished from administrative health care claims data;
3. Survey data;
4. Data from use of online platforms, especially social media; and
5. Qualitative data including observations, interviews, and focus groups with community members.

Administrative Data

Administrative data include public- and private-sector data, often from education, human services, criminal-legal, health care, and other systems (see Table 4-1). They are valuable because they generally cover large swaths of the population. They can capture critical domains of interest, such as risk factors (e.g., exposure to abuse) and outcomes (e.g., overdoses). Despite considerable challenges related to the interoperability of these systems, a number of initiatives have demonstrated that administrative data from different sources can be merged to study people's experiences over time and across different systems. They can be used to monitor many outcomes of interest in close to real time, a decided advantage over many other sources of data. They can miss many important outcomes, however, such as psychiatric symptoms, suicidal behavior, or untreated substance misuse. They also provide information only on preventive interventions implemented through the health care system. The use of large administrative linked data sets can help evaluate the returns on public investments in prevention through policy. Linking behavioral health (BH) outcomes data to tax records and public benefit receipt can be used for marginal value of public funds analysis, which, compared to cost–benefit analysis, can offer policy makers additional insights about policy effects (Hendren and Sprung-Keyser, 2020). It is crucial to note that the purpose of such research is not to identify specific individuals or to work with identified data. Economic researchers and other social scientists use different methods to link data sets, and multistep processes for de-identification have been developed to link data without compromising confidentiality (Jutte et al., 2011). For example,

TABLE 4-1 Examples of Sources and Types of Administrative Data Relevant to MEB Health

Sector	Relevant Variables
Education	Grade promotion, attendance, suspensions, expulsions, test scores
Health Care and Pharmacy	Well visits, diagnoses of psychiatric disorder, hospitalizations, emergency room visits, treatment for psychiatric and substance use disorders
Criminal Legal	Arrests, reason for arrest, incarceration
Medical Examiner	Deaths and causes of death
Emergency Services, such as 988	Calls, chats, texts that are routed, answered in-state, or abandoned; speed of answer average contact time

NOTE: MEB = mental, emotional, and behavioral.

linkages are made between people's health outcomes data and their tax records to inform research on the relationship between the Earned Income Tax Credit and a specific health outcome, such as anxiety. There are laws and regulations (e.g., Health Insurance Portability and Accountability Act (HIPAA) Privacy Rule) that are intended to safeguard people's privacy and confidentiality. Although many types of data needed for the prevention infrastructure are anonymized or aggregate (e.g., population surveys), there are circumstances where that is not the case, and careful stewardship and compliance with relevant laws and regulations are crucial.

EHRs

EHRs are distinct from administrative claims data in that they include a richer source of quantitative and qualitative documentation of health care encounters. Primary care clinicians could more frequently collect measures of MEB health, such as the Personal Health Questionnaire, and enter them into the EHR. They also could take advantage of the Z-codes to note health-related social needs (HRSNs). Natural language processing and other informatics approaches could be used to link social needs data to public health and clinical data (NASEM, 2019b; Hossain et al., 2023). The addition of HRSN fields in EHRs could be helpful in implementing preventive interventions in a variety of populations and predicting unmet HRSNs that have a bearing on BH outcomes or even risk of outcomes such as suicide to respond with indicated prevention strategies (He et al., 2023). The Minnesota EHR Consortium offers a good example for how aggregated EHR data can fill gaps in surveillance (i.e., high-level, timely population information on key public health indicators). It is a voluntary collaboration that uses a distributed data model. Data are held and analyzed by health systems, but summary data are aggregated at one site and available to all partners in the consortium (Raths, 2021).

Survey Data

Many federal, state, and local public health and other government agencies collect population-level and longitudinal survey data, which is reported to the public in the aggregate, and can convey the state of MEB health and provide estimates of population-level changes over time. Communities need to be able to measure and demonstrate the effectiveness of their prevention efforts, and this requires not only cross-sectional data (such as the four elements collected for the Drug-Free Communities grants) but also longitudinal cohort data, which are often available for larger geographic areas, such as county, state, and nation. Limitations and challenges of national surveys, such as the BRFSS, include the high cost of administering the survey, lack of estimates for smaller geographic areas, survey length (e.g., the BRFSS takes over 24 minutes), inadequate representativeness, and a "lack of community engagement in survey design, analysis, interpretation of results or dissemination" (Oregon Health Authority, 2021, p. 3). CDC's public health data modernization effort is a promising sign that these challenges will be considered and addressed.

To gather state- and local-level BH data, some states that do not participate in the YRBS implement their own surveys addressing MEB outcomes and their predictors of risk and protective factors (Chang, 2022). Examples include Washington State's Healthy Youth Survey (HYS), Pennsylvania's Youth Survey, and similar surveys in at least 5 states that are administered online to middle and high school students (Chang, 2022). Data from these surveys can be aggregated at state, local, and other relevant geographic levels. In some states, local data can be disaggregated by sex, race, and additional demographic characteristics. Several states have invested in dashboards that facilitate understanding trends over time and comparing community and state averages. Because of their granularity, data from the HYS and related surveys can facilitate local prevention planning by identifying locally specific strengths and areas of need and opportune points of intervention.

Requiring a common core of data elements in state surveys could address gaps left by state-specific surveys. Periodic investments by Substance Abuse and Mental Health Services Administration (SAMHSA) could also facilitate survey updates that incorporate new knowledge about risk and protective factors, changes in focal outcomes, and other realities in an ever-evolving prevention and health promotion landscape. Surveys administered to middle and high school students in over a dozen states are a valuable source of local data on risk, protection, and BH outcomes. To maximize their value in prevention planning, implementation, and monitoring, surveys benefit from periodic updates and psychometric validation. Investments in these activities would ensure surveys reflect state and community priorities and the latest prevention science.

Digital Platform Data

Big data is an emerging category that may include data from apps and social media that could contribute to real-time surveillance of public health concerns (Aebi et al., 2021). New and emerging technologies may provide future opportunities to identify at-risk populations with real-time data and deploy web-based interventions, such as identifying and preventing misinformation, developing "targeted communications to promote [behavior] change" and prediction and early intervention (WHO, 2022). More

> **BOX 4-1**
> **Elmo and the State of America's Well-Being**
>
> An event in 2024 illustrates both the potential of new technology to crowdsource or gather rapid subjective qualitative data and the utility of establishing a national measure of well-being. An official social media account of the Sesame Street character Elmo posted in January 2024: "Elmo is just checking in. How is everybody doing?" (Najib, 2024). The post went viral, with thousands replying and many conveying feelings of emotional distress. The anecdotal information resonated with data from major national surveys showing the reach and depth of the nation's mental health (MH) crises in adults and youth. Sesame Street launched an MH and well-being initiative with resources for children and families and later partnered with the Harris Poll on the inaugural Index on the State of America's Well-Being. The resulting August 2024 report showed that respondents to the online interview instrument ($N = 2,012$, plus an additional oversample of educators, $N = 289$) widely agreed that well-being is negatively affected by MH issues, lack of access to high-quality education/learning opportunities, and continuing aftereffects of the COVID-19 pandemic.
>
> SOURCE: Najib, 2024; Sesame Workshop, 2024.

research is needed to assess the utility and validity of relatively newer data sources, such as Internet search data and other big data (Knipe et al., 2021; Vaidyanathan et al., 2022; Wang et al., 2022) (see Box 4-1).

Qualitative data

Qualitative data include observations (e.g., to record behaviors, using standardized methods), interviews (e.g., to learn about people's experiences), and focus groups (e.g., to gather feedback, test out different options). Qualitative research methods can be useful in evaluating prevention programs, helping to assess progress and identify needed improvement (FRIENDS National Resource Center for CBCAP, 2009).

OVERVIEW OF EXISTING DATA SOURCES

Multiple sources of data and measures can help meet the needs of states, localities, and communities implementing preventive programs (see Table 4-2). The committee discusses the data elements needed by stage of

TABLE 4-2 Select Types and Examples of Data Relevant to MEB Health by Life Stage

Life Stage	Type of Data Will Depend on Setting	Source/What It Covers (a sampling)
Perinatal and early childhood stages	• Clinical system • Population-level survey data • Electronic health record (EHR) • Administrative (women, infants, and children, etc.)	• Clinical ages and stages questionnaire data, screening for maternal depression at prenatal and pediatric visits, and the population-level Centers for Disease Control and Prevention (CDC) Pregnancy Risk Assessment Monitoring System and health system claims data • State data from the Annie E. Casey Foundation Kids Count Data Book 2024
For elementary school ages	• School system administrative data • Survey data • EHR	• Early Development Instrument • National Survey of Children's Health Longitudinal Cohort • Medicaid Claims Data • Youth Risk Behavior Surveillance System (YRBSS) and state-specific surveys • Department of Education, Digest of Education Statistics[a] (e.g., percentage of schools; percentage of students suspended and expelled) • State data from the Annie E. Casey Foundation Kids Count Data Book 2024 • Education data sets from U.S. Department of Education (e.g., National Center for Education Statistics data (NCES, 2023a), including data about school environments; alcohol, illicit drugs,[b] and cigarettes (percentage of students, percentage distribution of students); school crime incidents, suspensions (Office of Civil Rights, School Survey on Crime and Safety; NCES, n.d.)) • National Survey of Child and Adolescent Well-Being (1997–2014 and 2015–2025) related to Child Protective Services investigations
Adolescents	• EHR • Hospital discharge data • Surveys	• Clinical sector (e.g., emergency department data) • YRBSS • National Survey of Children's Health (Health Resources and Services Administration) • Monitoring the Future[c] • Healthy Youth Survey (and state versions) • School Health Policies and Programs Study • School system and Department of Education data • Real-time survey data such as that collected by the MyVoice program (My Voice, n.d) (via SMS) • Drug-Free Communities (DFC) grant required data—every 2 years on the four core measures for alcohol, tobacco, marijuana, and prescription for three grades between 6th and 12th grades (CADCA, n.d.)[d]

Emerging adults	• Surveys • EHR • Administrative data	• YRBSS and Behavioral Risk Factor Surveillance System (BRFSS), National Survey on Drug Use and Health (NSDUH), clinical sector data • Data from educational settings (e.g., American College Health Association's Emotional Well-Being Survey) • Other sources of data for higher education settings, such as the Healthy Campus Inventory and parts of the National College Health Assessment[e]
Working-age adults	• Surveys • Clinical sector data	• BRFSS, NSDUH, National Health and Nutrition Examination Survey, National Health Interview Survey
Older adults	• Surveys • EHR • Administrative data (human services)	• National Health and Aging Trends Study (NHATS) (supported by the National Institute on Aging (NIA)) • National Social Life, Health, and Aging Project (NIA) • National Study of Caregiving (periodic survey of caregivers to NHATS participants)

[a] For example, "Number and percentage of public schools providing diagnostic mental health assessments and treatment to students and, among schools providing these services, percentage providing them at school and outside of school, by selected school characteristics: School years 2017–18, 2019–20, and 2021–22." (NCES, 2023b).

[b] For example, "Percentage of students in grades 9–12 who reported that illegal drugs were made available to them on school property during the previous 12 months, by selected student characteristics: Selected years, 1993 through 2021." (NCES, 2023c).

[c] https://monitoringthefuture.org/about/ (accessed 12/13/24)

[d] Those measures are (1) past 30-day use (the percentage of survey respondents who reported using alcohol, tobacco, or marijuana (prevalence of use) or misusing prescription drugs at least once within the past 30 days (prevalence of misuse)); (2) perception of risk (the percentage who perceived that the use of a given substance has moderate or great risk); (3) perception of parental disapproval (the percentage who perceived their parents would feel that regular use of alcohol (one or two drinks nearly every day) or use any tobacco or marijuana or misuse prescription drugs is wrong or very wrong); and (4) perception of peer disapproval (the percentage who perceived their friends would feel it would be wrong or very wrong for them to drink alcohol regularly (one or two drinks nearly every day) or use any tobacco or marijuana or misuse prescription drugs).

[e] "The report addresses the lack of a universally accepted definition of well-being and the inconsistencies in measuring well-being across campuses" and "focuses on five key dimensions: Community and Belonging, Coping and Stress Management, Purpose and Meaning, Subjective Well-being, and Institutional Environment." (ACHA, 2021). The survey has been piloted at nine universities with over 8,000 students, staff, and faculty. (Key findings included lower scores for students compared to staff and faculty across all scales of emotional well-being, higher levels of depression, loneliness, stress, and anxiety, and low perceptions of institutional support across all three groups.)

the life course. Data sources and metrics pertain to different levels of the socioecological model of health—illustrated by a wide variety of graphics that show the individual at the center of several concentric circles, with increasing influence and potential for impact in each larger circle: interpersonal relationship, community and institutional, and societal factors. If gathering data to inform an intervention for adolescents, for example, there are

- measures of risk and protective factors captured by different types of surveys, administrative, and other data (e.g., harmful drug use, interactions with criminal-legal system, suicide attempts);
- measures pertinent to interpersonal and family relationships (e.g., indicating support, connection);
- measures of the neighborhood level, such as physical/built environment factors that operate at the community level (e.g., related to alcohol and tobacco, neighborhood walkability, housing quality and housing instability);
- measures of institutional factors (e.g., teacher stress and job satisfaction, school climate) (NASEM, 2019a); and
- measures of the aspects of the social and economic environment associated with risk factors for BH disorders (e.g., poverty, firearm-related injuries, social support).

Federal agencies provide reports and data briefs that assemble relevant information by population groups and by state, county, planning area, ZIP code, and census tract. For example, the SAMHSA Behavioral Health Barometer, last published in 2020, provides key data from the 2019 National Survey on Drug Use and Health (NSDUH) and National Survey of Substance Abuse Treatment Services. Data are organized by youth, young adult, and adult age groupings (SAMHSA, 2020). CDC's National Center for Health Statistics provides data briefs, such as No. 467,[1] which is based on data from the National Health Interview Survey. The CDC WONDER Online Databases provide vital (birth and death) statistics. The National Survey of Children's Health is funded and directed by the Health Resources and Services Administration (HRSA) Maternal and Child Health Bureau and conducted by the Census Bureau annually. Data include items related to social factors, such as housing instability, which is correlated with a range of poor health outcomes. The National Health and Aging Trends Study is supported by the National Institute on Aging. A number of sources of data include all age groups, such as the multisource surveillance CDC National Violent Death Reporting System and the cross-sectional household National

---

[1] https://www.cdc.gov/nchs/data/databriefs/db467-tables.pdf (accessed January 17, 2025).

Health Interview Survey. The National Institute on Drug Abuse (NIDA) also provides several data resources, including the ongoing research study Monitoring the Future,[2] and the National Drug Early Warning System.[3]

The NIH All of Us Research Program offers a unique opportunity to learn about the health of millions of Americans and their experiences with specific risk factors and diagnoses. In 2023, the program launched new areas of mental health research. For example, researchers examined "what kinds of social support have the greatest positive impact on mental health and are most protective against depression," and potential future areas for research include exploring prevention strategies and early risk factors (NIH, 2024).

Public Health Surveillance Systems

Public health surveillance is a critical tool in keeping communities healthy and improving their health and well-being, and its uses are most evident with regard to infectious diseases, such as COVID-19. Public health surveillance relies on clinical care settings, ranging from primary care to hospital emergency departments, reporting infectious diseases to public health agencies. In recent years, other means of passive surveillance have emerged, including wastewater testing. During the early part of the COVID-19 pandemic, some public health agencies began such wastewater surveillance. Surveillance of BH status takes place through several avenues, including emergency department (could include firearm injuries, suicide attempts), 988 call, and pharmacy data. CDC's Drug Overdose Surveillance and Epidemiology System collects data about nonfatal overdose through syndromic surveillance by 46 states and the District of Columbia and discharge data from 34 states and DC. It also identifies information about overdose anomalies or outbreaks and changes in trends.

The Council of State and Territorial Epidemiologists has developed a list of 18 indicators for surveillance of substance misuse and mental health (MH) (CSTE, 2019). This indicator set draws on eight data sources: mortality data (death certificates), hospital discharge and emergency department data, the BRFSS, the YRBSS, prescription drug sales (opioids), state excise taxes for alcohol, the National Highway Transportation Safety Administration Fatality Analysis Reporting System, and SAMHSA's NSDUH (NHTSA, n.d.). These sources provide information about people, policies, and market data, such as drug sales. Public health surveillance data also provides insight into shifts in behavior, signals changes in products, and also helps detect an acute event.

---

[2] https://monitoringthefuture.org/ (accessed December 15, 2024).
[3] https://nida.nih.gov/research-topics/trends-statistics/national-drug-early-warning-system-ndews (accessed December 15, 2024).

Measurement Systems That Draw on Survey and Other Data

Nonprofit, academic, and government organizations manage these datasets and often create "dashboards" that provide a synopsis of the health of various communities. These organizations include America's Health Rankings, which is supported and overseen by the United Health Foundation and the American Public Health Association and provides yearly state rankings on specified measures; the County Health Rankings[4] at the University of Wisconsin—Madison Population Health Institute, which provides select measures for all U.S. counties; the City Health Dashboard[5] at NYU Langone Health, which provides dashboards for 750 of the largest cities; and the National Neighborhood Indicators Project (NNIP), an Urban Institute coordinated network of independent organizations in over 30 cities. NNIP's vision is that "by democratizing information, they could give residents and community organizations a stronger voice in improving their neighborhoods" (NNIP, 2024). In addition to these crosscutting sets, data sets are also produced by state and local government agencies (e.g., public health, metropolitan planning organizations, school districts) and hospitals and health systems. These metrics can inform communities about how cities or counties are performing on key metrics, counties compare to one another, their states compare to others, and their local indicators compare to their state averages.

In 2023, the U.S. Department of Health and Human Services (HHS) People and Places Thriving initiative adopted the Vital Conditions for Health and Well-Being framework, which lists seven domains that reflect key contributors to health and well-being: belonging and civic muscle, lifelong learning, meaningful work and wealth, humane housing, basic needs for health (safety), thriving natural world, and reliable transportation. These roughly map to the Healthy People 2030 framework that lists five categories of social determinants of health (SDOH): education access and quality, economic stability, social and community context, neighborhood and built environment, and health care access and quality.

The need for coordination and data integration across different government agencies, including tribal governments, and systems has been highlighted by National Academies and other reports. One National Academies report recommended that federal agencies collaborate with state and local counterparts and private-sector partners in philanthropy and business to "develop an integrated plan for longitudinal data collection and coordination and analysis of federal surveys, administrative data, and vital statistics that provides a comprehensive approach to measuring and tracking child and adolescent MEB health" (NASEM, 2019a, p. 6). Another asserted that

---

[4] https://www.countyhealthrankings.org/ (accessed December 15, 2024).
[5] https://www.cityhealthdashboard.com/ (accessed December 15, 2024).

"digitization in social care lags behind ... health care" and listed as barriers to integration "a lack of digital infrastructure, data standards, and modern technology architecture shared between and among organizations, as well as digital privacy and security concerns" (NASEM, 2019b). These barriers affect data sharing across a range of relevant systems and domains, including health care, public health, human services, and education. Solutions include legal arrangements and application program interfaces that can reduce risks to data owners (NASEM, 2023a), such as interfaces like those that allow ride-share providers to link to data from geomapping software on a user's smartphone.

FEDERAL AND NATIONAL DATA INITIATIVES AND GUIDELINES

Recent and ongoing examples of efforts to establish infrastructure for data exchange, linkage, or integration have relevance to promoting MEB health and well-being. These include high-level coordination within HHS to set standards, certify systems, and build a support infrastructure. The HHS Office of the National Coordinator for Health Information Technology (ONC) and CDC jointly lead the federal public health interoperability strategy (ONC, 2023; CDC, 2024b).

In 2022, the HHS Assistant Secretary for Planning and Evaluation launched the CHILDREN initiative to help public child welfare and Medicaid agencies "develop sustainable, integrated data systems with linked data, to support care coordination and oversight of prevention services and congregate care services" (Mathematica, n.d.-b; Greenfield et al., 2023). The first stage addresses data integration between the child welfare and Medicaid agencies in the District of Columbia, Iowa, Oregon, and Wyoming (Mathematica, n.d.-b). The initiative is intended to help states and tribes implement the Family First Prevention Services Act (FFPSA),[6] which reformed how funding under Title IV-E of the Social Security Act could be used to help keep children out of foster care (ACF, n.d.; Greenfield et al. 2023).

Between 2020 and 2021, the Robert Wood Johnson Foundation convened a National Commission to Transform Public Health Data Systems, which identified key challenges to the data infrastructure: limited funding, lack of federal–state coordination, and systemic hurdles (RWJF, 2021). It called for collecting better data stratified by population groups and geographic levels to provide better understanding of health disparities, the establishment of an interagency data council to "improve measures to assess equity and racial justice and bring together different agencies to

---

[6] *Family First Preventative Services Act of 2017*, HR 253, 115th Congress (accessed December 15, 2024).

create interoperable social and public health data," and ensuring "that community input is represented in data collection, interpretation and decision making" funding "to systems that are standards based and interoperable" (RWJF, 2021, p. 2).

In 2022, CDC launched its Public Health Data Strategy, and in 2024, it partnered with the Association of State and Territorial Health Officials, National Network of Public Health Institutes, and Public Health Accreditation Board to establish three Public Health Data Modernization Implementation Center Programs (Mathematica, n.d.-c). The effort includes "working with state, tribal, local, and territorial health departments to accelerate data exchange to reduce burden and improve public health threat detection and health outcomes across populations" (Mathematica, n.d.-a).

Better national coordination on prevention, such as the mechanisms recommended in the Governance and Partnerships chapter, could involve bringing together representatives from relevant agencies that play a role in preventing MEB disorders to extend or adapt interoperability standards to their data to enable integration that can better inform cross-sector work and meet the shared aims of improving MEB health.

State and Local Models and Examples

In addition to these national initiatives, state- and local-level efforts have brought together different data sources to inform decision making and the provision of health care and social services. The examples are not a comprehensive list but rather illustrate some ongoing efforts and innovations in states as geographically and demographically varied as Iowa, Oregon, California, New Jersey, Connecticut, and Minnesota and communities such as Hennepin County, Minnesota, and San Diego, California.

State Government–Academic Partnerships

The learning community training and technical assistance program at University of Pennsylvania Actionable Intelligence for Social Policy supported a partnership between Early Childhood Iowa and Iowa State University to form the state's Integrated Data System for Decision Making and a comprehensive statewide needs assessment in 2019 with a grant from the Administration for Children and Families. The Iowa Department of Health and Human Services has conducted a HRSA-supported assessment of family support, home visiting, and community risk, using the state's home-visiting data system and other types of data (e.g., child care subsidy, Early Head Start and Head Start, K–12 education) to ascertain "strengths and gaps among Iowa's home-visiting services for families with young children" (I2D2, 2021).

The Center for Evidence-Based Policy at Oregon Health and Science University operates the Oregon Child Integrated Dataset (OCID, 2020). The effort includes a dashboard that integrates the following indicators: health (birth, weight, and Medicaid well-child visits, ages 3–6); child welfare (foster care placement, early childhood, child maltreatment, early childhood); and education (kindergarten assessment, approaches to learning and early literacy, third grade assessment reading and math, ninth grade on track to graduate, student homelessness, school attendance).

In 2018, New Jersey enacted legislation that established the Integrated Population Health Data Project at Rutgers University. The project facilitates research and allows academics to support the state government in improving the health, safety, security, and well-being of state residents (Rutgers, n.d.). Its five foci are opioid misuse, maternal and infant health, SDOH, COVID-19 and other public health emergencies, and high-value care.

The University of Delaware prepares the annual State of Delaware Epidemiological Profile for substance use, MH, and related issues for the State Epidemiological Outcomes Workgroup, which promotes "the use of behavioral health data for prevention, strategic planning, decision-making, and evaluation." (University of Delaware, 2024). The profile draws on national data sources (NSDUH, BRFSS, and the Household Pulse Survey), Delaware School Survey and the state's YRBSS, data from the state's divisions of public health and of substance abuse and MH, the state's department of safety and homeland security, and crisis text line (Delaware State Epidemiological Outcomes Workgroup, 2023). The state uses Cantril's Ladder as a measure of well-being. This simple, self-reported measure asks respondents to place their state of being on a 10-step ladder to indicate where they stand in relation to the best possible life, with rungs from Suffering to Struggling to Thriving.

Data to Drive Resource Allocation and Evaluation

Data play a critical role in Washington State's Community Prevention Wellness Initiative (CPWI), a community- and school-based effort to prevent SUD (Mariani, 2024). Because of limited public prevention dollars, the Division of Behavioral Health and Recovery (DBHR), the single state agency for administering SAMHSA block grant dollars, prioritizes communities with higher need and greater risk for substance use problems. Eligibility is determined by a risk index developed with local data about crime, truancy, BH problems, and other factors. DBHR uses data from Washington State's HYS to evaluate the results of CPWI efforts.

Guidance for State-Level Health Information Sharing

California established the State Health Information Guidance, which supports information sharing among collaborators, including for BH. In April 2023, it expanded to include 22 scenarios derived from real user stories, which clarify how state laws govern the exchange of information about MH and SUD (Center for Data Insights and Innovation, n.d.).

Academic and Local Government Partnership

The University of Arizona has developed a dashboard that provides 36 specific health and SDOH measures for southern Arizona counties. It also allows Arizona cities to compare themselves with peer cities on key BH metrics, including number of poor MH days per month, percent of population with depression, percent of population who drink to excess, and SDOH measures, such as housing cost burden and poverty (Making Action Possible, n.d.).

Health Systems Data Integration Partnership

In Minnesota, the state's 11 largest health systems collaborate in its Electronic Health Record Consortium, which was launched in March 2020 to address gaps in traditional public health surveillance and support public health response to COVID-19. Hennepin County adapted it to inform the county's efforts to address substance use–related harms. The consortium collects timely health care use data that informs public health authorities and health care organizations about nonfatal overdoses and other relevant data, in addition to highlighting demographic patterns. One of its projects is Health Trends Across Communities, which provides a data dashboard with 24 priority health topics and technical assistance resources (MN EHR, n.d.). The consortium uses a master data use agreement (also known as a "data sharing agreement") that is amended for each new project (MN EHR, 2024).

State Government Data Effort

In Connecticut, DataHaven is a partner of the NNIP, and its largest program is the DataHaven Community Well-Being Survey, which is a source of information about quality of life, public health, economic development, and civic vitality for Connecticut communities and others in the region (DataHaven, n.d.). The survey "uses probability sampling to create highly reliable local information that is not available from any other public data source" (DataHaven and Siena College Research

Institute, 2024). Additionally, DataHaven produces a Community Index and the Connecticut Town. In 2023, DataHaven and its partners released the 2023 Community Well-Being Index at the State Capitol. A 2021 DataHaven report commissioned by the Quinnipiac Valley Health District explored root causes for a 40 percent increase in fatal overdoses in the New Haven area and recommended prevention strategies (Davlia, 2021).

These examples illustrate the breadth of capabilities that exist across different types of partnerships to support the collection and reporting of data from multiple sources to inform BH-related and other prevention efforts of states and localities. Although using, sharing, and integrating existing, new, and emerging data sources has challenges, especially with identified data, there are robust guidelines and frameworks to guide data sharing and integration, as well as methods for integrating multiple sources and systems (e.g., health care, housing, education, child welfare) not only for efficient service delivery to individuals but also to optimize the planning, implementation, and sustainment of population-level prevention strategies across a variety of settings and along the life course.

Privacy Standards

Privacy issues are largely relevant to health care contexts and, given that a considerable proportion of prevention services are delivered at the community level and not in clinical settings, there will be minimal risks to individual privacy. When health care providers share data with social services providers, such as using a single EHR to help serve individuals more seamlessly (e.g., case management, housing, food assistance) and an integrated data warehouse for analysis and reporting, the data collection and sharing are governed by both federal and state laws and policies (Owen, 2014). In educational settings, if a school is by the Health Insurance Portability and Accountability Act of 1996 (HIPAA) because it employs a health care provider that bills Medicaid electronically, health information maintained under "education records" is governed by Family Educational Rights and Privacy Act of 1974, and the school is not required to comply with the HIPAA Privacy Rule, though it must comply with the HIPAA Transactions and Code Sets Rule (HHS and ED, 2019). In many cases, however, health care systems can share deidentified data "to help public health departments and policy makers monitor and respond to emerging mental health issues" (Purtle et al., 2020). Also, health care systems along with public health agencies can advocate for evidence-supported public policy changes that can improve MEB health and well-being.

Building Community Capacity to Use Data

Some components of the systems needed to consistently collect and collate community data are already in place, but challenges remain. They include lack of skilled personnel to collect and analyze data, barriers to integration and interoperability, difficulty accessing data, and cost of some private-sector sources. Sources of data may include government agencies at all levels, including local health departments, schools, and area agencies on aging. Data collection (primary or secondary data) is necessary but not sufficient for communities to track their progress.

The prevention infrastructure in communities unfolds in a variety of settings, two of which are multisector community coalitions and primary care settings, beginning with community health centers and federally qualified health centers. Those working in and with communities to identify existing and collect new data inevitably need to partner with a variety of organizations, ranging from academic institutions to cooperative extensions.

Communities, partners, and prevention leaders and workers need not only the contextual data described (e.g., how a community or region compares to others and the averages in that state) but also hyperlocal or granular data. Local data (e.g., for census tract or zip code) are available from a variety of partners (public health agency, hospital, community health center, etc.) and sources. However, some data (e.g., program implementation and outcomes) must be collected and analyzed locally by the implementers of evidence-based interventions or their collaborators. These latter include data about local needs and assets, local capacity and other institutional or system features, and intervention- and implementation-specific features, such as reach and penetration and fidelity to design.

Community Coalitions

Data from the Office of National Drug Control Policy about the 2022 cohort of Drug-Free Communities–supported coalitions showed that "For all coalitions since inception, past 30-day use rates decreased significantly across all substances at both the middle and high school levels, evidence that DFC coalitions are meeting the goal of preventing youth substance use. That is, there were significant decreases in past 30-day use across substances. This same pattern held true for the FY 2021 cohort" (Drug-Free Communities Support Program and Executive Office of the President of the United States, 2023, p. 37). These data show that community coalitions can help improve key BH outcomes.

CADCA (formerly the Community Anti-Drug Coalitions of America) outlines the kinds of data collection or assessments that coalitions need to conduct to inform their work: quantitative, qualitative, and resource assessment. Data resources include surveys (available nationally, such as YRBSS, or at the state level and potentially also locally from partners and collaborators that collect data in the community) and archival or secondary data from other organizations, such as arrest data from local law enforcement or substance use treatment data from the state health department (CADCA, n.d.). Qualitative data collection methods include key informant interviews, focus groups, listening sessions, town hall or community meetings, observation, and environmental scans. Resource assessment includes identifying assets (broadly conceived), capacity, and a range of resources such as existing programs, initiatives, coalitions, laws and policies, and funding streams.

A growing body of research examines the relationship between different aspects of community coalition work and change in the outcomes of interest. One study of coalitions across multiple countries found that "perceptions of their community and their pride in community are closely linked to the way they talk about their life satisfaction and mental well-being and may be a key pragmatic measure for initiative success" (Powell et al., 2024). These data have been used to show that community coalitions can help improve key BH outcomes. Box 4-2 provides an example of a coalition's use of different kinds of data to inform planning.

Green and colleagues (2024) provide a noteworthy example of a finding about local capacity—an oversaturation of SUD prevention coalitions in a county in Montana, which indicated a risk of inefficient use of resources and diluted focus (Green et al., 2024). Researchers used the metric "program saturation," estimated with SAMHSA's Calculating an Adequate System Tool algorithm. Coalition Check-Up is another resource for coalitions.

BOX 4-2
Using Qualitative Data to Inform Selection of Preventive Strategies

A study in rural Georgia in a community where coalition development was in the early stages highlights the work of assessing "the feasibility and accessibility of implementing different rural suicide prevention efforts" (Roth et al., 2023 p. 3). Researchers identified data showing that the urban versus rural age-adjusted death rate due to suicide was 14.2 vs 18.4 per 100,000. Roth and colleagues (2023) examined county-level data (e.g., showing high poverty and unemployment rates), and collected qualitative data. They used in-depth one-on-one interviews and two focus groups to inform the community's efforts to "adapt the most appropriate preventive intervention to the population and context" (Roth et al., 2023, p. 3).

Data Equity and Data Ownership

Data equity considerations are needed to inform all aspects of data collection, use, and reporting. The Office of Management and Budget's report on the implementation of Executive Order 13985 Study to Identify Methods to Assess Equity: Report to the President states that "a broad range of assessment frameworks and data and measurement tools have been developed to assess equity, but equity assessment remains a nascent and evolving science and practice." (OMB, 2021, p. 14). Beyond measuring the implementation and outcomes of prevention programs, it is important to recognize that data belong to the communities from which they are collected, and communities need support in using their own data for planning and evaluation purposes.

The CDC Foundation has developed five equity principles for using public health data in partnership with the communities from which the data come: recognizing and defining systemic factors, paying attention to equity in language and action, making space for cultural modifications, developing a shared data agreement, and facilitating community governance of "the collection, ownership, dissemination and application of their own data." (CDC, 2024). Existing data may have biases and gaps, and the Rutgers Policy Lab notes that holding data producers accountable for data equity requires considering how data are collected, analyzed, interpreted, and shared and also "encourages further inspection into potential racial bias of research instruments, publication's role in the reinforcement of stereotypes, and marginalized communities' ability to control and access their own data. It also cautions against data misuse and inaccurately broad generalization. Data equity also considers issues regarding power and privilege between researchers and their targeted populations and concerns that harmful decisions might be justified through data" (Spiegel, n.d.). Implementation considerations are discussed in Box 4-3.

Using Data for Community Action

Several important resources inform variable and measure selection and data use and implementation considerations. The Prevention Technology Transfer Center (PTTC) Network has put forward a checklist of six data areas aligned with the SAMHSA Strategic Planning Framework to help communities identify data gaps: consequences, consumption, target populations, intervening variables (risk and protective factors), prevention resources, and community readiness (PTTC Network, 2021). For MH prevention work, other assessment data would be substituted for consequences and consumption.

> **BOX 4-3**
> **Implementation Considerations Related to MEB Health Data**
>
> **Expanding Opportunities for Health**
> - Build community capacity to use the data communities need.
> - Funders need to mandate usability of data produced from studies.
> - Implement the data recommendations of the National Academies report *Federal Policy to Advance Racial, Ethnic, and Tribal Health Equity*.[7]
> - Ensure collection and use of data that is disaggregated by race and ethnicity as required by OMB SPD-15.
> - Add (where needed) measures of systemic racism and the social determinants of health in existing national surveys.
> - Look at data by subgroups to track inequities.
> - Sample to ensure capture of underrepresented groups.

(continued)

---

[7] The report found that a "broad range of assessment frameworks and data and measurement tools have been developed to assess equity, but equity assessment remains a nascent and evolving science and practice" and made four recommendations on this topic:

Recommendation 5: The Office of Management and Budget (OMB) should require the Census Bureau to facilitate and support the design of sampling frames, methods, measurement, collection, and dissemination of equitable data resources on minimum OMB categories—including for American Indian or Alaska Native, Asian, Black or African American, Hispanic or Latino/a, and Native Hawaiian or Pacific Islander populations—across federal statistical agencies. The highest priority should be given to the smallest OMB categories—American Indian or Alaska Native and Native Hawaiian or Pacific Islander.

Recommendation 6: The Office of Management and Budget (OMB) should update and ensure equitable collection and reporting of detailed-origin and tribal affiliation data for all minimum OMB categories through data disaggregation by race, ethnicity, and tribal affiliation (to be done in coordination with meaningful tribal consultation), including populations who self-identify as American Indian or Alaska Native, Asian, Black or African American, Native Hawaiian or Pacific Islander, and Hispanic or Latino/a.

Recommendation 7: The Centers for Disease Control and Prevention should coordinate the creation and facilitate the use of common measures on multilevel social determinants of racial and ethnic health inequities, including scientific measures of racism and other forms of discrimination, for use in analyses of national health surveys and by other federal agencies, academic researchers, and community groups in analyses examining health, social, and economic inequities among racial and ethnic groups.

Recommendation 8: Congress should increase funding for federal agencies responsible for data collection on social determinants of health measures to provide information that leads to a better understanding of the correlation between the social environment and individual health outcomes. (NASEM, 2023b)

> **BOX 4-3 Continued**
>
> **Implementation Science**
> - Consider how this fits in the broader knowledge translation system.
> - Engage community in creating data infrastructure.
> - Ensure information is accessible, useful, and usable by community members
> - Ensure sampling goes beyond race and ethnicity, rural, class education, disability status, sexual orientation and gender identity, etc.

Communities and their collaborators in prevention require a parsimonious data set that describes outcomes of interest (e.g., substance use, psychological well-being, suicide rate) and measures that can inform them about sociodemographics, assets and resources, and data on risk (e.g., exposure to ACEs, such as abuse and violence) and protective (e.g., supportive family relationships) factors. Communities need to be able to use data to track and compare needs and outcomes against their own historical data (to assess impact, course correct), compare themselves against other communities, and determine the effectiveness of prevention efforts.

A key characteristic of effective data collection and integration efforts is that they occur in the context of multisector and community partnerships. The "Learning Health Care Communities" (Natafgi et al., 2021) model describes the relationship between the learning health care system (data are turned into knowledge that shapes patient care) and the learning health care community (health measures create awareness that help improve community health). Other public health and social or community change models exist that can inform and guide community-partnered MEB health promotion. One example is Mobilizing for Action through Planning and Partnership (MAPP and MAPP 2.0) from the National Association of County and City Health Officials that includes community partner assessment and both quantitative (community status) and qualitative (community context) assessments. Another is the collective impact model, which includes shared measurement systems as one of five conditions of collective success (with common agenda, mutually reinforcing activities, continuous communication, and backbone support organization) (Piff, 2021; Tamarack Institute, 2017). Communities also can learn from partnering with organizations about what measures and data are available to them (e.g., health department, schools, and area agencies on aging) to inform their planning, selection of interventions, implementation, and evaluation.

To support community data infrastructure, government agencies at all levels can provide funding for data sharing, analysis, and collection. While HHS agencies have a history of temporarily funding resources that provide local, small-area data, including on SDOH health elements, and mechanisms that allowed peer comparisons and collaboration, such federal efforts have fluctuated over time.

DATA ISSUES (CHALLENGES AND OPPORTUNITIES)

Some key issues related to data and measures in the prevention infrastructure for MEB health and well-being include the following:

1. The need to build a health equity focus into data and measurement systems themselves;
2. Community level—the role of communities in deciding what matters most and collecting and using data; frequency of collection and associated concerns, such as community burden/fatigue;
3. Related infrastructure and resource needs (i.e., workforce and funding); resources to address technical hurdles for integration and interoperability;
4. Regulatory and governance (e.g., data sharing and innovation); ownership and sovereignty; privacy and confidentiality when individual-level data are collected or needed;
5. Lack of hyperlocal/granular or small-area data; and
6. Inconsistencies in data.

Building an Equity Focus in Data Systems

Data are collected and used in the process of assessing and responding to the MEB health needs of populations and communities, so MEB health disparities are an important consideration. Data and measures may seem neutral in terms of their provenance, means of collection, and meaning, but that is not the case. Rather, they reflect values and norms and decisions about what matters and what does not, and they may hide or obscure important truths. Nancy Krieger described data as a two-edged sword: edge 1 is "no data, no problem," and edge 2 is "problematic data, big problem" (Krieger, 2021, p. 2). The former refers to the nonuse of data related to populations marginalized on the basis of race or ethnicity. That is exemplified in the inadequacy of data documenting the impact of COVID-19 in minoritized communities, notably in American Indian, Alaska Native, and Native Hawaiian populations (Douglas et al., 2021; Urban Indian Health Institute, 2021). The latter refers to the use of "problematic data in harmful ways" (Krieger, 2021, p. 2).

Community level

Communities have often been the locus for and subject of data collection. A long history exists of data collection (and research) approaches that exploit this resource, may be unaccountable to the community, and may not adequately engage or partner with, community members and organizations (Emmons et al., 2023). The Patient-Centered Outcomes Research Institute (PCORI) provides a good model for sharing research data with community members who contributed (PCORI, n.d.). Data to support MEB health promotion can be generated with the community and used to respond to its needs and priorities. As more community coalitions and organizations work with partners, including academic institutions, to implement preventive interventions and generate data, locally developed insights and implementation experiences could inform other communities, and efforts are needed to ensure the wide dissemination of information about intervention impact and other practice-based evidence.

Related infrastructure and resource needs

Financial resources are a challenge in establishing, operating, and sustaining data systems or data collection efforts. Braiding and blending of funding is often needed for data systems, given that many funding sources often lack robust support for data collection and measurement efforts (SAMHSA, 2024). But a patchwork of funding streams also has consequences, such as limiting data sharing, such as if data are associated with categorical programs that have narrowly constituted funding. There are workforce implications for data collection, too. For clinical, human services, education, and other types of metrics, data collection needs could overtax service providers.

Regulatory and Governance Issues

Solutions exist for most or all of these issues and challenges, including models and guidance, tools such as data use agreements, application programming interfaces, and other approaches that can be used to safeguard privacy and confidentiality whenever individual-level data are involved. An oft-raised concern is the perceived barriers to data sharing across systems and sectors, such as between state (or local) agencies or states and the federal government. The guidelines provided by the National Academies report *Toward a 21st Century National Data Infrastructure* include the following: "Data sharing is incentivized when all data holders enjoy tangible benefits valuable to their missions, and when societal benefits are proportionate to possible costs and risks" (NASEM, 2023a, p. 6).

Inconsistent or lack of state reporting

For some key metrics, there are inconsistent processes among states for collecting the same data. This may affect the ability to assess the effects of state policies on MEB outcomes (e.g., using quasi-experimental approaches that that compare states that do and do not adopt a preventive policy). For example, the counting of suicide deaths differs in county coroner-only states and coroner-only and state medical examiner states (Fernandez and Jayawardhana, 2024).

As noted above, some states opt out of the YRBSS and use their own youth survey, which in some cases may have data elements that align with the YRBSS. This is important to allow comparisons. However, there are cases, such as in Florida, where participation in a national state-level survey—the YRBSS—has been discontinued (Dollard 2023). That may impede the longitudinal tracking of MEB health, a crucial source of information for planning, implementation, and evaluation. James (2023) notes that unlike other federal surveys, states and local jurisdictions are only asked to use 60 percent of the survey, which "provides a lot of flexibility to state and local jurisdictions, and several states have exercised that flexibility to remove questions related to sexual orientation, gender identity, and sexual behaviors. The ability to adapt the YRBSS to meet local needs is another reason the complete withdrawal of a state is deeply concerning."

Need for small area data

One gap in the data infrastructure needed to inform MEB disorder prevention efforts is a federal community resource. HHS has had several efforts to create such a data repository, including the Community Health Status Indicators (CHSI) project, which operated for several years, with some interruptions, and the Health Indicators Warehouse. Both were ended in 2017. Phillips and colleagues (2021) outline the history of CHSI, which allowed counties to compare themselves to their peers (in 88 different strata that clustered counties according to several categories of similarity). The tool was moved from HRSA to CDC and terminated in 2017, along with several other federal community-level data resources: the Health Indicators Warehouse, Health Data Interactive, and BRFSS multiyear data roll-ups. In 2018, the National Committee on Vital Health Statistics partnered with the 100 Million Healthier Lives (100M Lives) network of communities, health coalitions, nonprofits, health care organizations, and others, in an effort that yielded the Well-Being in the Nation measurement framework and vetted measure sets. Five principles guided the collaboration:

- Codesign;
- Continual alignment (with Healthy People, with the County Health Rankings, etc.);

- Continual testing in the field with those who would use it;
- Flexibility and balance in measure selection, adaptation, and use; and
- A focus on creating a living library of measures (Saha et al., 2020, pp. 644–45).

The resulting measure sets (of overall well-being, of the well-being of people, and the well-being of places) are intended to "help communities access data that are already being connected," "connect what matters to create equitable well-being" and "drive their own change" (WIN Network, n.d.). They include nine core measures in three sets: well-being of people (e.g., Cantril's Ladder; life expectancy at birth); well-being of places (e.g., child poverty; healthy community indexes aligned with the framework); and equity (e.g., differences in well-being; years of life lost; income inequality; high school graduation rates; demographic variables to use in a standard way for equity analysis) (Saha et al., 2020).

The Federal Data Strategy is expected to create access to federal data assets that could help inform policy making in compliance with the provisions of the Evidence Based Policymaking Act of 2018 (Phillips et al., 2021). Its implementation includes the Population-Level Analysis and Community Estimates (PLACES) initiative, which provides "model-based estimates across 36 health measures, including seven disability measures added in 2023, for every county, city, and census tract in the U.S." (Wiltz et al., 2024). PLACES develops small-area estimates using BRFSS data, and data from the U.S. Census and American Community Survey.[8]

This is a good starting point, although more could be done to support the work of communities. Phillips and colleagues (2021) noted that PLACES "has limitations as a health planning tool as the imputed data can be at odds with locally collected data and cannot support tracking of intervention-related changes" (Phillips et al., 2021, p. 1871). They added that the importance of PLACES "for local health assessment and intervention efforts may be the platform and its functionality on which needed community data elements could be loaded" (Phillips et al., 2021, p. 1871). The result of the National Committee on Vital and Health Statistics collaboration with 100MLives, Philips and colleagues note, offers "a vetted framework for matching community measures to federal (and other) data assets, defining an automated routine for analyzing relevant data sets, and offering the analytic outputs publicly and equitably" (Phillips et al., 2021, p. 1871). Although PLACES may have some limitations, it can serve as an important tool for communities and could be strengthened or expanded to increase its usefulness. Earlier community data efforts could inform its continued development.

---

[8] https://www.cdc.gov/places/methodology/index.html (accessed December 13, 2024).

RECOMMENDATION 4-1: The Centers for Disease Control and Prevention (CDC) should sustain, enhance, and regularly update Population Level Analysis and Community Estimates (PLACES) as a data tool that communities can access for locally relevant, granular (i.e., census tract and ZIP code) data and the ability to compare themselves to peers. CDC should enhance PLACES in collaboration with the Substance Abuse and Mental Health Services Administration to add measures relevant to mental, emotional, and behavioral health and population well-being, and support functionalities to PLACES that allow community partnerships to layer their own data on PLACES data for their planning and evaluation efforts.

Communities will require funding to support data infrastructure and staffing, and identifying data elements will need to involve community expertise at every step. For example, the surveys of middle and high school students in over a dozen states are a valuable source of local data on risk, protection, and BH outcomes. Investments in these activities would ensure surveys reflect state and community priorities and the latest prevention science.

RECOMMENDATION 4-2: The Substance Abuse and Mental Health Services Administration, Centers for Disease Control and Prevention, and other federal agencies that provide resources for community-based prevention of behavioral disorders should include specific support for data infrastructure in all relevant grant programs, including funding for acquiring relevant data, data integrity and privacy, new data collection, data sharing, collaboration with relevant public- and private-sector partners, and obtaining training and technical assistance as needed.

Measuring Well-Being

HHS has made well-being a central concept in its Healthy People 2030 initiative's vision and adopted Overall Health and Well-Being Measures (OHMs), which it describes as "broad, global outcome measures intended to assess the Healthy People 2030 vision. OHMs can be used to summarize and evaluate progress toward achieving Healthy People objectives" (HHS, n.d.). HP2030 includes eight OHMs organized in three tiers: well-being (a measure of life satisfaction in the current year), healthy life expectancy, and summary mortality and health.

One noteworthy addition to the measurement of well-being is the development of an Indigenous measure of overall health and well-being (or *wicozani*), the Wicozani Instrument, by a Dakota community (Peters et al., 2019). This nine-item validated self-report measure applies Indigenous epistemology. Peters and colleagues (2019) noted that "[w]hile there is diversity among Native communities, the Wicozani Instrument may appeal to many Native communities because health is defined from an Indigenous perspective, in that it is viewed through a holistic lens and relies upon the understanding of relationality and interdependence between physical, mental, and spiritual health" (Peters et al., 2019).

NASEM panels have also made the case for using self-reported summary measures of population well-being as important signals as to how people in the nation and at state and community levels are doing. Such measures, by their nature, draw on peoples' mental and emotional assessment of their lives in the context of their social, economic, and environmental circumstances. One such measure is Cantril's Ladder (NASEM, 2020). It is used internationally, including by the Organisation for Economic Cooperation and Development, and has been demonstrated to have predictive validity for health outcomes. Scores of 7 and above indicate "thriving," while more than 4 and below 7 is considered "struggling"—with twice the number of sick days as those with higher well-being—and a score of 4 or below is considered "suffering" (WIN Network, n.d.). The most recent data on the United States averaged 6.7, with young people's scores bringing the average down.[9]

The committee asserts that measures of well-being, combining individual and structural-level factors, are critical constructs related to MEB health. A measure of population well-being would also provide a more expansive way to track and demonstrate progress, complementing specific national measures, such as for deaths of overdose and suicide, and framing a positive high-level target for the prevention infrastructure.

Such measures can be used to periodically ascertain, track, and report on population well-being and integrated into Healthy People and related state and tribal population health reports. The committee believes that a summary measure of well-being is needed at all levels of government that can be disaggregated by subpopulation to examine and track population-level inequities and progress in overcoming them.

RECOMMENDATION 4-3: To identify and adopt measures of population well-being that allow the nation to track progress and report on mental, emotional, and behavioral health, the Office of the Assistant Secretary of Health, National Center for Health Statistics, and the Substance Abuse and Mental Health Services Administration should convene and collaborate with relevant partners.

---

[9] Use cursor to view United States in https://ourworldindata.org/grapher/happiness-cantril-ladder (accessed December 15, 2024).

The measure(s) would be disaggregated by socioeconomic factors, race and ethnicity, age, and geography.

Relevant partners may include the HHS Office of the National Coordinator of Health Information Technology and national public health organizations, such as the Association of State and Territorial Health Officials and the National Indian Health Board.

The HHS Strategic Plan, to which ONC, SAMHSA, CDC, and NIH are contributors, includes Objective 4.4: "Improve data collection, use, and evaluation, to increase evidence-based knowledge that leads to better health outcomes, reduced health disparities, and improved social well-being, equity, and economic resilience" (HHS, 2024). In 2024, the Office of Management and Budget finalized revisions to Statistical Policy Directive No. 15 (SDP 15), which updates standards for maintaining, collecting, and presenting federal data on race and ethnicity. A National Academies report on federal policy effects of race, ethnicity, and tribal health equity discussed an early version of SDP 15 that was posted to the Federal Register in January 2023 (NASEM, 2023b).

Elevating prevention leadership to the White House Domestic Policy Council and a more robust BH Coordinating Council in HHS (see Governance chapter Recommendation 6-1) could include an initiative to create linkages among multiple data sources across the federal government, perhaps building on the CDC PLACES initiative. Such an effort could bring together administrative data (EHR, other system data such as education, child welfare), survey data (e.g., BRFSS), surveillance (reporting), big data (e.g., social media), and other types of data (including social sensing index using social media inputs to measure MH status in a specific geographic location) (Park et al., 2024). As noted, some states are already working with integrated or linked sets of measures that draw data from different systems.

HELPING COMMUNITIES WORK WITH DATA

Implementing evidence-based interventions that are well suited to a community and setting requires that communities, community coalitions, and their partners undertake a process to (1) choose what outcomes are of interest, (2) design feasible data collection and reporting, and (3) implement a method for using data to inform feedback/progress. State public health or BH agencies can help. For example, Washington State conducts state-level surveys, supports communities conduct surveys, administers a surveillance system (Community Outcome and Risk Evaluation Information System), and provides other data resources (Mariani, 2024). New York State has a state epidemiological workgroup to oversee the collection of data aligned with the SAMHSA Strategic Prevention Framework (e.g., risk and protective factor data) and also meets regularly with other relevant agencies in the state. Like Washington State, New York State works to make data more available and accessible, including to and through its community coalitions and state resource centers (Cunningham, 2024). Pennsylvania collaborates with counties in the process of needs assessment, using data primarily from the Pennsylvania Youth Survey (for most of the state) and YRBSS (Philadelphia and Pittsburgh), in addition to local surveys. The state works with multiple sources of data that have various limitations and caveats (e.g., NSDUH data are old and regional, many sources do not provide sufficiently local data) and has begun a recent effort to gather county-level evaluation (outcomes) data from counties.[10]

Technical Assistance for Communities

Although the prevention infrastructure is fragmented, robust resources are available to provide training and technical assistance to coalitions and organizations endeavoring to use data and indicators to inform their planning, implementation, and evaluation. Technical assistance is characterized by a focus on improving capacity of organizations or systems, and on targeted and tailored supports by subject matter experts (Scott et al., 2022). Although technical assistance is insufficiently reported on—and there is a lack of standard definition, objective measures, and reporting standards—existing research indicates that TA is more likely to be effective if it is intensive and there is fidelity of TA practices (Scott et al., 2022; Dunst et al., 2019; Anderson et al., 2021). TA sources include especially a range of partners, such as the PTTC Network (focused on SUD prevention) and previously a network of Mental Health Technology Transfer Centers (the MHTTC network was closed September 29, 2024). In place of the MHTTCs, SAMHSA has launched a new National Center for Mental Health: Dissemination, Implementation, and Sustainment, which will establish five bi-regional centers. PTTCs are available to provide technical assistance to public health departments, BH agencies, community coalitions, and other partners on prevention of substance use. The CDC-funded National Centers of Excellence for Youth Violence Prevention play a similar role, and some of CDC's Prevention Research Centers have, over the years, focused on aspects of preventing BH disorders (CDC, 2024c).

Kingston and colleagues (2016) provide detailed discussion for how academic institutions partnering with communities can help them use data and evidence to assemble packages of programs that are appropriate for their specific youth violence prevention needs. For example, a University of Colorado Boulder team worked with the Montebello community in Denver

---

[10] G. Kindt, personal communication, June 25, 2024.

to support them in using the Communities That Care model to establish community governance, review data about community risk factors, and consider EBPs (using an existing clearinghouse of EBPs). The university team gathered baseline data through parent and youth surveys and worked with neighborhood partners to prioritize a small set of risk and protective factors.

Virginia Tech and Iowa State University collaborated to create a model for data-driven community engagement and community-based research, the Community Learning Through Data Driven Discovery (CLD3) (Keller et al., 2018). One pillar is the Cooperative Extension System funded through the U.S. Department of Agriculture. Cooperative extension professionals work with university researchers to "translate their science-based research results into language and decision tools appropriate for targeted audiences" (Keller, 2018). Another pillar is the network of four Regional Rural Development Centers that "serve as sources of economic and community development data, decision tools, education, and guidance in rural communities" (Keller, 2018).

The University of Pennsylvania Community Engagement and Research Core could be helpful to communities in building their own approach to identifying and using data to inform action (CEAR, n.d.). Participating institutions can collaborate with community leaders "to understand community needs and improve community health" (NCATS, 2023).

CDC Prevention Research Centers (PRCs) can support communities in gathering data to inform their efforts. For example, the Fayette County Integrated Community Engagement Collaborative has collaborated with the local school district and West Virginia University's PRC to collect data to inform "what can be done to reduce risk and protect children and adolescents" (ICE Collaborative, 2020, p. 4). With the help of their academic partner, the collaborative collected data through a 2023 high school and middle school surveys that drew on several sources, including the YRBSS, National Institutes of Health Monitoring the Future survey of youth substance use, and European School Survey Project on Alcohol and Drugs (ICE Collaborative, 2023a-b).

Using Community Evaluation and Outcomes Data to Inform Planning

The work of implementing EBPs to promote MEB health and well-being is cyclical (see Figure 4-2), with data such as needs assessments informing initial decisions about the outcomes of interest and selection of interventions and evaluation data indicating progress and informing next steps. It is important for community knowledge generated during implementation to be shared with others systematically, similar to the post-marketing surveillance (also known as Phase IV clinical trials) conducted once a drug begins to be widely prescribed and used. Communities collect data for their own local partnerships' continuous improvement and monitoring, but there are

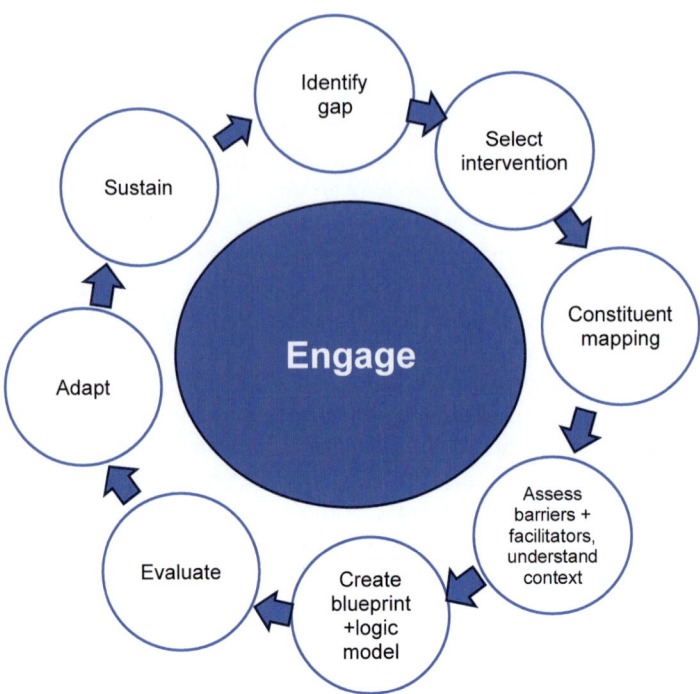

FIGURE 4-2 Eight steps toward implementation to promote MEB health equity.
NOTE: MEB = mental, emotional, and behavioral.
SOURCE: Inspired by Graham et al., 2006.

broader implications. The learnings and findings that result from implementation of EBPs outside of research settings need to be shared widely and make their way into the practice-based knowledge that informs other communities and could be used to spread and scale programs.

Data Systems Require Funding

The cost for a community data system will vary depending on community size, available in-kind resources (such as free data infrastructure support), and the data needs. Local data intermediaries are one type of model for the core of a community's data system. Local data intermediaries serve as "mediator between data and local stakeholders—nonprofit organizations, governments, foundations, and residents . . . are data translators, educators, conveners, collaborators, and voices for change. They use data to describe their communities, and they empower communities to use data in their activities, from community building to advocacy and program planning, to policymaking" (Hendey et al. 2016). Data intermediaries can be used to derive rough estimates for the cost of operating a data system in a community. The cost of launching a data intermediary will require at least one full time employee at $100,000–150,000 (Hendey et al, 2016).

Another model is the community data infrastructure, as found in the work of the National Neighborhood Indicators Project. An analysis of the membership of 35 partners shows that the range of budgets for partners in NNIP ranges from $200,000 to $604,000, with a median budget of $325,000 (Kingsley et al., 2015). That provides a rough figure for the cost of community data infrastructure. Multiplying $325,000 by 3,142 counties (U.S. Census figure), it would cost nearly $1 billion dollars for every county to have a community data infrastructure.

REFERENCES

ACF (Administration for Children & Families). n.d. *Family first prevention services act (FFPSA)*. https://capacity.childwelfare.gov/about/cb-priorities/family-first-prevention (accessed December 16, 2024).

ACHA (American College Health Association). 2021. *Measuring well-being in a college campus setting*. https://www.acha.org/resource/measuring-well-being-in-a-college-campus-setting/ (accessed January 2, 2025).

Aebi, N. J., D. De Ridder, C. Ochoa, D. Petrovic, M. Fadda, S. Elayan, M. Sykora, M. Puhan, J. A. Naslund, S. J. Mooney, and O. Gruebner. 2021. Can big data be used to monitor the mental health consequences of Covid-19? *International Journal of Public Health* 66:633451. https://doi.org/10.3389/ijph.2021.633451.

Anderson, M. A., K. Conroy, A. Mastri, A. Benton, and G. Lehman. *Improving the design, targeting, and effectiveness of training and technical assistance: A learning agenda*. Mathematica Policy Research. https://aspe.hhs.gov/sites/default/files/migrated_legacy_files//198136/Training-TA-Learning-Agenda.pdf (accessed December 14, 2024).

CADCA (Community Anti Drug Coalitions of America). n.d. *Describing your community, collecting data, analyzing the issues and establishing a road map for change*. https://www.cadca.org/wp-content/uploads/2019/02/community_assessmentcompressed.pdf (accessed September 2, 2024).

CDC (Centers for Disease Control and Prevention). 2024a. *About the public health approach to violence prevention*. https://www.cdc.gov/violence-prevention/about/about-the-public-health-approach-to-violence-prevention.html (accessed November 8, 2024).

CDC. 2024b. *Implementing public health interoperability*. https://www.cdc.gov/data-interoperability/php/public-health-strategy/index.html (accessed October 15, 2024).

CDC. 2024c. *National centers of excellence in youth violence prevention*. https://www.cdc.gov/youth-violence/php/yvpcs/index.html (accessed September 29, 2024).

CDC. 2024d. *National violent death reporting system*. https://www.cdc.gov/nvdrs/about/index.html (accessed October 15, 2024).

CDC. 2024e. *Data: the building blocks of health*. https://www.cdcfoundation.org/HealthEquity/data-equity-principles (accessed December 16, 2024).

CDC. 2024f. *Methodology*. https://www.cdc.gov/places/methodology/index.html (accessed December 13, 2024).

CEAR (University of Pennsylvania Community Engagement and Research Core). n.d. *FAQ*. https://cear-itmat-upenn.org/about-2/faqs/ (accessed December 17, 2024).

Center for Data Insights and Innovation. n.d. *State health information guidance (SHIG)*. https://www.cdii.ca.gov/compliance-and-policy/state-health-information-guidance-shig/ (accessed October 15, 2024).
Chang, D. 2022. States opting out of a federal program that tracks teen behavior as youth mental health worsens. *KFF Health News*. https://kffhealthnews.org/news/article/states-opt-out-federal-teen-mental-health-survey/ (accessed December 31, 2024).
ICE Collaborative (Integrated Community Engagement). 2020. *County report: Fayette County middle schools*.
ICE Collaborative. 2023a. *Deidentified county report: Fayette and Wyoming high schools*.
ICE Collaborative. 2023b. *Deidentified county report: Fayette and Wyoming middle schools*.
Community Learning through Data-Driven Discovery. n.d. *Community learning through data-driven discovery*. https://cld3.org/ (accessed November 8, 2024).
CSTE (Council of State and Territorial Epidemiologists). 2019. *Recommended CSTE surveillance indicators for substance abuse and mental health, version 3*.
Cunningham, C. 2024. State-level infrastructure to support prevention, presented to the Committee on Blueprint for a National Prevention Infrastructure for Behavioral Health Disorders, Meeting 3. https://www.nationalacademies.org/event/42281_04-2024_blueprint-for-a-national-prevention-infrastructure-for-behavioral-health-disorders-meeting-3.
DataHaven. n.d. *Datahaven: Home*. https://www.ctdatahaven.org/ (accessed September 30, 2024).
DataHaven and Siena College Research Institute. 2024. *Datahaven community wellbeing survey*. https://www.ctdatahaven.org/reports/datahaven-community-wellbeing-survey (accessed September 30, 2024).
Davlia, K. 2021. Fatal overdoses in the New Haven area increased by 40 percent in 2020: New report explores root causes and recommends prevention strategies: DataHaven. https://www.ctdatahaven.org/blog/fatal-overdoses-new-haven-area-increased-40-percent-2020-new-report-explores-root-causes-and (accessed December 31, 2024).
Delaware State Epidemiological Outcomes Workgroup. n.d. *The Delaware 2023 epidemiological profile: Substance use, mental health, and related issues*. https://bpb-us-w2.wpmucdn.com/sites.udel.edu/dist/9/12983/files/2023/11/COMPANION-GUIDE_The-Delaware-2023-Epidemiological-Profile.pdf (accessed April 30, 2025).
Dollard, N. 2023. *It's time to reinstate the Youth Risk Behavior Survey*. FPI (Florida Policy Institute) https://www.floridapolicy.org/posts/its-time-to-reinstate-the-youth-risk-behavior-survey (accessed December 17, 2024).
Douglas, M. D., E. Respress, A. H. Gaglioti, C. Li, M. A. Blount, J. Hopkins, P. T. Baltrus, R. J. Willock, L. S. Caplan, D. E. Dawes, and D. Mack. 2021. Variation in reporting of the race and ethnicity of Covid-19 cases and deaths across US states: April 12, 2020, and November 9, 2020. *American Journal of Public Health* 111(6):1141–1148. https://doi.org/10.2105/ajph.2021.306167.
Drug-Free Communities Support Program and Executive Office of the President of the United States. 2023. *Drug-free communities support program end-of-year 2022 report national cross-site evaluation*. https://www.cdc.gov/overdose-prevention/media/pdfs/DFC-NATIONAL-EVALUATION-EOY-REPORT_2022_Report_2023_AUG_28_FINAL_ONDCP-APPROVED.pdf (accessed December 31, 2024).
Dunst, C. J., K. Annas, H. Wilkie, and D. W. Hamby. 2019. Scoping review of the core elements of technical assistance models and frameworks. *World Journal of Education* 9(2):109–122. https://doi.org/10.5430/wje.v9n2p109.
Emmons, K. M., S. Mendez, R. M. Lee, D. Erani, L. Mascioli, M. Abreu, S. Adams, J. Daly, B. E. Bierer, and R. A.-M. Partners. 2023. Data sharing in the context of community-engaged research partnerships. *Social Science & Medicine* 325:115895. https://doi.org/10.1016/j.socscimed.2023.115895.
Fernandez, J. M., and J. Jayawardhana. 2024. Are suicides underreported? The impact of coroners versus medical examiners on suicide reporting. *Health Services Research*. https://doi.org/10.1111/1475-6773.14381.

FRIENDS National Resource Center for CBCAP (Community-Based Child Abuse Prevention). 2009. *Using qualitative data in program evaluation: Telling the story of a prevention program.* https://friendsnrc.org/wp-content/uploads/Using-Qualitative-Data-in-Program-Evaluation_-Telling-the-Story-of-a-Prevention-Program.pdf (accessed January 14, 2025).

Graham, I. D., J. Logan, M. B. Harrison, S. E. Straus, J. Tetroe, W. Caswell, and N. Robinson. 2006. Lost in knowledge translation: Time for a map? *Journal of Continuing Education in the Health Professions* 26(1):13–24. https://doi.org/10.1002/chp.47.

Green, B., Q. Cao, R. McCloskey, and F. Kim. 2024. Recovery support and capacity assessment using the calculating an adequate system tool: Two case studies. *Substance Use & Addiction Journal* 45(1):136–143. https://doi.org/10.2105/AJPH.2024.307582.

Greenfield, B., L. Chadwick, E. Madden, and M. Abbott. 2023. *Project update: Child welfare and health infrastructure for linking and data analysis of resources, effectiveness, and needs (CHILDREN) initiative.* https://aspe.hhs.gov/sites/default/files/documents/3f2c25d488d4f2f80a00cfca25e4ff02/CHILDREN-Updated-Description-11-27-2023.pdf (accessed December 31, 2024).

He, Z., E. Pfaff, S. J. Guo, Y. Guo, Y. Wu, C. Tao, G. Stiglic, and J. Bian. 2023. Enriching real-world data with social determinants of health for health outcomes and health equity: Successes, challenges, and opportunities. *Yearbook of Medical Informatics* 32(1):253–263. https://doi.org/10.1055/s-0043-1768732.

Hendey, L., J. Cowan, G. T. Kingsley, and K. L. Pettit. 2016. *NNIP's guide to starting a local data intermediary.* https://www.urban.org/sites/default/files/publication/80901/2000798-NNIP%27s-Guide-to-Starting-a-Local-Data-Intermediary.pdf (accessed December 17, 2024).

Hendren, N., and B. Sprung-Keyser. 2020. A unified welfare analysis of government policies. *The Quarterly Journal of Economics* 135(3):1209–1318. https://doi.org/10.1093/qje/qjaa006.

HHS (Department of Health and Human Services). n.d. *Overall health and well-being measures.* https://odphp.health.gov/healthypeople/objectives-and-data/overall-health-and-well-being-measures#:~:text=to%20search%20results-,Overall%20Health%20and%20Well%2DBeing%20Measures,toward%20achieving%20Healthy%20People%20objectives. (accessed November 8, 2024).

HHS. 2024. *Objective 4.4: Improve data collection, use, and evaluation, to increase evidence-based knowledge that leads to better health outcomes, reduced health disparities, and improved social well-being, equity, and economic resilience* https://www.hhs.gov/about/strategic-plan/2022-2026/goal-4/objective-4-4/index.html (accessed December 16, 2024).

HHS and ED (Department of Education). 2019. *Joint guidance on the application of the Family Educational Rights and Privacy Act (FERPA) and the Health Insurance Portability and Accountability Act of 1996 (HIPAA) to student health records.* https://studentprivacy.ed.gov/sites/default/files/resource_document/file/2019%20HIPAA%20FERPA%20Joint%20Guidance%20508.pdf (accessed December 31, 2024).

Hossain, E., R. Rana, N. Higgins, J. Soar, P. D. Barua, A. R. Pisani, and K. Turner. 2023. Natural language processing in electronic health records in relation to healthcare decision making: A systematic review. *Computers in Biology and Medicine* 155:106649. https://doi.org/10.1016/j.compbiomed.2023.106649.

I2D2 (Iowa's Integrated Data System for Decision-Making). 2021. *Family support, home visiting, and community risk.* https://i2d2.iastate.edu/blog/portfolio_page/familys-support-home-visiting-and-community-risk/ (accessed December 31, 2024).

James, C. V. 2023. *We can't fix what we don't measure: Why the Youth Risk Behavior Survey is critical* https://www.gih.org/from-the-president/we-cant-fix-what-we-dont-measure-why-the-youth-risk-behavior-survey-is-critical/ (accessed December 16, 2024).

Johnson, K. Personal communication, September 13, 2024.

Jutte, D. P., L. L. Roos, and M. D. Brownell. 2011. Administrative record linkage as a tool for public health research. *Annual Review of Public Health* 32(1):91–108. https://doi.org/10.1146/annurev-publhealth-031210-100700.

Keller, S., S. Nusser, S. Shipp, and C. E. Wotek. 2018. Helping communities use data to make better decisions. *Issues in Science and Technology* 34(3). https://issues.org/helping-communities-use-data-to-make-better-decisions/ (accessed December 31, 2024).

Kingsley, G. T., S. M. Kandris, and M. Woluchem. 2015. *A picture of NNIP partner finances*. National Neighborhood Indicators Partnership and Urban Institute. https://www.neighborhoodindicators.org/sites/default/files/publications/2000505-A-Picture-of-NNIP-Partner-Finances.pdf (accessed December 17, 2024).

Kingston, B. E., S. F. Mihalic, and E. J. Sigel. 2016. Building an evidence-based multitiered system of supports for high-risk youth and communities. *American Journal of Orthopsychiatry* 86(2):132. https://doi.org/10.1037/ort0000110.

Knipe, D., D. Gunnell, H. Evans, A. John, and D. Fancourt. 2021. Is Google Trends a useful tool for tracking mental and social distress during a public health emergency? A time-series analysis. *Journal of Affective Disordorders* 294:737–744. https://doi.org/10.1016/j.jad.2021.06.086.

Krieger, N. 2021. Structural racism, health inequities, and the two-edged sword of data: Structural problems require structural solutions. *Frontiers in Public Health* 9:655447. https://doi.org/10.3389/fpubh.2021.655447.

Making Action Possible. n.d. *Health & social well-being*. https://mapazdashboard.arizona.edu/health-social-well-being/behavioral-health (accessed October 1, 2024).

Mariani, S. 2024. State-level infrastructure to support prevention, presented to the Committee on Blueprint for a National Prevention Infrastructure for Behavioral Health Disorders, Meeting 3. https://www.nationalacademies.org/event/42281_04-2024_blueprint-for-a-national-prevention-infrastructure-for-behavioral-health-disorders-meeting-3.

Mathematica. n.d.-a. *A new collaboration to modernize public health data*. https://www.mathematica.org/news/a-new-collaboration-to-modernize-public-health- (accessed November 8, 2024).

Mathematica. n.d.-b. *Projects: Children initiative*. https://www.mathematica.org/projects/child-welfare-and-health-infrastructure-for-linking-and-data-analysis-of-resources (accessed December 30, 2024).

Mathematica. n.d.-c. *Projects: Public health data modernization implementation center program*. https://www.mathematica.org/projects/public-health-data-modernization-implementation-center (accessed December 16, 2024).

MN HER (Minnesota Electronic Health Record Consortium). n.d. Health trends across communities in Minnesota. https://mnehrconsortium.org/health-trends-across-communities-minnesota-dashboard (accessed December 31, 2024).

MN HER. 2024. About the MN EHR Consortium. https://mnehrconsortium.org/about-mn-ehr-consortium (accessed December 17, 2024).

MTF (Monitoring the Future). 2024. *About MTF*. https://monitoringthefuture.org/about/ (accessed December 13, 2024).

My Voice. n.d. *Mental health presentations and publications*. https://hearmyvoicenow.org/research/mental-health/ (accessed September 30, 2024).

Najib, S. 2024. Elmo shares mental health help after 'how is everybody doing' question goes viral. *ABC News*. https://abcnews.go.com/GMA/Wellness/amid-mental-health-crisis-kids-elmo-steps/story?id=109948499 (accessed December 31, 2024).

NASEM (National Academies of Sciences, Engineering, and Medicine). 2019a. *Fostering healthy mental, emotional, and behavioral development in children and youth: A national agenda*. Washington, DC: The National Academies Press. https://doi.org/10.17226/25201.

NASEM. 2019b. *Consensus study report highlights: Integrating social care into the delivery of health care: Moving upstream to improve the nation's health*. Washington, DC: The National Academies Press. https://nap.nationalacademies.org/resource/25467/09252019Social_Care_highlights.pdf (accessed December 17, 2024).

NASEM. 2020. *Leading Health Indicators 2030: Advancing Health, Equity, and Well-Being.* Washington, DC: The National Academies Press. https://doi.org/10.17226/25682.
NASEM. 2023a. *Toward a 21st century national data infrastructure: Mobilizing information for the common good.* Washington, DC: The National Academies Press. https://doi.org/10.17226/26688.
NASEM. 2023b. *Federal policy to advance racial, ethnic, and tribal health equity.* Washington, DC: National Academies Press. https://doi.org/10.17226/26834.
Natafgi, N., O. Ladeji, Y. D. Hong, J. Caldwell, and C. D. Mullins. 2021. Are communities willing to transition into learning health care communities? A community-based participatory evaluation of stakeholders' receptivity. *Qualitative Health Research* 31(8):1412–1422. https://doi.org/10.1177/1049732321998643.
NCATS (National Center for Advancing Translational Sciences). 2023. *Turning science into health: Clinical and Translational Science Awards (CTSA) Program.* https://ncats.nih.gov/sites/default/files/2023-10/NCATS-CTSA-Fact-Sheet-2023-508.pdf (accessed December 31, 2024).
NCES (National Center for Education Statistics). n.d. *School Survey on Crime and Safety (SSOCS).* https://nces.ed.gov/surveys/ssocs/ (accessed September 30, 2024).
NCES. 2023a. *List of 2023 digest tables.* https://nces.ed.gov/programs/digest/2023menu_tables.asp (accessed August 30, 2024).
NCES. 2023b. *Table 233.69a. Number and percentage of public schools providing diagnostic mental health assessments and treatment to students and, among schools providing these services, percentage providing them at school and outside of school, by selected school characteristics: School years 2017–18, 2019–20, and 2021–22* https://nces.ed.gov/programs/digest/d23/tables/dt23_233.69a.asp (accessed January 2, 2025).
NCES. 2023c. *Table 232.70.Percentage of students in grades 9–12 who reported that illegal drugs were made available to them on school property during the previous 12 months, by selected student characteristics: Selected years, 1993 through 2021* https://nces.ed.gov/programs/digest/d23/tables/dt23_232.70.asp (accessed January 2, 2025).
NHTSA (National Highway Traffic Safety Administration). n.d. *Fatality Analysis Reporting System (FARS).* https://www.nhtsa.gov/research-data/fatality-analysis-reporting-system-fars (accessed August 30, 2024).
NIDA (National Institute on Drug Abuse). n.d. *Research, data, measures, & resources.* https://nida.nih.gov/research/research-data-measures-resources (accessed December 15, 2024).
NIH (National Institutes of Health). 2024. All of us participants are fueling mental health research. https://allofus.nih.gov/news-events/announcements/all-us-participants-are-fueling-mental-health-research (accessed December 13, 2024).
NNIP (National Neighborhood Indicators Partnership). 2024. *NNIP partners' guide to the network.* https://www.neighborhoodindicators.org/library/guides/nnip-partners-guide-network (accessed September 30, 2024).
OCID (Oregon Child Integrated Dataset). 2020. *Oregon's data-driven resource on the well-being of the state's* children https://www.ocid-cebp.org/ (accessed December 16, 2024).
OMB (Office of Management and Budget). 2021. *Study to identify methods to assess equity: Report to the President.* https://www.whitehouse.gov/wp-content/uploads/2021/08/OMB-Report-on-EO13985-Implementation_508-Compliant-Secure-v1.1.pdf (accessed December 13, 2024).
OMB SPD 15 (Statistical Policy Directive No. 15 on Race and Ethnicity Data Standards). 2024. *U.S. Office of Management and Budget's Statistical Policy Directive No. 15: Standards for maintaining, collecting, and presenting federal data on race and ethnicity.* https://spd15revision.gov/ (accessed December 14, 2024).
ONC (Office of the National Coordinator for Health Information Technology) 2023. *Social determinants of health information exchange toolkit.* https://www.healthit.gov/sites/default/files/2023-02/Social%20Determinants%20of%20Health%20Information%20Exchange%20Toolkit%202023_508.pdf (accessed December 31, 2024).

Oregon Health Authority. 2021. *Engaging communities in the modernization of a public health survey system.* https://www.oregon.gov/oha/PH/ABOUT/TASKFORCE/Documents/Engaging-Communities-in-Public-Health-Survey-Modernization.pdf (accessed December 31, 2024).

Owen, R. 2014. *Improving care, ensuring patient privacy: Hennepin health data-sharing case study.* Center for Health Care Strategies. https://www.chcs.org/improving-care-ensuring-patient-privacy-hennepin-health-data-sharing-case-study/ (accessed December 31, 2024).

Park, J., M.-H. Tsou, A. Nara, S. Cassels, and S. Dodge. 2024. Developing a social sensing index for monitoring place-oriented mental health issues using social media (Twitter) data. *Urban Informatics* 3(1). https://doi.org/10.1007/s44212-023-00033-5.

PCORI (Patient-Centered Outcomes Research Institute). n.d. *Awardee resources: Policies & guidelines.* https://www.pcori.org/funding-opportunities/applicant-and-awardee-resources/awardee-resources/policies-guidelines (accessed August 30, 2024).

Pennsylvania Department of Drug and Alcohol Programs n.d. *AISP Network: Iowa's integrated data system for decision making (I2D2).* https://aisp.upenn.edu/network-site/iowa/ (accessed October 15, 2024).

Peters, H. J., T. R. Peterson, and C. Dakota Wicohan. 2019. Developing an Indigenous measure of overall health and well-being: The Wicozani Instrument. *American Indian and Alaska Native Mental Health Research Journal* 26(2):96–122. https://doi.org/10.5820/aian.2602.2019.96.

Phillips, R. L., N. F. Kanarek, and V. L. Boothe. 2021. Rebuilding a US federal data strategy after the end of the "community health status indicators." *American Journal of Public Health* 111(10):1865–1873. https://doi.org/10.2105/ajph.2021.306437.

Piff, J. 2021. Data in collective impact: Focusing on what matters. *Stanford Social Innovation Review.* https://ssir.org/articles/entry/data_in_collective_impact_focusing_on_what_matters (accessed December 31, 2024).

Powell, N., H. Dalton, J. Lawrence-Bourne, and D. Perkins. 2024. Co-creating community wellbeing initiatives: What is the evidence and how do they work? *International Journal of Mental Health Systems* 18(1):28. https://doi.org/10.1186/s13033-024-00645-7.

Prevention Technology Transfer Center (PTTC) Network. 2024. *PTTC: Ditching the discomfort with data.* https://www.preventionnetwork.org/resources/pttc-ditching-the-discomfort-with-data/ (accessed December 14, 2024).

PTTC Network. 2021. *Checklist for Identifying Data Gaps.* https://pttcnetwork.org/products_and_resources/checklist-for-identifying-data-gaps/ (accessed October 12, 2024).

Purtle, J., K. L. Nelson, N. Z. Counts, and M. Yudell. 2020. Population-based approaches to mental health: History, strategies, and evidence. *Annual Review of Public Health* 41(1):201–221. https://doi.org/10.1146/annurev-publhealth040119-094247.

Raths, D. 2021. Minnesota's EHR consortium helps inform statewide vaccine equity efforts. *Healthcare Innovation.* https://www.hcinnovationgroup.com/analytics-ai/big-data/article/21218974/minnesotas-ehr-consortium-helps-inform-statewide-vaccine-equity-efforts (accessed December 30, 2024).

Roth, K. B., E. Gaveras, F. Ghiathi, E. K. Shaw, M. S. Shoemaker, N. A. Howard, M. Dhir, G. R. Caiza, and H. S. Szlyk. 2023. A community-engaged approach to understanding suicide in a small rural county in Georgia: A two-phase content analysis of individual and focus group interviews. *International Journal of Environmental Research and Public Health* 20(24):7145. https://doi.org/10.3390/ijerph20247145.

Rutgers. n.d. *Integrated population health data project.* https://iphd.rutgers.edu/ (accessed September 28, 2024).

RWJF (Robert Wood Johnson Foundation). 2021. *Charting a course for an equity-centered data system: Federal policy recommendations.* National Commission to Transform Public Health Data Systems. https://www.rwjf.org/en/insights/our-research/2021/10/charting-a-course-for-an-equity-centered-data-system.html (accessed September 1, 2021).

Saha, S., B. B. Cohen, J. Nagy, P. M. Mcpherson, and R. Phillips. 2020. Well-being in the nation: A living library of measures to drive multi-sector population health improvement and address social determinants. *Milbank Quarterly* 98(3):641–663. https://doi.org/10.1111/1468-0009.12477.

SAMHSA (Substance Abuse and Mental Health Services Administration). 2020. *Behavioral health barometer: United States, volume 6.* Rockville, MD.

SAMHSA. 2024. Substance Abuse and Mental Health Services Administration: Examining the Use of Braided Funding for Substance Use Disorder Services. Publication No. PEP23-06-07-002 Rockville, MD: Center for Substance Abuse Treatment. Substance Abuse and Mental Health Services Administration. https://store.samhsa.gov/sites/default/files/cfri-braided-funding-report-pep23-06-07-002.pdf (accessed April 30, 2025).

Scott, V. C., Z. Jillani, A. Malpert, J. Kolodny-Goetz, and A. Wandersman. 2022. A scoping review of the evaluation and effectiveness of technical assistance. *Implementation Science Communications* 3(1):70. https://doi.org/10.1186/s43058-022-00314-1.

Sesame Workshop, 2024. *Sesame workshop and the Harris Poll unveil inaugural index on the state of America's well-being.* https://sesameworkshop.org/about-us/press-room/sesame-workshop-and-the-harris-poll-unveil-inaugural-index-on-the-state-of-americas-well-being/ (accessed December 14, 2024).

Spiegel, J. n.d. *Applying an equitable lens to evidence-based research.* https://policylab.rutgers.edu/data-equity/ (accessed March 11, 2025).

Swedo, E. A., M. V. Aslam, L. L. Dahlberg, P. H. Niolon, A. S. Guinn, T. R. Simon, and J. A. Mercy. 2023. Prevalence of adverse childhood experiences among U.S. adults—behavioral risk factor surveillance system, 2011–2020. *MMWR Morbidity and Mortality Weekly Report* 72(26):707–715. https://doi.org/10.15585/mmwr.mm7226a2.

Tamarack Institute. 2017. *Tool: Five conditions of collective impact.* https://www.tamarackcommunity.ca/hubfs/Collective%20Impact/Tools/Five%20Conditions%20Tools%20April%202017.pdf (accessed December 16, 2024).

University of Delaware. 2024. *Epidemiological reports and products.* https://cdhs.udel.edu/seow/epidemiological-reports-and-products/ (accessed December 16, 2024).

Urban Indian Health Institute. 2021. *Data genocide of American Indians and Alaska Natives in Covid-19 data.*

Vaidyanathan, U., Y. Sun, T. Shekel, K. Chou, S. Galea, E. Gabrilovich, and G. A. Wellenius. 2022. An evaluation of internet searches as a marker of trends in population mental health in the US. *Scientific Reports* 12(1):8946. https://doi.org/10.1038/s41598-022-12952-5.

Vought, R. T. 2020. *Memorandum for heads of executive departments and agencies, March 10, 2020: Phase 4 implementation of the Foundations for Evidence-Based Policymaking Act of 2018: Program evaluation standards and practices.* https://www.whitehouse.gov/wp-content/uploads/2020/03/M-20-12.pdf (accessed December 31, 2024).

Wang, A., R. McCarron, D. Azzam, A. Stehli, G. Xiong, and J. DeMartini. 2022. Utilizing big data from Google trends to map population depression in the United States: Exploratory infodemiology study. *JMIR Mental Health* 9(3):e35253. https://doi.org/10.2196/35253.

Washington State Department of Health. n.d. *Healthy youth survey.* https://doh.wa.gov/data-and-statistical-reports/data-systems/healthy-youth-survey (accessed December 16, 2024).

WHO (World Health Organization). 2022. *Big data analytics and artificial intelligence in mental health.* https://www.who.int/europe/news-room/events/item/2022/12/07/default-calendar/big-data-analytics-and-artificial-intelligence-in-mental-health (accessed September 29, 2024).

Wiltz, J. L., B. Lee, R. Kaufmann, T. J. Carney, K. Davis, and P. A. Briss. 2024. Modernizing CDC's practices and culture for better data sharing, impact, and transparency. *Preventing Chronic Disease* 21:230200. https://doi.org/10.5888/pcd21.230200.

WIN Network. n.d. *Well-being in the nation (WIN) measures.* https://www.winmeasures.org/ (accessed July 14, 2024).

Winkelman, T. 2024. Personal communication, August 14, 2024.

5

Governance and Partnerships

Governance[1] is a component of the prevention infrastructure at all levels—from the array of federal agencies that fund research and practice, to state agencies that channel federal funding to communities and provide workforce support, certification, and other resources, to local government, community-based organizations, community members, and a wide array of academic, association, and other partners. The infrastructure supports the delivery of evidence-based programs (EBPs) and policies to reduce risk factors and strengthen protective factors (both upstream and downstream) along the life course. This infrastructure needs to bring together various sectors at different levels of government (federal, state, tribal, and local) and other partners, connect these components, and be guided by a vision of health equity—"the state in which everyone has a fair opportunity to attain their full potential for health and well-being, and no one is disadvantaged from doing so because of social position or other socially defined circumstances" (NASEM, 2023). As in programs and in policies, implementation science (IS) approaches are key to making governance effective.

The national mental, emotional, and behavioral (MEB) disorder prevention infrastructure is embedded in existing systems, including the public health, health care, and human services infrastructures (the latter includes

---

[1] Governance, as defined by the United Nations, is "participatory, consensus oriented, accountable, transparent, responsive, effective and efficient, equitable and inclusive, and following the rule of law" (WHO, 2021).

child welfare and aging services). Partnerships with other sectors also are crucial, including with education and criminal-legal settings. The guiding principles of implementation science and health equity (in the context of governance, the latter refers to tailoring to local and cultural contexts and prioritizing community-driven partnerships) are necessary to inform each component, i.e., reach each "gear" by "flowing" throughout the infrastructure as illustrated in Figure 1-1. Attention to these principles will drive each gear forward and ensure that this infrastructure will meet the needs—and integrate the experience and voice—of all communities, including those that have been historically excluded or marginalized.

This chapter provides an overview of federal, state, territorial, tribal, and local governance mechanisms (government leadership focus) and governance supports, including those from the private sector to the work of delivering interventions that prevent MEB disorders and promote MEB health. Governance in public health has been described through six functions (Carlson et al., 2015), which apply broadly to governance in the prevention domain examined in this report:

1. Policy development (e.g., Substance Abuse and Mental Health Services Administration (SAMHSA) or state agency regulations),
2. Resource stewardship (e.g., block grants and other grant programs),
3. Continuous improvement (through well-supported evaluation, e.g., via government–academic and community–academic partnerships),
4. Partner engagement (e.g., through the National Prevention Network, relationships with national associations of state directors),
5. Legal authority (derived from Title V of the Public Health Act), and
6. Agency oversight.

Funding and sustainability—of both financing and effective programming—are crucial outputs of an effective governance structure. The committee asserts that to explore and make recommendations about strengthening funding and sustaining resources and efforts, it is necessary to articulate a vision of the attributes of governance that are needed: more connected, more cohesive, better coordinated, and integrated where appropriate.

Governance of the prevention infrastructure for MEB disorders is primarily shared by U.S. federal and state government agencies, although a wide range of public-sector entities at the federal, state and territorial, tribal, and local levels perform functions that include funding, providing oversight, regulating, setting standards and holding accountable, and collaborating with varied private-sector entities. Any discussion of governance also requires attention to a list of partners, exploration of centralized authority/leadership, and the meaning of leadership in this complex context and considering federalism and how it operates with regard to the MEB infrastructure. Federalism refers to "the division and sharing of power between the national and state governments."[2] In the context of prevention, the federal role is one of funding, supporting, advising, and interacting with states as partners with primary responsibility for their populations. The federal government also interacts with states' sometimes-divergent approaches, which can create both challenges (e.g., too much flexibility that leads to gaps in coverage) and opportunities (e.g., testing innovations) (Willison et al., 2021).

This chapter also discusses the issue of parity in the context of health care and how leadership action is needed to fulfill the promise of the Mental Health Parity and Addiction Equity Act of 2008 (MHPAEA), which "generally prevents group health plans and health insurance issuers that provide mental health or substance use disorder (MH/SUD) benefits from imposing less favorable benefit limitations on those benefits than on medical/surgical benefits" (CMS, 2024a). However, the Act only required that health plans and insurers avoid less favorable or more limited MH/SUD benefits; it did not require that they provide coverage for MH and SUD. That requirement was added by the Affordable Care Act of 2010 (ACA), included as part of a package of 10 essential benefits, leaving it up to the states to interpret this. While the U.S. health care delivery sector acknowledges the importance of BH parity, the reality does not align with the aspiration. In September 2024, the Departments of Health and Human Services (HHS), Labor (DOL), and Treasury released final rules on implementing MHPAEA to further improve parity, although outcomes of these changes remain to be seen (CMS, 2024a).

This resembles the value ascribed to prevention but the lack of follow-through with commensurate investment. On a more positive note, in the context of prevention, the spirit of parity seems to inform the integration of screening for MEB disorders in the Early Periodic Screening, Diagnosis, and Treatment benefit provided to children under 21 enrolled in Medicaid, and in Screening, Brief Intervention, Referral, and Treatment services delivered in primary care settings, emergency departments, and other community settings (Medicaid.gov, n.d.; SAMHSA, 2024a).

Examining the prevention infrastructure highlights the many levels of authority and responsibility characterizing federal, state, and local governance and difficulties in bringing them into coordinated, long-term efforts. Not only must key actors be identified; their existing spheres of influence and powers must be reconciled toward a common purpose. Overlapping,

---

[2] https://constitution.congress.gov/browse/essay/intro.7-3/ALDE_00000032/ (accessed April 30, 2025).

sometimes competing, sources of authority and distinct organizational structures that should (but do not always) work in concert with local communities and actors can make large-scale preventive interventions difficult.

FEDERAL GOVERNANCE STRUCTURE

Federal departments, including HHS, Department of Veterans Affairs (VA), and the Department of Defense (DoD), support, oversee, and sometimes operate programs offering preventive interventions, or programs that might be adapted to integrate prevention components at the state and local levels. At federal, state, and local levels, the existing BH infrastructure is primarily in health care services (NASEM, 2024). Health care services examples can range from primary care settings where people may be screened for early signs of MEB disorders, such as anxiety, depression, or alcohol or substance use disorders, as well as clinicians providing cognitive behavioral therapy (which could serve as primary or secondary prevention). The infrastructure for preventing MEB disorders overlaps with the public health infrastructure and parts of the human services infrastructure (e.g., child welfare systems at the state and local levels, aging services). At the federal government level, governance of the prevention infrastructure is fragmented, with greater centralized attention and support for SUD compared to MH. The substance use domain has a central point of coordination in the White House Office of National Drug Control Policy (ONDCP), which works closely with other executive branch entities focused on substance use, while the MH domain has no central coordination.

HHS has several agencies with responsibilities relevant to MH and SUD. These include the Substance Abuse and Mental Health Services Administration (SAMHSA), the National Institutes of Health (NIH), Centers for Disease Control and Prevention (CDC), Health Resources and Services Administration (HRSA), and the Indian Health Service. SAMHSA's administrator is also the assistant secretary for MH and SUD, an important but perhaps insufficient point of connection between the two sides of the agency, which has the Center for Substance Abuse Prevention (CSAP) and Center for Substance Abuse Treatment (CSAT) but only one Center for Mental Health Services (CMHS), which oversees both treatment and prevention. SAMHSA's major funding outlays (discussed in Chapter 6)—its Substance Use Prevention, Treatment, and Recovery Services Block Grant (SUBG) and Community Mental Health Services Block Grant (MHSBG)—are similarly asymmetrical. Congress requires that 20 percent of the former be set aside for prevention, while the latter is entirely devoted to addressing serious mental illness (SMI) and may not be used for prevention (SAMHSA, 2017). In addition to the block grants, all three centers also provide discretionary grant programs known as the Programs of Regional and National

Significance (PRNS). PRNS grants from the CMHS are largely secondary/tertiary prevention and treatment oriented but include suicide prevention and Project LAUNCH (on child resiliency). PRNS for substance use prevention include the Strategic Prevention Framework and Sober Truth on Preventing Underage Drinking (STOP) grants. SAMHSA's support for SUD is strengthened by ONDCP grant programs, such as the Drug Free Communities support program managed through an ONDCP partnership with CDC.

CDC includes the National Center for Injury Prevention and Control, whose priorities include preventing adverse childhood experiences, overdose and substance use–related harms, and suicide. It also focuses on preventing community violence—a risk factor for MEB disorders (McDonald and Richmond, 2008).

Multiple institutes, centers, and offices in NIH contribute to the research that informs the prevention infrastructure. These include National Institute on Drug Abuse, National Institute on Mental Health, National Institute on Alcohol Abuse and Alcoholism, National Institute on Child Health and Human Development, and the Office of Behavioral and Social Sciences Research, for example. The history of NIH is intertwined with the nation's shifting views of mental illness, and the pendulum swinging between two ways of addressing these issues, from the biomedical approach to the psychosocial and public health approach. The historian Anne Harrington (2023) noted that the National Mental Health Act of 1946 marked a milestone in the nation's recognition of mental illness as a public health problem, which began with the mental hygiene movement, and a shift from direct care to affected individuals toward prevention across the entire population. The act established National Institute of Mental Health, initially as a part of the Public Health Service. Reorganizations of the service, training, and research functions of federal agencies that focused on MH and SUD reflected broader societal preoccupations with these issues. Although the 1963 Community Mental Health Act fell short of fulfilling its promise, it reframed the focus from state psychiatric hospitals and toward community care settings (BPC, 2019). The 1965 launch of the first neighborhood health centers, later community health centers, supported by President Johnson's War on Poverty, funded by the Office of Economic Opportunity, and offering comprehensive, community-based health care (including MH and SUD care) along with other social services, provided an early glimpse of health care services that prioritized closing the gaps in health affecting poor, rural, and minoritized communities, and were responsive to health-related social needs (e.g., for food, housing).

The history of the MH and SUD components of HHS is complex and multidimensional. It includes the War on Drugs, which, like President Kennedy's Community Mental Health Act (intended to solve the problems with state mental hospitals), sought to fix the problem of drug use and associated criminal activity. As the dialogue about prevention developed and federal resources grew considerably, an ecosystem of agencies and organizations (see Table 1-1) emerged and developed, representing services and research components, along with advocacy for prevention research, support for community engagement, and other extensive networks and interactions. The ecosystem includes the Society for Prevention Research, National Prevention Network, and CADCA—the membership organization for national (and some international) substance use prevention coalitions. This robust network is largely oriented around preventing substance use, while the ecosystem around MH issues is almost entirely devoted to treatment. While the Prevention Technology Transfer Centers (PTTCs) are the prevention counterpart to the Addiction Technology Transfer Centers, the analogous Mental Health Technology Transfer Centers (MTTCs) (ended in September 2024) focused almost entirely on treatment of MH.

Interagency Coordination

There are several examples, both historic and current, of interagency entities established for the purpose of furthering aspects of prevention or well-being. Federal interagency coordinating entities on behavioral health, such as the Federal Executive Steering Committee for Mental Health, last active in 2009, can play an essential role in improving coordination (GAO, 2014). The existing Interagency Task Force on Trauma-Informed Care established in 2018 and chaired by the Assistant Secretary for Mental Health and Substance Use, includes in its membership multiple departments, including the Departments of Justice (DOJ), the Interior, Education (ED), VA, and Housing and Urban Development. The following problem statement and outcomes statement have been articulated for the Task Force:

> Problem Statement: Childhood trauma, including exposure to substance misuse, is a serious public health problem in the United States. It has potentially long-lasting negative impacts on physical and mental health. Communities need support to build infrastructure and capacity to prevent trauma, respond to those impacted by trauma, and enhance resilience. A robust evidence base for a continuum of interventions (e.g., prevention of traumatic exposures, early intervention to address acute reactions and responses, treatments for 2 identified health, education and other adverse conditions) at the individual, system, and community levels are needed to promote the provision of best practices.
>
> Outcome Statement: A national, trauma-informed, and coordinated federal strategy to build community capacity to identify, disseminate, foster, and refine evidence-based, evidence-informed, and best practices regarding childhood trauma to reduce the incidence of trauma, improve the response

to families with exposure to substance misuse, enhance recognition of and response to trauma, strengthen resilience, and improve outcomes for children, youth, and families.

Because trauma is a risk factor for MEB disorders, the Task Force has clear relevance to the coordination functions discussed below, including in Recommendation 5-1.

In the broader prevention domain, the ACA established the National Prevention, Health Promotion, and Public Health Council (National Prevention Council or NPC), which, with its National Prevention Strategy and led by the U.S. Surgeon General, provided "coordination and leadership among 20 executive departments and agencies with respect to prevention, wellness, and health promotion activities" (NPC et al, 2014, p. 3). Although it concluded its work in 2015, its examples of interagency coordination and partnership have lasting relevance. These include the Sustainable Communities Initiative (Lushniak et al., 2015), which was a partnership among the Departments of Housing and Urban Development and of Transportation and the Environmental Protection Agency that included coordinating on policies and programs and, even more germane to the topic of this report, how ED partnered with DOJ and HHS to launch a School Climate Transformation Grant Program in FY 2014 (HUD Exchange, n.d.; NPC et al., 2014).

In 2022, HHS spearheaded an interagency effort in response to the COVID-19 pandemic and a shared recognition of the need for coordination and partnership. The Office of the Assistant Secretary launched the Equitable Long-Term Recovery and Resilience (ELTRR) initiative and plan. Although it does not have an NPC-like "body" associated with it, it has an interagency coordination group. Its recommendations include, in the category of "Basic Needs for Health and Safety," several that are relevant to promoting MEB health and well-being (see Box 5-1).

As noted, since the disbandment of the National Prevention Council (whose remit was public health and prevention, broadly conceived), there has been no equivalent whole-of-government effort to coordinate and collaborate on a prevention agenda—either broad or specific to MEB health. The ELTRR initiative is promising in its focus on the societal factors that shape health and well-being (e.g., education, housing), but its priorities go well beyond improving MEB health.

There is a "drug czar" in the public official who leads ONDCP, but no BH leader (with combined focus on MH and SUD) or entity that represents an organized "whole-of-government" effort across the federal executive branch to prevent BH disorders. HHS is the main department devoted to supporting and overseeing the delivery of BH interventions, with some siloing between MH and SUD activities in both SAMHSA and CDC. But multiple agencies across the federal government have prevention functions

> **BOX 5-1**
> **Recommendations from Federal Plan for Equitable Long-Term Recovery and Resilience for Social, Behavioral, and Community Health**
>
> *Freedom from Trauma, Violence, and Addiction*
> - Increase cross-agency coordination of complementary federal resources to support community-led prevention, reduction, and elimination of individual and collective victimization and trauma for groups placed at increased risk of victimization and exposure to trauma
> - Leverage cross-agency federal support (e.g., policies, waivers, funds) to permit the use of funds for and increase the availability of qualified and/or credentialed peer support professionals integrated with prevention, treatment, and recovery services
> - Invest in the development of collaborative networks extending from education settings (e.g., Head Start, childcare, and schools) to respond to social, emotional, and physical needs of children and their families
>
> *Related to Physical and Mental Health*
> - Enhance policies and programs that increase availability and integration of patient- and family-centered primary care and behavioral health (BH) services
> - Expand family-centered and multigenerational approaches across federal agency programs and resources (e.g., policy, funding, programs, technical assistance, and research) to foster the healthy development and wellness of children, youth, and families as a whole
> - Increase federal cross-agency coordination to integrate community-based BH services within broader health care, public health, and human service systems (ODPHP, 2022)

and would benefit from coordination. These include the DoD, ED, DOJ, and VA. Given the fact that the prevalence of behavioral disorders is a national crisis, it requires top federal leadership to avoid higher economic and health care costs of MEB disorders. Furthermore, White House leadership is needed to spearhead and support coordination across departments.

Related to promoting better governance of the prevention infrastructure and interagency coordination across the federal government, the Foundations of Evidence-Based Policymaking Act of 2018[3] requires federal

---
[3] Foundations of Evidence-Based Policymaking Act, Public Law 115–435, 115th Cong., 2nd sess (January 14, 2019).

agencies to develop evidence-building plans, called "Learning Agendas." A 2024 search of these across the federal government for mentions of BH found that, besides HHS, four agencies and two cross-agency plans included priorities relevant to MEB health (Evaluation.gov, n.d.; Tsai, 2024). The analysis provides two insights relevant to preventing MEB disorders. First, the Learning Agendas underscore "a focus on promoting social and emotional well-being, particularly among school children (ED), veterans with disabilities, and veterans with military sexual trauma" (Tsai, 2024, p. 15). Second, they largely overlook the relationship between physical and mental health, "aside from the [USDA] which briefly mentioned the link between food security and mental health" (Tsai, 2024, p. 15). The Learning Agenda developed by executive branch agencies may offer a point of connection across agencies on promoting MEB health that could inform coordination and collaboration (see Box 5-2).

Intradepartmental Coordination

The committee notes the existence of an HHS Behavioral Health Coordinating Council (BHCC) announced in 2021 and described as an intradepartmental effort to "facilitate collaboration and strategic planning" on behavioral health issues.[4] However, the committee has found little information about BHCC and its work, and the few references suggest the focus is primarily to address behavioral treatment needs.[5,6] Based on publicly available information, the committee was not able to ascertain the extent to which the BHCC focuses on BH prevention. The BHCC or a similar body is needed to ensure a greater focus on MEB prevention, for example, in integrating MH promotion and substance use prevention objectives in the way funding opportunities are developed, and in the technical assistance and other support provided to states. An earlier iteration of the BHCC was in existence in 2009 and 2011, with indications that it included subcommittees, such as a subcommittee on primary care and behavioral health integration.[7]

In 2023, CDC established a Behavioral Health Coordinating Unit, whose mission is to "elevate, advance, and coordinate CDC's public health approach to promote mental well-being and prevent mental distress, substance use,

---

[4] https://www.samhsa.gov/newsroom/press-announcements/202105181200 (accessed January 13, 2025).

[5] https://www.apa.org/news/press/releases/2021/05/hhs-behavioral-health-coordinating-council (accessed January 13, 2025).

[6] https://www.naatp.org/advocacy/public-policy/hhs-creates-behavioral-health-coordinating-council/may-18-2021 (accessed January 13, 2025).

[7] https://crs.od.nih.gov/CRSPublic/View.aspx?Id=5278; https://crs.od.nih.gov/CRSPublic/View.aspx?Id=2501 (accessed January 13, 2025).

> **BOX 5-2**
> **Mental, Emotional, and Behavioral Health Elements in Three Departmental "Learning Agendas"**
>
> As part of its Learning Agenda developed to comply with the Evidence Based Policymaking Act of 2018, each department in the executive branch identified and outlined a response to priority research questions. A small sample from among many plans that addressed MEB issues illustrates the possibilities for greater coordination and even for a whole-of-government effort on prevention of MEB disorders.
>
> **Department of Agriculture**
> The department's response to its priority question about food security included
>
> "This study will identify measures of poverty and well-being associated with household food security status among SNAP-eligible participants and nonparticipants in persistent poverty counties, defined as counties where 20 [percent] or more of their population lived in poverty in the last four decennial Censuses. Moving beyond household income, policy-actionable elements of well-being and material deprivation such as mental health, depression, health-related quality of life, disablement, medical expenditures, alcohol or opioid addiction, place of residence, and unequal sharing of resources within the household may impact food security status and SNAP participation" (USDA, n.d., pp. 17–18).
>
> **Department of Education**
> One National Center for Special Education Research project "involves evaluating the efficacy of a coaching intervention to determine whether it improves paraprofessionals' behavioral intervention practices and the behavioral and academic outcomes of students with or at risk for externalizing behavior disorders" (ED, n.d., p. 105).
>
> **Department of Housing and Urban Development**
> The evaluation of the Indian Housing Block Grant Competitive Program "would include an assessment of community-level impacts from the resulting units built and rehabilitated, including the number of families assisted, the impact on homelessness and overcrowding, physical and mental health, accessible housing provided for persons with disabilities, and economic and educational outcomes" (HUD, 2022, p. 44).

overdose, and suicide. This includes a focus on behavioral health as a necessary component of well-being across the life course, particularly during early childhood and adolescence" (Abad, 2024, p. 12). This mechanism suggests a focus in CDC to integrate disparate prevention-oriented BH efforts into a more cohesive and coordinated whole. With regard to community partner engagement, the agency's Centers for Substance Abuse Prevention, Substance Abuse Treatment, and Mental Health Services each have advisory committees, but all members appear to be federal officials or professionals in the BH field; none of the committee members were identified as community members with lived experience (SAMHSA, n.d.-a).

The federal government lacks coordination on MEB disorder prevention, both between agencies with separate and somewhat siloed units on MH and substance use and among all federal entities with a role in MEB health. Establishing a central point for improving coordination—at the highest level of the federal government, at the department level, and at the agency level, i.e., in SAMHSA—will be helpful across multiple dimensions of prevention, from research, to funding, to supporting the workforce development and functioning.

The committee found that it is a coordination challenge that SAMHSA, like the entire BH enterprise, is asymmetrical in its structure, with greater attention to preventing substance use than promoting MH. It has separate centers for substance use prevention and SUD treatment but only one center for MH with functions in both treatment and to a far lesser extent, prevention; there is a 20 percent prevention set-aside from the SUBG but no analogous set-aside from the MHBG, which is devoted to treating SMI. For a well-functioning prevention infrastructure, greater integration or at least collaboration is needed between the MH and SU prevention functions of SAMHSA.

A multi-layered approach is needed to strengthen coordination, collaboration, and support for prevention. The committee believes it is reasonable to assume that a stronger locus in SAMHSA for prevention efforts related to MH would be helpful, including for the purpose of (at a minimum) greater coordination and (ideally) integration between prevention efforts in mental health and substance use, and ultimately, for creating conditions for improving population level MEB outcomes. In the current structure, the governance for MEB disorder prevention is uneven, with greater attention in SAMHSA and elsewhere in the ecosystem to prevention of substance use than to promotion of mental health. An integrated prevention infrastructure requires similar level of attention to substance use and mental health along with greater collaboration and ideally integration, with better interagency coordination among all agencies working on aspects of MEB disorder prevention, and with top federal leadership to drive change.

RECOMMENDATION 5-1: To strengthen capacity and coordination to promote mental, emotional, and behavioral (MEB) health and population well-being, governance structures for prevention should be added at each level in the Executive Branch.

a. The White House could establish a central point for MEB prevention capacity and coordination. There are two options for doing this: appointing a special assistant on MEB disorder prevention to the president who serves on the Domestic Policy Council, or establishing a new office on MEB prevention in the White House. Either the special assistant or the new office would coordinate with the Office of National Drug Control Policy and the Office of Management and Budget, and convene all executive branch departments with a role in prevention, perhaps through an interagency task force. An office would require more resources than a special assistant, but could support a more robust portfolio of efforts to streamline and enhance coordination throughout the Executive Branch. There is a history of interagency task forces spearheaded or called for by an Administration to help implement a strategic objective. The relevant executive branch departments include Health and Human Services (HHS), Department of Education, Veterans Affairs, Department of Defense,[8] U.S. Department of Agriculture, Department of Justice, and Department of Labor and Department of Treasury;
b. The HHS Behavioral Health Coordinating Council (or similar intra-departmental entity) could establish a workgroup on promoting MEB health and preventing MEB disorders and adopt strategies to engage individuals with lived experience; and
c. Congress could expand the Substance Abuse and Mental Health Services Administration's (SAMHSA's) ability to support state, tribal, and local MEB disorder prevention efforts by either establishing a Center for Prevention of Behavioral Disorders that integrates the agency's prevention activities, or by establishing a Center for Mental Health Promotion (equal to and working closely with the existing Center for Substance Abuse Prevention). In addition, the SAMHSA administrator, who is also the Assistant Secretary for Mental Health and Substance Use, should appoint a prevention advisor to support and report on state efforts to prioritize prevention.

Given the societal and economic costs of behavioral disorders and the existence of many evidence-based programs to prevent them, elevating MEB

---

[8] DoD's prevention integration initiative is illustrative of high-level attention to prevention in domains external to HHS. https://www.prevention.mil/ (accessed October 1, 2025).

disorder prevention in this manner could have a profound impact. Also, the Domestic Policy Council comprises all domestic cabinet secretaries and advises the President on domestic and economic initiatives important to a given administration (Troy, 2025), and special assistants to the President play a key role in advising the President on a given issue of national importance.[9] For example, President Bill Clinton's DPC "led the effort to develop and pass welfare reform and the crime bill," while President George W. Bush's DPC "was the leading force behind the enactment of 'No Child Left Behind'" education reform effort (Weinstein, 2008, p. 67-68). Clearly DPC leadership on an issue can drive policy change.

Past and current examples of federal interagency task forces, on which a task force for MEB disorder prevention could be modeled, are discussed above.

Regarding (b), an entity such as the Behavioral Health Coordinating Council (BHCC) could facilitate coordination among multiple agencies in HHS that conduct and fund a variety of activities related to behavioral health prevention. Coordination could help address fragmentation in addressing this topic of great national interest, and could improve efficiency of programs (GAO, 2014).

Regarding (c), CSAP[10] works with state, tribal, local, and private sector organizations engaged in prevention efforts, and serves as a central point for thought leadership on substance use prevention, technical assistance, oversight of prevention-focused grants, and development of prevention strategy. For mental health promotion, it is not evident that the Center for Mental Health Services is able to play the same range of roles. The CMHS[11] has a division of Children and School Mental Health which includes a Mental Health Promotion Branch, but there is no other mental health promotion unit, suggesting limited capacity to support mental health focused prevention for other age groups and settings. Establishing a CSAP-equivalent Center for Mental Health Promotion or a joint Center for Behavioral Disorder Prevention would help ensure that prevention of mental illnesses is being at least well-coordinated with prevention of substance use, and ideally, that these are integrated. Finally, the SAMHSA prevention advisor's role could include using the levers of the block grants to incentivize state health agencies to enhance prevention efforts, supporting (e.g., through funding, technical assistance) prevention leaders in states. As noted later, it is important that this strengthened governance structure be linked with state-level leadership for prevention.

If establishing a new center—which requires an amendment to Title V of the Public Health Service Act—proves unfeasible, other approaches could

---

[9] For examples, see The American Presidency Project https://www.presidency.ucsb.edu/ (accessed January 13, 2025).

[10] https://www.samhsa.gov/about/offices-centers/cmhs (accessed January 13, 2025).

[11] https://www.samhsa.gov/about/offices-centers/cmhs (accessed January 13, 2025).

be considered to strengthen coordination and collaboration between promotion of mental health and efforts to prevent substance use disorders. Also, it is important to note that the SAMHSA National Mental Health and Substance Use Policy Laboratory (Policy Lab) could play a role in the coordination and to some extent, integration, of mental health and substance use prevention efforts in SAMHSA. The Policy Lab "coordinates cross-SAMHSA and inter-agency policy efforts and promotes coordination and collaboration of SAMHSA programs" (GAO, 2024). It has two teams relevant to this issue: the Evidence-Based Practices Innovation and Dissemination Team and the Policy Analysis, Development, and Implementation Team.

The leaders to be appointed in Recommendation 5-1 will need training and expertise in identifying and addressing health disparities and in implementation science. Establishing a Center for Mental Health Promotion will require attention to functions and capabilities analogous to those of CSAP and a mandate and resources for coordination and collaboration with CSAP—including in grant requirements, guidance for data collection, integration, and reporting (including sharing with communities). Like CSAP, the new center could have divisions for primary prevention, targeted prevention, workplace or community programs, prevention communications and public engagement, innovation, and program analysis and coordination (SAMHSA, n.d.-b).

The alternative option of a joint Center for (MEB Disorder) Prevention would need to bring together existing functions of CSAP with equivalent functions for mental health promotion. A center that integrates prevention functions related to both mental health and substance use would present some advantages, such as potential for true integration and not just coordination both internally in SAMHSA and in relationship to the state agencies working on substance use and mental health. The siloed funding channels for mental health and substance use would be a considerable barrier to overcome, as would the requirements associated with the funding (e.g., limited ability to use substance use prevention funds for mental health promotion) (SAMHSA, 2017).

There are some advantages and disadvantages to the two options proposed. Organizations and individuals who champion substance use prevention may fear that integrating MH and SU could mean decreased attention to SU. On the other side, there may be people or organizations that worry that having a center for promoting MH in SAMHSA and taking a set aside from the Community Mental Health Services Block Grant may decrease attention to serious mental illness. Dialogue among all partners and constituencies could address concerns, but it must be emphasized that the status quo is suboptimal for a coherent and well-coordinated national prevention infrastructure.

STATE GOVERNANCE STRUCTURE

Given the U.S. federalist system of government, the federal government cannot compel states to work in furthering prevention or any other health improvement efforts. Federal agencies partner with states, providing funding, technical assistance, and other incentives to engage in best practices, follow standards, or coordinate with various partners. The structure of state and local governance of prevention varies (SAMHSA, 2017). Some states have a public health agency and a separate BH agency; in others, public health agencies include BH functions, such as assessment of risk factors and partnerships with relevant community organizations, such as anti-drug coalitions.

State public health agencies can play an important role in establishing baseline infrastructure in localities in the state. Funding for public health efforts needs to include attention to promoting BH and preventing MEB disorders. Public health agencies integrate MEB health promotion efforts in collaboration with schools at the state and local level.

States play a central role in delivering prevention services along the life course and providing or contracting with other entities for extensive and ongoing technical assistance. However, as with other components of the existing infrastructure, state oversight and support of MH and SUD differ markedly, with the latter being far more prevention oriented in focus, funding, organization, oversight, and supports to local providers and workforces. Presentations to the committee by the National Association of State Alcohol and Drug Agency Directors (NASADAD) and the National Association of State Mental Health Program Directors highlighted those differences. The former's remarks highlighted aspects of a robust multilevel prevention infrastructure for SUD, while the latter reflected a focus on mental illness (including community and carceral care settings) and crisis care and suicide prevention (supporting the implementation of the 988 Suicide and Crisis Lifeline).

Single state authorities (the state agencies that received SAMHSA funding for substance use prevention) provide oversight of regional, county, and local providers (NASADAD, 2023). State health authorities oversee the allocation of federal grants, but states vary in their capacity and resources to provide regional oversight, coordination, and training and technical assistance. The committee reviewed three state-level examples: New York, Pennsylvania, and Washington. These each provide robust support to the state's SUD infrastructure through a range of activities, including Pennsylvania's partnership with the Evidence-Based Prevention and Intervention Support Center, which includes supporting a staff position;[12] New York's

---

[12] Personal communication, Grace Kindt, May 2024.

six regional prevention resource centers; and Washington's State Prevention Enhancement Policy Consortium, which hosts the Athena Forum, a resource that provides training and technical assistance to prevention providers and communities (The Athena Forum, 2024; PSU, 2020; OASAS, n.d.).

As a condition of SAMHSA prevention funding, states could be asked to appoint prevention leads (both SUD and MH) to ensure funding is used effectively and coordination and collaboration between the SUD and MH silos is maximized in program delivery. This would allow the governance structure described in Recommendation 5-1 to expand beyond the federal government. As noted in Chapter 6, SAMHSA prevention funding is primarily for SUD prevention, and includes the 20 percent prevention set-aside in the SUBG and the Strategic Prevention Framework—Partnerships for Success Grant Program.

State departments of BH and/or public health play a key role in what Wandersman and colleagues call the "Interactive Systems Framework for Dissemination and Implementation" (Wandersman et al., 2012). This three-part framework outlines the roles and relationships among the entities that develop, select, and support the implementation of evidence-based preventive interventions. This includes the Prevention Synthesis and Translation system that "designs interventions and creates tools for their widespread implementation" by the "Prevention Delivery System" (e.g., local health department, community organizations), which is in turn supported by and receives technical assistance from the "Prevention Support System" (e.g., state health department, universities). The prevention support system includes research institutions that have created models to build, support, and evaluate the effectiveness and implementation of community coalitions and prevention programming that are well positioned to support these training needs. These models include the network of PTTCs[13] that can provide implementation support and technical assistance on SUD prevention and the network of CDC-funded prevention research centers,[14] some of which have an MEB health promotion focus. In government–academic partnerships, universities support state efforts to promote MEB health—providing research support and using state funding to provide training and technical assistance. The MHTTCs offered training and technical assistance largely for providers of MH treatment services and, to a lesser extent, those in education, child welfare, and law enforcement systems (MHTTCN, 2024).[15]

---

[13] https://pttcnetwork.org/ (accessed January 13, 2025).
[14] https://www.cdc.gov/prevention-research-centers/php/index.html (accessed January 13, 2025).
[15] Personal communication, H. Gotham, July 26, 2024.

TRIBAL GOVERNANCE

The United States' complex relationship with the American Indian and Alaska Native (AIAN) population is relevant to the infrastructure for MEB disorders for two reasons. One is functional, given the fact that 574 federally recognized AIAN tribes are recognized sovereign nations—allowing self-governance—and their interactions with the federal government are government-to-government interactions (NCAI, 2020). The other reason is the historic trauma that has affected generations of AIAN people (NASEM, 2023). Different departments (HHS, Interior, and Justice) and health agencies (e.g., IHS, SAMHSA, CDC) in the federal government interact with tribal leaders. HHS has a Tribal Advisory Committee, and SAMHSA has an Office of Tribal Affairs and Policy and an Office of Indian Alcohol and Substance Abuse (SAMHSA 2024b; 2024c). Also, the Indian Health Service Division of Behavioral Health interacts with tribal governments, and it initiates Tribal Consultation and Urban Confer events to solicit comments on the distribution of annual behavioral health initiative funding. The Division's National Tribal Advisory Committee on Behavioral Health convenes regularly to make recommendations based on the input IHS receives from the Tribal Consultation and Urban Confer.

In 2016, SAMHSA and IHS developed a National Tribal Behavioral Health Agenda (NTBHA) with extensive input from tribal leaders with the assistance of the National Indian Health Board (SAMHSA and IHS, 2016). At the department level, HHS has a Tribal Advisory Committee, which also played a role in informing the NTBHA. The agenda's three components include the American Indian and Alaska Native Cultural Wisdom Declaration (CWD), sections that provide background information, and a section that articulates the substance of the agenda (SAMHSA and IHS, 2016). Notably, and echoing the discussion provided in Chapter 2 about attention to cultural context and practice-based evidence, the CWD's purpose is to "ensure that cultural wisdom and traditional practices are taken into account and supported as fundamental elements of programs, policies, and activities that are designed, or contribute, to improvements in behavioral health" (SAMHSA and IHS, 2016). The TBHA consists of five foundational elements (see Figure 5-1): historical and intergenerational trauma, sociocultural-ecological approach, prevention and recovery support, behavioral health systems and support, and national awareness and visibility. Community engagement and collaboration is a throughline in the report.

The research component of the tribal governance ecosystem is the Native American Research Centers for Health (NARCH) program, a collaboration between NIH and IHS. With greater engagement in both research and practice, "a growing number of tribes have initiated their own Tribal review processes to

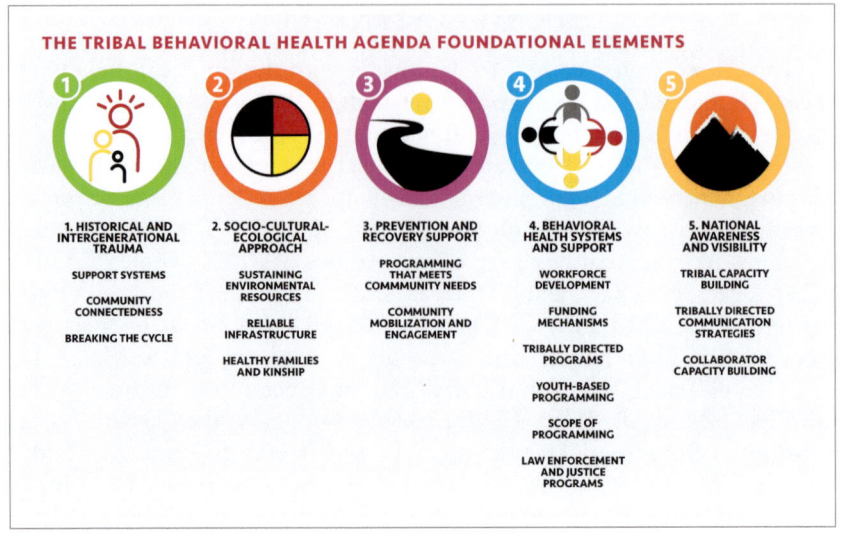

FIGURE 5-1 Tribal behavioral health agenda foundational elements.
SOURCE: SAMHSA and IHS, 2016.

govern research efforts undertaken on Tribal lands and with Tribal members" to further Tribal knowledge and public health (SAMHSA and IHS, 2016).

In addition to federal collaboration with Tribal governments, there are multiple examples of states partnering with tribes to deploy funding to improve behavioral health. For example, the Oregon Health Authority partners with tribes to support and expand access to behavioral health services, and to an array of resources that include Tribal Behavioral Health Resource Networks (Gooding et al., 2024). Oregon, along with three other states (HHS, 2024), has received CMS approval for a section 1115 demonstration amendment that allows "Medicaid and Children's Health Insurance Program (CHIP) coverage of traditional health care practices provided by I/T/U [Indian Health Service, Tribes and Tribal organizations, and urban Indian organizations] facilities" (CMS, 2024b). In Oklahoma, 13 tribes partnered with the state's Department for Mental Health and Substance Abuse Services to use SAMHSA Tribal 988 grant funding for suicide prevention programs (SAMHSA, 2024d; Gooding et al., 2024). Although no details about these programs were easily accessed, the IHS website provides an overview of funded tribal Substance Abuse and Suicide Prevention programs by state and indicates that several Oklahoma tribal authorities have implemented evidence-based, practice-based, strengths-focused, culturally sensitive suicide prevention programs.[16]

---

[16] https://www.ihs.gov/sasp/fundedprojects/oklahoma/ (accessed January 13, 2025).

REGIONAL AND LOCAL GOVERNANCE STRUCTURE

At regional and local levels, public agencies can and do play key roles in preventing MEB disorders, though the way these efforts are organized may differ substantially across different jurisdictions. For example, while San Francisco and Philadelphia are similar as both cities and counties, San Francisco's BH services are located within the public health department, while the City of Philadelphia's Department of Behavioral Health and Intellectual disAbility Services is distinct from public health. The latter model affords the BH department an unobstructed focus on MEB issues, including prevention, but for all city residents to enjoy optimal MEB health, collaboration and coordination between two separate departments is required. Many communities also have a variety of nonprofit organizations, government agencies, coalitions or partnerships, and community entities, including congregations, that work together to promote MEB well-being. Also, organizations that play the role of community integrator may serve as both a governance mechanism for collective impact initiatives and facilitator for partnerships, capacity building, and funding (McHale, 2014).

Implementation, Partnerships, and Collaboration

Multisector community partnerships can weave together efforts to develop and implement interventions to prevent MEB disorders and promote population well-being. Some examples of partnerships are found in accountable communities for health, which are "multisector, community-based partnerships that bring together health care, public health, social services, other local partners, and residents to address the unmet health and social needs of the individuals and communities they serve" (FFAH, n.d.). The Funders Forum on Accountable Health at the George Washington University Milken School of Public Health hosts a database of 185 accountable communities for health. Table 5-1 offers examples of governance approaches among these partnerships.

Models of Shared Governance

Models of governance articulated by various experts are applicable to the prevention infrastructure for MEB disorders. Fishbein and Sloboda (2023) describe a community-based comprehensive prevention service system that delivers evidence-based SU prevention services by certified providers in a variety of settings—they identify micro-level environments in which interventions may take place as family, school, peer, faith-based, and workplace. They describe the importance of matching community need to accessibility of services, ensuring quality, addressing ethical issues in research, and conducting cost–benefit assessment and analysis. These highlight key

TABLE 5-1 Governance Arrangements and Partnerships in Example Accountable Communities for Health

Example	Governance	Partners	Focus	Funding Sources
Chicanos Por La Causa Arizona	Community advisory board	Businesses, philanthropic organizations, area agency on aging, community-based organizations, financial institution	Parenting classes Home visitation Drug use prevention	Owns and manages mission driven for-profit subsidiaries that help fund the nonprofit initiatives
Humboldt County Health Trust California	Backbone organization: North Coast Health Improvement and Information Network Governance board	Family resource center, health system, Yurok Tribe, community health centers, First Five Humboldt, community leaders, Medicaid health plan	Portfolio of interventions Goal to increase access to prevention and treatment for families, improve policies and systems, etc.	California Accountable Communities for Health Initiative
Jackson Care Connect Oregon	Community Advisory Council	Public health agencies, community health centers, Oregon State University Extension Service	Strong Families program; mental health and substance use disorders; traditional health workers	Oregon Health Authority

SOURCE: Adapted from the Inventory of Accountable Communities for Health from the Funders Forum on Accountable Health (FFAH, n.d.)

aspects of governance. Fishbein and Sloboda propose a system with an advisory council that represents a mechanism not only for "interagency-institution coordination" but also for engaging key organizations and communities (see Figure 3 in Fishbein and Sloboda [2023]). The ecosystem they describe around that advisory entity includes Drug-Free Communities grantees, the PTTCs, NASADAD and the National Prevention Network, the Society for Prevention Research, and the National Prevention Science Coalition.

The Bipartisan Policy Center has made recommendations related to public health governance, and many have relevance to the prevention infrastructure for MEB disorders. The report defined governance as the "legal authority and responsibility to protect and promote the health of populations" that sets "the structure and boundaries in which public health interventions and policies are developed, implemented, and evaluated"

(Armooh et al., 2021, p. 38). Public health governance varies, the report noted, with both centralized (state) and decentralized (local) authority models. The report recommended collaboration with communities, calling for funding "public health departments for community collaboration and develop[ing] output measures that account for progress toward building trust and working in partnership" (Armooh et al., 2021, p. vii). It also calls for public health leaders to "engage in routine Tribal consultation to support intergovernmental public health planning that recognizes Tribal authority, autonomy, and self-governance" (Armooh et al., 2021, p. vii). The committee notes that engaging with tribes in consultation also applies to the behavioral health context, as discussed above.

Additional resources and discussion of the role of community input and expertise in informing federal policy, including specific guidance for integrating community representation and advisory practices in accountability measures and enforcement mechanisms, are provided in NASEM, 2023 (a relevant recommendation from that report is highlighted in Box 5-3).

BOX 5-3
Endorsing a Recommendation on Community Input and Expertise (NASEM, 2023)

The federal government should prioritize community input and expertise when changing or developing federal policies to advance health equity. Specifically,

1. The president of the United States should require federal agencies relevant to the social determinants of health to generate and sustain community representation and advisory practices that are integrated with accountability measures and enforcement mechanisms.
2. Congress should request a Government Accountability Office report to document across federal agencies whose work impacts the social determinants of health, as well as federal statistical agencies, that
    a. Assesses how community advisory boards are positioned within their agencies, whom they are composed of, how often they meet, how they report back, and how that work influences the agencies' policies and programs; and
    b. Identifies promising and evidence-based practices, gaps, and opportunities for community advisory boards that could be applied by other agencies (NASEM, 2023, p. 424).

Models of Collaboration

Over the past 2 decades, the attention to cross-sector partnerships has grown, along with some examples of government initiatives that support this, such as the proliferation of health in all policies efforts and projects. These range from the short-lived but important National Prevention Council and ongoing Health in All Policies Taskforce of the California Strategic Growth Council, to the Accountable Care Act and Internal Revenue Service (IRS) requirement that tax-exempt hospitals provide a community benefit equivalent to their tax exemption. IRS also calls for a description of community health improvement and community building activities that hospitals and health systems in IRS Schedule H (Form 990) along with conducting a triennial community health needs assessment.

Long-standing models and frameworks from the public health and population health fields outline the structure and processes for community-based health planning and population health improvement efforts. These include the Mobilizing for Action Through Planning and Partnership from the National Association of County and City Health Officials and accountable communities for health multisector partnership models being used around the country to link and generate collective impact among health care, public health, and social sector organizations. Community-based participatory research and related approaches have been fruitful.

Several community coalition–based prevention models work as delivery systems or implementation support systems for preventive interventions in MEB health and related issues. These include Communities That Care, PROmoting School-community-university Partnerships to Enhance Resilience, Getting to Outcomes, and the Icelandic Model (Blueprints for Healthy Youth Development, n.d.; RAND, 2024.; Kristjansson et al., 2020; Miller, 2017; Spoth et al., 2013). These models provide structured processes and resources for working with community and cross-sector partners to assess needs, identify solutions (i.e., evidence-based interventions), and implement, evaluate and improve, and sustain the interventions over time. Each of these models is evidence based and has evidence of its effectiveness in the implementation of interventions for specific outcomes, either MEB health related or other health risk topics (e.g., teen pregnancy) (Chinman et al., 2018).

Models for Involving Communities People with Lived Experience in Governance

Local communities are the places where the work of prevention unfolds, and community members use their lived expertise to co-create and contribute to the success of prevention efforts. Building community capacity should be a central guiding principle by which federal, state, and tribal entities aim to implement EBPs and practices and identify community-defined evidence. Even with a robust and supportive infrastructure, people on the ground need the skills and knowledge to drive and support community coalitions, inform the identification of EBPs and practices and community-defined evidence, enable fidelity to implementation, maintain integrity to data collection and sharing principles, and review data along with communities to support quality improvement (NACCHO, 2023).

Good governance is shared governance, which requires sharing power. It includes community partnerships and people with lived expertise, and, as noted, there are many models and examples of community governance in health promotion, public health, and community health settings, ranging from state-level advisory councils that include community members and people with lived expertise to federally qualified health centers that are required to have at least 51 percent of board members drawn from their patients. The Youth Wellness Hub is a "community governance model for integrating delivery and financing systems for youth behavioral health and wellness services" using three social policy tools that are evidence-based or promising: community governance, public health education campaigns, and blending of funding sources for service delivery (SFA, 2023). Another model is the community coalition board that governs the Morehouse School of Medicine Prevention Research Center. It comprises neighborhood residents (who are the majority and hold all leadership seats), academic institutions, and social service providers. The board oversees the school of medicine's community health needs assessment, and community members develop research questions and identify health strategies (Henry Akintobi et al., 2020). Another example is found in the State of Maryland Behavioral Health Advisory Council, which includes "individuals who are consumers, family members, professionals, and involved community members" (MDH, n.d.).

Including community members and people with lived expertise in governance of the prevention infrastructure is an important strategy for ensuring that resources are flowing to areas with greatest need—such as communities with higher rates of MEB disorders and high level of risk factors and low levels of protective factors (see Box 5-4 for implementation considerations relevant to governance and partnerships). Community members are also crucial to conducting effective community health needs assessments. The many excellent examples include Chicago's West Side United, which is a collaboration of multiple hospitals, health systems, and community members and organizations. In 2017, when the effort was launched, the assembled community members called for shared governance. The resulting 16-member collaborative planning committee was designed to include eight community members, four institutional representatives, two

> **BOX 5-4**
> **Implementation Considerations in Governance and Partnerships for MEB Disorder Prevention**
>
> - **For federal funders and state leaders:** Communities and organizations need support for capacity building, including resources to engage with partners and conduct implementation with a focus on sustainment and impact for communities that are most affected by MEB disorders.
> - **For communities:** Agree on and assign clear roles (pre-implementation concepts): Who is in charge? Who monitors/evaluates? Who delivers? (For communities, see Box 2-8 for more details about implementation planning, and for constituents focused on implementing policies, see Box 7-4.)
> - **For all partners:** Funders must be accountable to communities and other constituents, and partners working together must be accountable to one another.

government officials, and two citywide nonprofit leaders (RUMC, 2017). The partnership has contributed to community health needs assessments. In 2020, partners learned that 10 percent of Chicago adults surveyed said they were experiencing serious psychological distress, an increase from 7 percent 2 years earlier, and MH was a major concern in every focus group. In response to the need, partners added two new school-based health centers to provide primary care and MH services and conducted community-based training for faith communities that provided MH first aid training to 300 people (RUMC, 2022).

REFERENCES

Abad, N. 2024. *CDC's behavioral health coordinating unit: Mental health is public health: CDC's strategic approach to mental health.* https://www.cdc.gov/injury/media/pdfs/2024/06/Neetu_Abad.pdf (accessed January 2, 2025).

Armooh, T., T. Barton, G. Castillo, S. Cinnick, S. Clark, B. Giles-Cantrell, and Q. Nav. 2021. Public health forward: Modernizing the US public health system. Washington, DC: Bipartisan Policy Center.

The Athena Forum. 2024. *State Prevention Enhancement (SPE) policy consortium.* https://theathenaforum.org/prevention-priorities/state-prevention-enhancement-spe-policy-consortium (accessed December 13, 2024).

Blueprints for Healthy Youth Development. n.d. *Communities that care.* https://www.blueprintsprograms.org/programs/444999999/communities-that-care/ (accessed December 16, 2024).

BPC (Bipartisan Policy Center). 2019. *Integrating clinical and mental health: Challenges and opportunities*. https://bipartisanpolicy.org/download/?file=/wp-content/uploads/2019/03/Integrating-Clinical-and-Mental-Health-Challenges-and-Opportunities.pdf (accessed December 13, 2024).

Carlson, V., M. J. Chilton, L. C. Corso, and L. M. Beitsch. 2015. Defining the functions of public health governance. *American Journal of Public Health* 105(S2):S159–S166. https://doi.org/10.2105/ajph.2014.302198.

Chinman, M., J. Acosta, P. Ebener, P. S. Malone, and M. E. Slaughter. 2018. A cluster-randomized trial of getting to outcomes' impact on sexual health outcomes in community-based settings. *Prevention Science* 19(4):437–448. https://doi.org/10.1007/s11121-017-0845-6.

CMS (Centers for Medicare & Medicaid Services). 2024a. *The Mental Health Parity and Addiction Equity Act (MHPAEA)*. https://www.cms.gov/marketplace/private-health-insurance/mental-health-parity-addiction-equity (accessed September 24, 2024).

CMS. 2024b. *Letter to Emma Sandoe, Medicaid Director Oregon Health Authority*. https://www.medicaid.gov/medicaid/section-1115-demonstrations/downloads/or-health-plan-dmnstrtn-aprvl-10162024.pdf.

DOD (Department of Defense). n.d. *Prevention*. https://www.prevention.mil/ (accessed January 2, 2024).

ED (Department of Education). n.d. *Fiscal years 2022–2026 learning agenda*. https://ies.ed.gov/sites/default/files/ncee/document/2025/02/ED_FY22-26_Learning_Agenda_v2.pdf (accsessed July 2, 2024).

Evaluation.gov. n.d. *Evidence plans: Learning agendas*. https://www.evaluation.gov/evidence-plans/learning-agenda/ (accessed July 2, 2024).

FFAH (Funders Forum on Accountable Health). n.d. *Accountable Communities for Health*. https://accountablehealth.gwu.edu/ (accessed December 12, 2024).

Fishbein, D. H., and Z. Sloboda. 2023. A national strategy for preventing substance and opioid use disorders through evidence-based prevention programming that fosters healthy outcomes in our youth. *Clinical Child and Family Psychology Review* 26(1):1–16. https://doi.org/10.1007/s10567-022-00420-5.

GAO (Government Accountability Office). 2024. Behavioral health: Activities of the National Mental Health and Substance Use Policy Laboratory. GAO-24-106760. https://www.gao.gov/assets/gao-24-106760.pdf (accessed December 31, 2024).

Gooding, N. D., R. Falkner, N. Kaye, and K. Greene. 2024. *How states and tribes can partner to improve the access of American Indians and Alaska Natives to behavioral health Care Services*. NASHP. https://nashp.org/how-states-and-tribes-can-partner-to-improve-the-access-of-american-indians-and-alaska-natives-to-behavioral-health-care-services/ (accessed December 31, 2024).

Harrington, A. 2023. Mental health's stalled (biological) revolution: Its origins, aftermath & future opportunities. *Daedalus*. 2023;152(4):166–185. https://doi.org/10.1162/daed_a_02037.

Henry Akintobi, T., T. Jacobs, D. Sabbs, K. Holden, R. Braithwaite, L. N. Johnson, D. Dawes, and L. Hoffman. 2020. Community engagement of African Americans in the era of COVID-19: Considerations, challenges, implications, and recommendations for public health. *Preventing Chronic Disease* 17:E83. https://doi.org/10.5888/pcd17.200255.

HHS (Department of Health and Human Services). 2024. Biden-Harris Administration Takes Groundbreaking Action to Expand Health Care Access by Covering Traditional Care Practices. News Release. https://www.hhs.gov/about/news/2024/10/16/biden-harris-administration-takes-groundbreaking-action-expand-health-care-access-covering-traditional-health-care-practices.html (accessed January 2, 2025).

HUD (Department of Housing and Urban Development). 2022. *Learning agenda: Fiscal years 2022–2026*. https://www.huduser.gov/portal/sites/default/files/pdf/HUD-Learning-Agenda.pdf (accessed January 2, 2025).

HUD Exchange. n.d. *Sustainable communities library*. https://www.hudexchange.info/programs/sci/ (accessed October 18, 2024).

Kristjansson, A. L., M. J. Mann, J. Sigfusson, I. E. Thorisdottir, J. P. Allegrante, and I. D. Sigfusdottir. 2020. Development and guiding principles of the Icelandic model for preventing adolescent substance use. *Health Promotion Practice* 21(1):62–69. https://doi.org/10.1177/1524839919849032.

Lushniak, B. D., D. E. Alley, B. Ulin, and C. Graffunder. 2015. The national prevention strategy: Leveraging multiple sectors to improve population health. *American Journal of Public Health* 105(2):229–31. https://doi.org/10.2105/AJPH.2014.302257.

McDonald, C. C., and T. R. Richmond. 2008. The relationship between community violence exposure and mental health symptoms in urban adolescents. *Journal of Psychiatric and Mental Health Nursing* 15(10):833–849. https://doi.org/10.1111/j.1365-2850.2008.01321.x.

McHale, B., and N. O. Andrews. 2014. Community development needs a quarterback. *Stanford Social Innovation Review*. https://doi.org/10.48558/T9FA-1932.

MDH (Maryland Department of Health). n.d. *Maryland behavioral health advisory council*. https://health.maryland.gov/bha/pages/maryland-behavioral-health-advisory-council.aspx (accessed December 13, 2024).

Medicaid.gov. n.d. *Early and periodic screening, diagnostic, and treatment*. https://www.medicaid.gov/medicaid/benefits/early-and-periodic-screening-diagnostic-and-treatment/index.html (accessed December 13, 2024).

MHTTCN (Mental Health Technology Transfer Center Network). 2024. *Mental health technology transfer center network*. https://mhttcnetwork.org/ (accessed December 13, 2024).

Miller, M. 2017. PROSPER program reduced young adult substance abuse by up to 41 percent. https://www.psu.edu/news/research/story/prosper-program-reduced-young-adult-substance-abuse-41-percent (accessed January 2, 2025).

NACCHO (National Association of County and City Health Officials). 2023. *Intro to MAPP 2.0*. https://www.naccho.org/uploads/card-images/public-health-infrastructure-and-systems/MAPP-2.0-Launch-V3.pdf (accessed December 13, 2024).

NASADAD (National Association of State Alcohol/Drug Abuse Directors). 2023. *Role of state alcohol and drug agencies*. https://nasadad.org/role-of-ssas/ (accessed December 13, 2024).

NASEM (National Academies of Sciences, Engineering, and Medicine). 2023. *Federal policy to advance racial, ethnic, and tribal health equity*. Washington, DC: National Academies Press. https://doi.org/10.17226/26834.

NASEM. 2024. *Expanding behavioral health care workforce participation in Medicare, Medicaid, and marketplace plans*. Washington, DC: The National Academies Press. https://doi.org/10.17226/27759.

NCAI (National Congress of American Indians. 2020. Tribal nations and the United States: An Introduction. https://archive.ncai.org/about-tribes (accessed January 2, 2025).

NPC (National Prevention Council), National Prevention Strategy, and CDC. 2014. *National Prevention, Health Promotion, and Public Health Council Annual Health Status Report 2014*. https://stacks.cdc.gov/view/cdc/24071 (accessed October 18, 2024).

OASAS (New York State Office of Addiction Services and Supports). n.d. *Regional offices*. https://oasas.ny.gov/providers/regional-offices (accessed December 13, 2024).

ODPHP (Office of Disease Prevention and Health Promotion). 2022. *Federal plan for equitable long-term recovery and resilience for social, behavioral, and community health: Recommendations*. https://odphp.health.gov/our-work/national-health-initiatives/equitable-long-term-recovery-and-resilience (December 13, 2024).

PSU (Penn State Unviersity). 2020. *EPIS*. https://epis.psu.edu/ (accessed December 13, 2024).
RAND. 2024. *Getting to Outcomes™*. https://www.rand.org/health-care/projects/getting-to-outcomes.html (accessed December 13, 2024).
RUMC (Rush University Medical Center). 2017. *What we heard: Coming together to improve health and wellness on the West Side*. https://www.rush.edu/sites/default/files/2020-09/what-we-heard-july-2017%283%29.pdf (accessed December 13, 2024).
RUMC. 2022. *Stronger together: Advancing equity for all*. https://www.rush.edu/sites/default/files/chna-chip-2022.pdf (accessed December 13, 2024).
SAMHSA (Substance Abuse and Mental Health Services Administration). n.d.-a. *Advisory councils*. https://www.samhsa.gov/about-us/advisory-councils (accessed September 25, 2024).
SAMHSA. n.d.-b. *Center for Substance Abuse Prevention*. https://www.samhsa.gov/about-us/who-we-are/offices-centers/csap (accessed September 26, 2024).
SAMHSA. 2024a. *Screening, brief intervention, and referral to treatment (SBIRT)*. https://www.samhsa.gov/sbirt (accessed April 30, 2025).
SAMHSA 2024b. *Contact the Office of Tribal Affairs and Policy (OTAP)*. https://www.samhsa.gov/tribal-affairs/contact-otap (accessed December 16, 2024).
SAMHSA 2024c. *Office of Indian Alcohol and Substance Abuse*. https://www.samhsa.gov/tribal-affairs/oiasa (accessed Decmber 16, 2024).
SAMHSA. 2024d. *Support for 988 Tribal Response Cooperative Agreements*. https://www.samhsa.gov/grants/grant-announcements/fg-23-005 (accessed January 1, 2025).
SAMHSA. 2017. *Funding and Characteristics of Single State Agencies for Substance Abuse Services and State Mental Health Agencies, 2015*. HHS Pub. No. (SMA) SMA-17-5029. Rockville, MD: Substance Abuse and Mental Health Services Administration. https://store.samhsa.gov/sites/default/files/sma17-5029.pdf (accessed January 2, 2025).
SAMHSA and IHS (Indian Health Service). 2016. *The national tribal behavioral health agenda*. https://store.samhsa.gov/sites/default/files/pep16-ntbh-agenda.pdf (accessed December 16, 2024).
SAMHSA and IHS (Indian Health Service). 2015. National Tribal Behavioral Health Agenda. https://store.samhsa.gov/product/national-tribal-behavioral-health-agenda/pep16-ntbh-agenda (accessed January 2, 2025).
SFA (Systems for Action). 2023. *Achieving reach in youth behavioral health and wellness through catchment-area community governance*. https://systemsforaction.org/achieving-reach-youth-behavioral-health-and-wellness-through-catchment-area-community-governance (accessed December 13, 2024).
Spoth, R., C. Redmond, C. Shin, M. Greenberg, M. Feinberg, and L. Schainker. 2013. PROSPER community-university partnership delivery system effects on substance misuse through 6 1/2 years past baseline from a cluster randomized controlled intervention trial. *Preventative Medicine* 56(3–4):190–196. https://doi.org/10.1016/j.ypmed.2012.12.013.
Troy, T. 2025. How the White House makes policy. *National Affairs* 62(Winter). https://www.nationalaffairs.com/publications/detail/how-the-white-house-makes-policy (accessed April 30, 2025).
Tsai, J. 2024. Beyond the usual players: Evidence-building priorities for behavioral health among all U.S. federal agencies. *Administration and Policy in Mental Health* 51(1):14–16. https://doi.org/10.1007/s10488-023-01313-7.
USDA (U.S. Department of Agriculture). n.d. *U.S. Department of Agriculture—learning agenda*. https://www.usda.gov/sites/default/files/documents/usda-learning-agenda.pdf (accessed January 2, 2025).
Wandersman, A., V. H. Chien, and J. Katz. 2012. Toward an evidence-based system for innovation support for implementing innovations with quality: Tools, training, technical assistance, and quality assurance/quality improvement. *American Journal of Community Psychology* 50(3–4):445–459. https://doi.org/10.1007/s10464-012-9509-7.

Wandersman, A., J. Duffy, P. Flaspohler, R. Noonan, K. Lubell, L. Stillman, M. Blachman, R. Dunville, and J. Saul. 2008. Bridging the gap between prevention research and practice: The interactive systems framework for dissemination and implementation. *American Journal of Community Psychology* 41(3–4):171–181. https://doi.org/10.1007/s10464-008-9174-z.

Weinstein, P. 2008. White House Policy Councils. In *Getting It Done: A Guide for Government Executives*. Lanham, MD: Rowman & Littlefield Publishers, Inc. https://www.businessofgovernment.org/sites/default/files/Getting%20It%20Done.pdf (accessed January 13, 2025).

WHO (World Health Organization). 2021. *Guidance for health information system governance*. Copenhagen. https://iris.who.int/bitstream/handle/10665/342572/WHO-EURO-2021-1999-41754-57182-eng.pdf? (accessed December 13, 2024).

Willison, E. C., M. P. Singer, and L. K. Grazier. 2021. Double-edged sword of federalism: Variation in essential health benefits for mental health and substance use disorder coverage in states. *Health Economics, Policy and Law* 16(2):170–182. https://doi.org/10.1017/S1744133119000306.

6

Funding for Prevention of Mental, Emotional, and Behavioral (MEB) Disorders

To date, approaches to addressing mental, emotional, and behavioral (MEB) health and well-being in society have focused on providing clinical services to individuals rather than focusing on factors that promote positive mental, emotional, and behavioral health outcomes. This is reflected in the U.S. funding landscape for behavioral health (BH), where a modest number of preventive services delivered in health care settings are sometimes reimbursable by insurers, while the majority of preventive interventions delivered in communities (e.g., schools, community centers, human services settings) is supported by a patchwork of federal grants, state and local funding, and smaller amounts of private-sector support. Better and more sustainable funding for prevention of MEB disorders could lead to better outcomes (e.g., healthy MEB development in children, prevention of some mental illnesses, of suicide, and of substance use disorders), help lessen the need for treatment and recovery services, and reduce the societal and economic cost of these disorders. As an example, investing $1 in the Good Behavior Game school-based, teacher-delivered intervention returns $64 dollars in benefits (WSIPP, 2024a). Benefits of investing in children through evidence-based interventions may include gained lifetime earnings, averted involvement with the juvenile criminal legal system, and saved health care costs (PTTC, 2024). Most compelling, research on the adolescent brain shows its greater vulnerability to the negative effects of substance use (nicotine, alcohol, and drugs) and greater likelihood of long-term consequences (Hsiung et al., 2022). This underscores the importance of primary prevention (i.e., before any symptoms of MEB disorders).

The sources of funding for MEB health are siloed between mental health (MH) and substance use disorders (SUDs) spread out across multiple agencies and not well coordinated (especially for MH, which has no central point of federal coordination). Chapter 5 highlights the array of agencies that support MEB health research and services, with separate units in the Substance Abuse and Mental Health Services Administration (SAMHSA) providing support to address SUDs or MH. Similarly, most BH funding sources are focused on treatment and recovery rather than prevention. The status quo must be changed because the need to prevent MEB disorders is substantial and growing. Sustained investment and enhanced coordination to lessen the administrative burdens on federal grant recipients (e.g., state BH agencies) are needed to build and maintain the other components of the infrastructure described in this report. For example, coordination among different funders of school-based prevention services—including SAMHSA, Centers for Disease Control and Prevention (CDC), Health Resources and Services Administration (HRSA), and Centers for Medicare & Medicaid Services (CMS)—could lead to aligning and simplifying performance measurement, reporting, and other requirements (see for example Brown et al., 2019). The gap between research and practice, especially with a focus on improving outcomes for underserved communities or groups and enhanced implementation support, as discussed in Chapter 2, also requires a much higher level of funding commitments.

This chapter provides an overview of the funding available to prevent MEB disorders, drawing in part on a comprehensive review of primarily federal funding sources developed by a consultant and provided in Appendix C. The funding approaches discussed would largely support and scale universal (i.e., directed at the entire population) policies and programs—those that have a broad reach and are intended to reduce risks and strengthen protective factors widely (see for example PTTC Network, 2024; Stelmach et al., 2022). Some of these may be more cost effective (i.e., lower cost for equivalent greater gains) than treating a diagnosed disorder, but the benefits associated with prevention go beyond health care savings and include economic productivity and improved quality of life. There are also cost-effective selective interventions—targeted at families of or directly at children with behavioral problems (McDaid et al., 2019). Funding is also needed to support all aspects of their implementation, and ensure necessary resources for workforce, data systems, governance and partnerships.

The chapter also discusses economic analyses of MEB disorder prevention, describes the range of funding needs and gaps relevant to the various components of the prevention infrastructure, and identifies potential sources to generate sustainable funding for it.

VALUE OF PREVENTION IN BEHAVIORAL HEALTH

Usually, no one knows that a problem was averted because of a preventive service. Undervaluing of prevention may explain in part why the Prevention and Public Health Fund established by a provision of the 2010 Affordable Care Act (ACA) has not been spent as intended, but used for nonprevention and non-public health purposes (CRS, 2024; Fraser, 2019). The underfunding of the nation's public health infrastructure has been detailed in reports from the National Academies and others (IOM, 2012; TFAH, 2024). In general, the funding devoted to prevention and population health improvement efforts, including promoting BH, has been estimated at approximately a few cents per dollar spent on treatment (Martin et al., 2023[1]), e.g., just under 5 percent of health spending reflected in the 2022 National Health Expenditure Accounts (CMS, 2024-b).

It is well established that population-based prevention of chronic health conditions is cost effective in broad terms and can even yield positive return on investment (ROI) (TFAH, 2017). Despite a robust evidence base for the effectiveness of preventive interventions in BH, evaluation of their *economic impact* is more limited and generally uses measures different from those in other areas of health care and public health (Kaplan et al., 2019; WSIPP, 2024b; The Pew Charitable Trust, 2024). Benefits of applying cost-effectiveness analysis and ROI studies to BH interventions include expanding funding sources, encouraging reimbursement by third-party payors, and spurring new funding opportunities. Cost-utility analysis (CUA)—which compares the incremental cost of a program to the incremental value in terms of quality adjusted life years—is uniquely well suited to comparing approaches as varied as school-based, clinical care, and social determinants of health (SDOH) interventions. Chapter 7 provides a broad discussion of social and economic policies that shape trajectories toward BH disorders (macrolevel interventions), and Chapter 2 discusses the evidence for interventions at the individual, family, and community levels. CUA permits comparing investments in a wide range of interventions to guide public policy.

Both programs and policies can provide ROI, making the case for the value of investing in prevention broadly and prevention of MEB disorders in particular (Le et al., 2021). Moreover, investing with health equity in mind is needed, given the economic cost of racial and ethnic health disparities. LaVeist and colleagues estimated the cost of health disparities in 2018 to be $451 billion (using Behavioral Risk Factors Surveillance System data) or $421 billion (using Medical Expenditure Panel Survey data) (LaVeist et al., 2023).

---

[1] $187.6 billion in public health activity is just over 3.6 percent of the $4,255 trillion national health expenditure (Martin et al., 2023).

A systematic review of economic analyses of BH interventions along the life course found that school-based screening plus psychological interventions, such as cognitive behavioral therapy, were highly cost effective at preventing MEB disorders in children and adolescents, and parenting and workplace interventions were effective for adults (Le et al., 2021). School-based substance use prevention programming also has considerable evidence of cost effectiveness. For example, LifeSkills Training had an ROI of $21 for every $1 spent delivering it (Miller, 2012). Expanded diagnosis and treatment of depression returns $7 for every $1 invested (Miller, 2012). Clear interconnected benefits are yielded by investing in prevention with a public health focus: improving health and well-being, preventing onset of mental illness and substance use (and the associated suffering and loss of human potential), and saving resources. More economic analyses are needed to inform investments in protective factors that support MEB health.

One challenge with public- and private-sector investments is that savings from investing in proven interventions in one domain may accrue to a different sector or agency—the wrong pockets problem—but there are potential solutions (see Box 6-1).

FEDERAL FUNDING FOR PREVENTION OF MEB DISORDERS

Most federal prevention funding for MEB disorders comes from the Department of Health and Human Services (HHS), primarily in SAMHSA and Centers for Disease Control and Prevention (CDC). It is harder to identify the funding available for preventing MH disorders compared to that for substance use prevention. Some reasons for this asymmetry are discussed in Chapter 5 (Governance and Partnerships): unlike MH, substance use has a central point of coordination in the White House Office of National Drug Control Policy (ONDCP). Moreover, it is far easier to define, characterize, test for, and measure substance use. The line between normal and pathological in the MH domain is less clear-cut and can be viewed as a continuum from mental emotional well-being to mental illness, thus complicating identification of the relevant programs and interventions and the funding available for them (see Appendix C for further discussion). The committee worked with a consultant to gain a clearer understanding of federal government spending on MH and SUD—both treatment and prevention.

Appendix C provides calculations that show the federal amounts spent on MH ($2.7 billion) and SUD ($1.8 billion) prevention. Also, it is likely that private-sector funding for MH and SUD prevention is small—likely from philanthropic sources. For context, total U.S. spending across the health care sector, public and private, on BH treatment tripled between 2000 and 2021, from $40 billion to $140 billion according to the Bureau of

> **BOX 6-1**
> **Solving the Wrong Pockets Problem**
>
> A challenge of successfully implementing prevention programs is that it may yield its savings in a different domain—this is known as the "wrong pockets" problem. For example, very often, the government agency that invests in a preventive intervention is not the one that reaps the benefit in the form of saved money and lives, or lower costs for a specific service or need.
>
> Butler (2018) has outlined four potential solutions to the wrong pockets problem, beginning with more research on return on investment and a cataloguing of studies for use by state and local government.
>
> Second, there are strategies to break down budgetary silos in government agencies. For example, Butler (2018) found that two-thirds of states had children's cabinets, and many counties had local management boards that could support braiding and blending of funding to allow more flexibility.
>
> The third strategy is to integrate all the pockets in one budget process, such as by having hospitals or clinics respond to health-related social needs in house—and bringing that spending into their business model (e.g., as made possible by capitated payment models that incentivize keeping patients healthy by addressing a wide range of nonmedical needs).
>
> Fourth, Butler (2018) suggested creating and testing "new organizational models that would mitigate the wrong pocket problem by creating procedures for the costs and benefits of cross-sector collaboration to be identified and built into decision making" (Butler, 2018). One such example is Collaborative Approach to Public Goods Investing, which provides a mechanism for stakeholders to invest in a service from which they stand to benefit (with facilitation by a trusted intermediary) (Nichols, 2020; Taylor and Nichols, 2024).

Economic Analysis (BEA, 2021).[2,3] Although the Bureau of Economic Analysis data[4] are not broken down by public and private sources, SAMHSA

---

[2] See here for a more detailed discussion of how the BEA Blended Account data in the Health Care Satellite Account are gathered: https://apps.bea.gov/scb/pdf/2015/01%20January/0115_bea_health_care_satellite_account.pdf (Dunn, Rittmeuller, and Whitmire, 2015).

[3] Note that the Bureau of Economic Analysis uses a different methodology from that used by SAMHSA (2019) in its Behavioral Health Spending and Use Accounts (Dunn, A., personal communication, December 11, 2024). The estimate for total behavioral health spending in 2015 provided in the SAMHSA report was $212 billion.

[4] See Bureau of Economic Analysis data visualization for "mental disorders," including mood disorders, anxiety disorders, alcohol-related disorders, substance-related conditions, and other disorders: https://apps.bea.gov/data/special-topics/health-care/viz/diseases/ (accessed January 2, 2025).

TABLE 6-1 SAMHSA Breakdown of Spending on Treatment Services for Substance Use Disorders and Mental Health in 2015

Treatment of	Out of pocket	Medicaid	Medicare	Private Insurance	Other Private	Other Federal	Other State and Local
SUD	10%	25%	<5%	29%	5%	11%	17%
MH	11%	24%	16%	28%	4%	5%	12%

SOURCE: SAMHSA, 2019.

did include such breakdowns in their calculations for 2015 (the last year for which SAMHSA seems to have provided behavioral health spending and use accounts). (See Table 6-1 for an overview of the total spending on treatment services in 2015.)

The 2023 drug control budget overseen by ONDCP indicates that $21.6 billion and $2.7 billion went to SUD treatment and prevention, respectively (other spending is largely on interdiction and law enforcement) (ONDCP, 2023). However, the committee was unable to identify equivalent figures for the federal portion of spending on MH treatment and prevention, as discussed in more detail in Appendix C.

Appendix C shows that when setting aside prevention research funding and Department of Defense drug interdiction activities from the $2.7 billion above, approximately $1.8 billion (6 percent) of the ONDCP budget was devoted to substance use prevention, with roughly four-fifths allocated to SAMHSA and CDC and one-fifth for SUD prevention programs delivered by the Departments of Defense, Education, Interior (Bureau of Indian Affairs), Justice (e.g., Bureau of Prisons), Labor (e.g., Office of Workers' Compensation Programs), and Transportation (Appendix C). For federal-level prevention of MH disorders in 2023, Appendix C provides an estimate of $2.7 billion.

Substance Abuse and Mental Health Services Administration

SAMHSA provides both nondiscretionary (e.g., its two block grants—the Substance Use Prevention, Treatment, and Recovery Services Block Grant (SUBG) and Community Mental Health Services Block Grant (MHSBG)—which allocate funding to states according to a formula), and discretionary funding through a variety of grants for MH, substance use treatment, and SUD prevention programs (e.g., Strategic Prevention Framework—Partnerships for Success, Tribal Behavioral Health).

SAMHSA's total funding in 2023 was $7.5 billion, and Appendix C estimates that $638 million of that was devoted to SUD prevention—composed of the $236 million for the Center for Substance Abuse Prevention (CSAP) and the required 20 percent prevention set-aside from the SUBG administered by the Center for Substance Abuse Treatment in collaboration with CSAP. Notably, CSAP funding rose from $200 million in 2009 to only $236 million in 2023, not even keeping up with inflation, let alone meeting the need for adequate and sustained support for prevention efforts in communities.

The funding for prevention of mental disorders is more difficult to calculate for the reasons noted; the committee's estimate, based on Appendix C, is $912 million, although $617 million is devoted to suicide prevention, so only $395 million is available to fund (primary) preventive interventions. The SAMHSA Mental Health Services Block Grant is solely devoted to funding treatment for serious mental illness. Calls for creating a set-aside for prevention out of the MHBG have been made in the 2019 NASEM report, and in the 2024 Early Action and Responsiveness Lifts Youth (EARLY) Minds Act[5] introduced by Representative August Pfluger of Texas calling for a 5 percent set-aside from the Mental Health Services Block Grant to fund prevention and early intervention for children and youth.

Centers for Disease Control and Prevention

"CDC does not have a single enabling statute that defines its overall mission and structure" (CRS, 2023, p. 1). Because many CDC programs are based in general authorities, Congress often uses the appropriations process to fund CDC's programs and would therefore be in a position to direct more funding to BH prevention through the appropriation process.

Trust for America's Health (TFAH) has called for increases to CDC's FY 2025 budget for programs important to promoting MEB health (TFAH, 2024):

- Division of Adolescent and School Health (DASH): increase from $57 million to $100 million
- Suicide Prevention: increase from $30 million to $80 million
- Adverse Childhood Experiences (ACEs): increase from $9 million to $33 million

DASH supports the implementation of school-based programs to improve parent engagement and increase access to health services, but DASH programs only reached 7 percent of middle and high school students in 2022 (TFAH, 2024). Suicide prevention efforts target the highest levels of suicide since 1941 (49,000 deaths in 2022), but funding did not increase from 2023 and the Comprehensive Suicide Prevention program needs to

---

[5] *EARLY Minds Act*, HR 7808, 118th Congress, 2nd sess., (March 22, 2024).

be strengthened to achieve intended reductions in suicide and in suicide attempts "among populations that are disproportionately affected by suicide, including veterans and rural communities" (TFAH, 2024, p. 38). Increasing the investment in prevention and mitigation of ACEs would contribute to preventing 21 million cases of depression and would enable the program's expansion to 30 new states, territories, tribes, and localities (TFAH, 2024).

Other called-for increases would also benefit prevention of SUD and mental disorders, including increases to the public health infrastructure and capacity, public health data modernization, social determinants of health (from $6 million to $100 million), and Racial and Ethnic Approaches to Community Health and Healthy Tribes (from $69 to $103 million) (TFAH, 2024).

The TFAH report also underscored the importance of the Prevention and Public Health Fund to CDC's budget (13 percent of CDC's budget comes from the Prevention Fund) with a smaller outlay for SAMHSA. But the fund's resources have been halved from the original $2 billion per year, and also directed to nonprevention purposes, such as offsetting a cut in Medicare physicians' payments and cutting $3.5 billion over 7 years to pay for the 21st Century Cures Act (APHA, n.d.).

Administrations for Children and Families and for Community Living

The Older Americans Act funds agencies, such as area agencies on aging, through the Administration for Community Living (ACL), that can directly provide or purchase BH services for their clients under Title III-D (Disease Prevention and Health Promotion). Recipients of Title III-D funding are required to implement evidence-based programs (EBPs) to address chronic disease and diabetes management, BH, and falls prevention (which can avert injuries that can contribute to poor MH outcomes) (Benson, 2024). The funding level for ACL was $2.76 billion in FY 2024, which, if divided by the 11.4 million people served, amounts to less than $240 per person. It is not sufficient to fund training, supervision, and support of lay MH workers interacting with older adults or support eliminating digital obstacles by enabling computer or tablet ownership and an Internet subscription. ACL employs 30,000 staff and works with hundreds of thousands of volunteers, many of whom are family caregivers.

The Administration for Children and Families (ACF), whose overall budget is $70 billion, oversees a considerable portion of the $2.7 billion federal government MH investment (not including Centers for Medicare & Medicaid Services CMS)—$1.126 billion for the prevention of child maltreatment (ACF, 2023; see Appendix C). But this funding is inadequate in the face of an ongoing workforce crisis in children's services systems— low pay and high stress lead to high turnover, and the pandemic has considerably exacerbated these challenges (Quality Improvement Center for Workforce Development, 2022; DiLorenzo and Lukich, 2020). Stressed and overworked providers may be less able to support the MEB health needs of children in the system.

Other Federal Funding

In 1999, the federal government began to provide funding under the Safe and Drug Free Schools and Communities program for drug prevention and school safety program coordinators, a specific category of prevention workers focused on middle schools; funding ended in FY 2004 (NCES, 2024). Per Appendix C, school-based prevention efforts are funded by a mix of Medicaid, block grants, such as the Title V Maternal and Child Health (HRSA), Social Services Block Grant (ACF), and Preventive Health and Health Services Block Grant (CDC), SAMHSA's Project Advancing Wellness and Resilience Education, and the U.S. Department of Education Project Prevent. Recent legislation, including the American Rescue Plan Act and Bipartisan Safer Communities Act, provided funding to support and expand MH services in schools. Even so, over half of U.S. schools report that they experience staffing and funding constraints in responding to the MH needs of students (NCES, 2024).

School-based MH services can facilitate early identification and treatment of MH issues in a safe environment. It can also increase access for underserved populations, particularly children from low-income and minoritized communities. The 2022 Bipartisan Safer Communities Act[6] allocated $500 million each for the School-Based Mental Health Services Grant (SBMH) Program and Mental Health Services Professional (MHSP) Demonstration Grant Program to increase the number of MH providers in schools and the necessary training for them.

In FY 2022 and 2023, the Department of Education provided $255 million to 264 grantees for the SBMH and MHSP programs, which were expected to help communities hire approximately 5,400 school-based MH professionals and train an estimated 5,500 more, doubling the workforce of social workers, counselors, and other MH providers (ONDCP, 2024). The pandemic-era and post-pandemic increases in funding are temporary, however, and the enhanced programming and workforce will not be sustained if funding declines to earlier levels, especially if the decline is precipitous and does not allow state and local health and education agencies to secure long-term funding.

Given the public health burden of BH disorders on the lives of individuals and their families and, more broadly, on the nation's productivity, the committee finds that adequate, stable, and sustained funding for the

---

[6] Bipartisan Safer Communities Act, Public Law 117-159, 117th Cong. (June 25, 2022).

prevention infrastructure is needed, while preserving current levels of funding for treatment and recovery and adapting to follow the data.

> CONCLUSION 6-1: *Descriptions of major programs pair the words "prevention" and "treatment," suggesting that prevention funding is more robust than it is. Also, additional research on funding needs for the prevention of MEB disorders could better inform funding decisions. Most of the funding for behavioral health services is currently directed toward treatment and addressing the opioid crisis; more is needed to support primary prevention.*

It is critical to invest now in explicit prevention of acute and chronic MEB disorders; to stem the current crisis in behavioral health; and to strategically build and fund current and future infrastructure for governance, operations, workforce development, capital improvements and growth, standby capacity, and development and implementation of policies and programs targeted for general and special populations. It is imperative to seek federal funding and mobilize partners in government to move quickly, collaborate, marshal resources, permit regulatory flexibility, and expedite creative solutions. As noted earlier, expenditures may not reflect cost of actual or potential delivery of preventive initiatives or cross-agency collaboration that may be underappreciated for the complexity of their implementation and the full scope of the value they return.

Estimates of total federal expenditures for MEB prevention in this report are a compilation of expenditures reported by publicly available funding sources. In the committee's view, the available information on funding and its use in MEB disorder prevention is fragmented, uneven, and incomplete. However, what is known indicates there are important unmet needs and gaps in funding. As seen in Appendix C, the contributions over time for individual programs and initiatives in different HHS agencies vary in absolute and relative amounts, over time, and are dependent themselves on financial resources available for reporting and data integrity. They are often unrelated to prior expenditures and are seldom adjusted for inflation measures, population characteristics, or need. Precision in funding estimates can be compromised by the number of sources of data, methods of collection, standardization of measures, and intensity of oversight of validity over time.

Given the public health burden and economic costs of MEB disorders and the importance of preventing them, the federal government could approach the problem in a transformative manner or a more incremental manner.

Increasing funding for prevention could be focused on the four agencies that provide the most support for prevention of MEB disorders: Administration for Children and Families (ACF), CDC, HRSA, and SAMHSA. More dependable funding could support implementation of evidence-based programs (EBPs) and technical assistance from pre-implementation to sustainment as described in Chapter 2. More funding could also help strengthen the workforce as discussed in Chapter 3, facilitate greater access to and work with data to inform prevention work and show improved outcomes, as outlined in Chapter 4, and nurture greater coordination and collaboration through governance and partnerships at the state, tribal, and local levels discussed in Chapter 5. But improved governance is also a tool for better coordination, less fragmentation, and greater efficiency—which illustrates a feedback loop, or even a virtuous cycle, between governance and funding (two "gears" in the infrastructure graphic provided in Figure 1-1).

A substantial, transformative investment across federal agencies delivering preventive services to children and youth (up to 18 years old) would include but would not be limited to ACF, CDC, HRSA, and SAMHSA. Why the focus on children? The onset for more than half of mental health conditions is before age 18 (Solmi et al., 2022). Also, intervening in early life offers the best opportunities for prevention and associated benefits (NASEM, 2019). The cost of mental health treatment in children has been estimated at approximately $4,361 (Loo et al., 2024). The public health and prevention portion of the 2021 National Health Expenditure Accounts (all health care spending) is approximately 5 percent (Martin et al., 2023). Five percent of $4,361 is $218 per individual. If $218 were spent on each of 73.2 million U.S. children 10 to 18 years old for a package of interventions that met their needs (from Nurse Family Partnership to family and school-based interventions), that would cost approximately $14 billion in new funding. This is a large investment but is potentially transformative given the evidence about intervening in early life on risk factors for MEB disorders. Such a commitment could ensure that every child in every community receives the package of interventions needed to address risk factors and support positive trajectories to MEB health.

Given the current challenging fiscal environment, the federal government could also consider funding increases that are more modest, such as inflation-adjusting specific funding streams, increasing the main sources of prevention funding in HHS. At a more modest level, providing a new additional outlay of $1.8 billion to the four key federal agencies responsible for prevention of MEB disorders includes adjusting for inflation for specific ACF and SAMHSA programs, and expanding the capacity of specific programs in CDC and HRSA. As shown in Appendix F, this amounts to a 40 percent increase from $4.57 billion to $6.37 billion. New funding would allow greater capacity of service delivery in settings across the life course, from preconception through older adulthood.

RECOMMENDATION 6-1: To secure adequate, sustainable, and locally responsive funding for the mental, emotional, and behavioral (MEB)

disorder prevention infrastructure, Congress should consider a range of funding options that include:
a. Providing $14 billion in new funding to the Department of Health and Human Services for interventions on early life risk factors for MEB disorders for all children birth to 18 years old.
b. At a time of funding constraints, providing $1.8 billion in new funding to the Administration for Children and Families, Centers for Disease Control and Prevention, Health Resources and Services Administration, and Substance Abuse and Mental Health Services Administration would help to increase capacity for MEB disorder prevention.

Detailed calculations describing each of the options above are provided in Appendix F. Some of the increases above can be achieved partly by restoring the Prevention and Public Health Fund to its original amount of $2 billion per year (it was $1.3 billion for 2024 (TFAH, 2024]) to support SAMHSA and CDC prevention programs.

Centers for Medicare and Medicaid Services

CMS is the nation's largest payer and a key source of reimbursement for BH services (CMS, 2024c). It has long provided opportunities for states and providers to innovate. This includes a wide range of 1115 Medicaid waivers (referring to the authorizing section of the Social Security Act, the enabling statute for Medicaid and Medicare) that allow states to test novel approaches, and the work of the Center for Medicare and Medicaid Innovation (CMS, 2024a), which develops population health and alternative payment models (CMS, n.d.-a; CMS, 2024a; KFF, 2024). In April 2024, the Innovation Center issued a new Behavioral Health Strategy, which "focuses on three key areas: 1) substance use disorders prevention, treatment and recovery services, 2) ensuring effective pain treatment and management, and 3) improving mental health care and services" (CMS, n.d.-a.).

However, primary prevention, especially given the population-level interventions that are required, is generally not reimbursable by Medicaid (screening is one exception). One speaker noted at one of the committee's public meetings that universal prevention, which is population-, not individual-, based, is routinely funded with appropriated dollars through SAMHSA block grants or through discretionary funding mechanisms. Thau (2024) added that universal prevention is not part of the medical care paradigm, and thus it generally has no diagnostic or billing codes and does not qualify for fee-for-service payment.

Screening is an important universal prevention strategy. The U.S. Preventive Services Task Force recommends screening adults for behavioral disorders—depression, alcohol abuse, and drug abuse—in primary care settings. However, screening rates are low, perhaps due to lack of financing for behavioral health and inadequate behavioral health infrastructure for referral and follow up (NASEM, 2021; Mulvaney-Day et al, 2018; USPSTF, 2024). There is evidence that value-based payment reform has a positive association with improved behavioral health outcomes (e.g., reduced emergency department visits). Integrating screening in all value-based purchasing programs under Medicare and Medicaid could further prevention goals and also could serve as a health care quality metric.

Medicaid reimbursement is used for prevention services in clinical and other settings, including schools, but challenges include obtaining billable codes and securing enhanced reimbursement for group counseling. Medicaid and the Children's Health Insurance Program play an important role in supporting BH services by reimbursing providers, but, as discussed in Appendix C, federal and state regulatory constraints on how Medicaid funds can be used affect application to a broader range of prevention activities. However, recent or emerging models exist for expanding the ability to use Medicaid to support primary prevention in community settings:

- Interventions to prevent the onset of diabetes occurred in clinical settings between patients and their health care providers, but in 2008, a research study demonstrated that the YMCA was a "promising channel" for delivering the evidence-based Diabetes Prevention Program (DPP) in group settings (Ackermann, 2008). Over the decade that followed, CDC developed the National DPP program, and further evidence emerged. Implementation was rolled out with several organizations delivering the interventions with CDC or state Medicaid funding (e.g., Montana and Minnesota). In 2018, CMS began covering the DPP program under Medicare.
- A second example of prevention services delivered in a group format, and with Medicaid reimbursement, is group prenatal care. Centering Pregnancy is the best-known and most extensively studied model (Liu et al., 2021; Rising, 1998), and eight states provide enhanced reimbursement (to cover more than just per-participant reimbursement and include provider preparation, etc.) for the group sessions. The EleVATE program (Washington University in St. Louis, Missouri) was successful in securing reimbursement for group prenatal care that incorporates trauma-informed care and BH services (Cohen Marill, 2022).

Barriers to obtaining Medicaid reimbursement for BH services have been described as a persistent issue in the field that contributes to access challenges (providers unavailable because of reimbursement issues). For example, one study found that some providers listed in Medicaid directories had not seen any Medicaid patients in the previous year. Thus, including them in the directories may have given an inaccurate picture of provider availability (Giliberti, 2023).

Schools are one kind of community-based, non-health care setting of great importance to the infrastructure for delivering BH prevention (Panchal and Guth, 2023). In many states, school settings are a main site for primary prevention and participate in Medicaid for specific preventive services, including MH and BH services, primary care, and screenings. Federal Medicaid funding supports BH services in schools under the Individuals with Disabilities Education Act (IDEA) and for children who are Medicaid or Children's Health Insurance Program beneficiaries, but only 16 states have Medicaid plans that allow reimbursement for Medicaid-eligible students in addition to those who qualify under IDEA (ED, 2024). School-based health centers (SBHCs) can play an important role in delivering BH services to children, but they only reach approximately 8 percent of students, and funding is a persistent challenge (Haeder, 2021; Heinrich et al., 2023). The Guide to Community Preventive Services recommends SBHCs as a strategy to improve child health (including reducing health risk behaviors) and school performance in low-income communities (Community Guide, 2015).

Medicaid Reimbursement for Health-Related Social Needs (HRSNs)

Over the past decade, CMS and private-sector payers and health care organizations have come to recognize that nonmedical factors, such as housing and food security, play important roles in shaping health status (Tsega et al., 2019) and have begun to explore financing strategies to cover related services and providers. CMS under both Medicare and Medicaid has developed models for providing reimbursement or other types of financing for services that address beneficiaries' nonmedical needs, such as housing, food, and transportation.

Medicaid funding is available for both the point of care (reimbursement for secondary prevention, e.g., screening) and, more recently, HRSNs, such as assistance with finding housing (MACPAC, 2021). In 2017, CMS put forward a tool for screening for HRSNs, including housing, transportation, and exposure to interpersonal violence. The lens on the latter has widened to include community violence, in recognition of the fact that Medicaid is the largest payer for firearm-related injuries that create lifelong "medical and psychological complications" as discussed in Chapter 7 (CMS, n.d.-b; CHCS, 2023). In 2024, California, Colorado, Connecticut, Illinois, Maryland, New York, and Oregon allowed Medicaid to reimburse for violence prevention services (Barna, 2024). New York enacted legislation directing the state Department of Health to apply to the federal government for including community violence prevention among the services available to Medicaid beneficiaries.[7] The program would train violence prevention specialists and require training and certification in violence prevention through the state department of health.

There are arrangements under capitation or value-based purchasing where a community-based organization (CBO) works with a health care provider to support meeting a health or health care target by meeting an HRSN (e.g., enrolling person for Supplemental Nutrition Assistance Program, supporting a meal plan to control blood sugar). Medicaid can be said to indirectly pay for linkage (e.g., help with finding housing), although such a claim may be more difficult to file and have reimbursed.

CMS increasingly targets adverse social conditions (e.g., housing instability, homelessness, nutrition insecurity) that contribute to poor health (Hinton and Diana, 2024). Because fee-for-service arrangements do not permit federal Medicaid funds to pay the direct costs of nonmedical services, billing flexibility is needed. Movement away from these restrictions is evident: "The U.S. Playbook to Address Social Determinants of Health" proposed, as "Pillar 2" to "Support Flexible Funding for Social Needs" through Medicare and Medicaid (DPC and ONDCP, 2023).

Opportunities to fund HRSNs include state Medicaid programs using existing "state plan and waiver authorities (e.g., 1905(a), 1915(i), 1915(c), or Section 1115) to add certain non-clinical services to the Medicaid benefit package" (Hinton and Diana, 2024). CMS has approved 1115 waiver demonstrations focusing on flexible funding in seven states.

Another route to addressing HRSNs is through Medicaid managed care federal authorities (Hinton, 2024). This opportunity could reach many beneficiaries: more than 70 percent of beneficiaries have their benefit administered through Managed Care organizations (MCOs) providing comprehensive, risk-based managed care (KFF, 2021).

Through "in-lieu-of" authority, Medicaid MCOs can be given flexibility to pay for nonmedical services: services or settings when they act as substitutes for standard Medicaid benefits (Hinton and Diana, 2024). Recent CMS guidance clarifies that Medicaid MCOs can, within certain guidelines, pay for housing, nutrition support and certain other HRSN services as substitutes for standard Medicaid benefits (CMS, 2023).

Federal rules allow Medicaid MCOs to pay for nonmedical services when these are designated as "value added." Value-added services are provided voluntarily outside of covered contract services and paid for from

---

[7] New York State Senate Bill S580, 2023-2024 Legislative Session. Relates to the provision of and payment for violence prevention programs. https://www.nysenate.gov/legislation/bills/2023/S580/amendment/A (accessed February 28, 2025).

contract administrative funds; however, they are sometimes counted in the MCO's favor in calculating its "medical loss ratio" (Hinton and Diana, 2024).

MCO contracts can call for HRSN-related performance targets, with incentive payments for investments made in support of meeting these targets. For example, some states provide incentive payments for HRSN screening and establishing partnerships to ensure beneficiaries receive housing or other needed services. Incentive payments can be included in capitated rates, allowing MCOs to receive additional funding to address HRSNs (Hinton and Diana, 2024).

As MCOs contract with provider organizations, many negotiate flexible financing of value-based care that encourages addressing HRSNs to overcome barriers to effective delivery. About one-quarter of state Medicaid programs contract with Accountable Care Organizations (ACOs), long popular with Medicare as a delivery model (Kaufman et al., 2019).

ACOs are provider and health organization networks with shared responsibility to care for a defined population meeting agreed quality-of-care standards. Financing is incentive based, and this encourages addressing HRSNs as part of care meeting spending targets or within capitation rates (Rosenthal et al., 2023). Spending is flexible and can address HRSNs. Preliminary evidence indicates that 85 percent of ACOs report addressing some form of HRSNs (Niles et al., 2019).

These options exist within a wider push toward flexible financing. Through its Innovation Center, CMS has sought development of models reorienting Medicare and Medicaid payment from fee-for-service billing to pay for achieving mutually agreed-upon performance objectives even when attained by activities beyond office-based clinical practice (CMS, 2024a). The center has launched over 50 model tests between 2018–2020, reaching hundreds of thousands of providers and covering millions of patients. Its objectives call for, by 2030, all Medicare Part A and B beneficiaries to be cared for in a relationship defined by accountability, quality, and total cost rather than traditional billing practices.

Reimbursement for Different Types of Community Workers

CMS reimburses providers, including non-licensed, non-master's-level SUD service providers (peers, counselors, etc.), to deliver group BH therapy and counseling, and there is a Medicaid reimbursement category for "Behavioral health prevention education" (H0025) (NASHP, 2019). However, it is unclear what proportion of the services these workers provide could be classified as primary or secondary prevention.

Options for reimbursement of community health worker (CHW) services—and potentially other types of unlicensed workers delivering preventive interventions—could include Section 1115 demonstration waivers (under Medicaid) and payment reform structures, such as bundled payments for episodic or encounter-based payments for conditions. Several states have received approval for reimbursement of CHW services (D'Alessandro et al., 2024).

Alternative payment models

In addition to expanded opportunities for CHW reimbursement, CMS has a history of testing alternative payment models and allowing waivers that test novel approaches for improving outcomes. States' experiences with 1115 waivers offers several examples of experimentation relevant to both population-based prevention and universal approaches that lead to improvements for non-Medicaid beneficiaries:

- In 2015, CMMI approved an 1115 waiver for Texas, and the San Antonio Metropolitan Health District partnered with health care entities and nonprofit organizations to invest in population-level changes that supported health, including built environment interventions (Schlenker and Huber, 2015).
- The Maryland Total Cost of Care 1115 waiver included "population health credits" the state could earn based on total population health improvements anticipated to save Medicare dollars, and measures included diabetes incidence in all Marylanders aged 45 years and older (HSCRC, 2017).
- North Carolina's program, NCCARE 360, paid for infrastructure for screening and referral for HRSNs that is available to everyone, not just Medicaid beneficiaries (NCCARE360, 2024).

Medicaid reimbursement is a crucial source of funding for BH services, but there are barriers related to staffing, setting, benefits, and eligibility. Specifically, some types of workers, community settings, and population-level preventive interventions are difficult or impossible to pay with Medicaid dollars. Medicaid does not pay for population-level preventive interventions, such as public health communication campaigns. However, Medicaid amendments, authorities, flexibilities, and waivers offer opportunities for greater adaptability and experimentation.

CONCLUSION 6-2: *Interventions to prevent mental, emotional, and behavioral (MEB) disorders and promote MEB health and well-being could be supported through a range of approaches that create more sustainable, coordinated, and adequate funding beginning with greater flexibility and innovation in the use of federal funding.*

RECOMMENDATION 6-2: The committee recommends that the Centers for Medicare & Medicaid Services should

a. Encourage states to use Medicaid 1115 waivers to implement evidence-based approaches for prevention of mental, emotional, and behavioral (MEB) disorders. Potential approaches could focus on school-based strategies and the work of multisector partnerships in other community settings (e.g., accountable communities for health, faith-based, aging services) and that are implementing population-based universal interventions (e.g., environmental change, media campaigns).
b. Prioritize specific quality metrics relevant to prevention of MEB disorders, e.g., screening for alcohol misuse, depression, and anxiety in all value-based purchasing programs under Medicaid and Medicare.
c. Facilitate reimbursement of non-licensed non-clinical MEB prevention workers (e.g., prevention specialists, community health workers) considered qualified to deliver such interventions.

CMS could invest in states to support scale-up of evidence-based programs, similar to the Innovation Accelerator Program (2014) or integrate prevention of behavioral disorders as part of all-payer models that also involve Medicaid state agency buy-in, like the AHEAD (States Advancing All Payer Health Equity Approaches and Development) Model. Notably, CMS already encouraged states to submit waivers that involve billing on the basis of risk rather than diagnosis for MEB prevention in children, and as noted, for the use of CHWs. Also, prevention measures and incentives could focus on true prevention. One potential model is Maryland's Diabetes Incidence Outcomes-Based Credit Methodology,[8] which allows the state to compare its performance averting cases of diabetes and realize an outcomes-based credit.

State and Local Funding

State agencies support a variety of BH prevention activities with state funds and pass-through funding from SAMHSA. States have the ability to reimburse providers for Screening, Brief Intervention, and Referral to Treatment for substance use and alcohol, and in 2023, 38 states did so, in addition to providing reimbursement for other health education and counseling.

A noteworthy example of state funding innovations is found in the prevention of Adverse Childhood Experiences, major risk factors for

---

[8] See https://hscrc.maryland.gov/Documents/Modernization/OBC/Diabetes%20OBC%20Methodology%20Summary%209182019.pdf (accessed December 11, 2024).

BH disorders. States are doing this by braiding or layering funding from multiple sources, sometimes including private-sector support, to implement programming that addresses these risk factors (ASTHO, 2021). For example, South Carolina's Nurse-Family Partnership Pay-for-Success program braids 1915(b) waiver funds with private philanthropic funding (ASTHO, 2021). The funds are safeguarded from changes in leadership by being held in escrow by an external trustee, and if the program is successful in achieving improvements across several outcomes, the state makes success payments to fund further services (Harvard, n.d.). However, recent findings from a study of the relationship between the Nurse-Family Partnership and a composite of adverse birth outcomes found that the program did not lead to improvement in those outcomes, and researchers noted several limitations (e.g., factors that affect pregnancy outcomes may be set in motion well before the intervention). Study is ongoing on other outcomes, but the financial structure in South Carolina is noteworthy for creating a potentially sustainable funding model of performance-based contracts. The literature on pay-for-success (or social impact bond) financing models has shown that the programs that succeed financially are ones that implement a proven intervention (Lantz and Iovan, 2018).

Tax policy offers another conduit to funding prevention more sustainably. Purtle and colleagues (2023) mapped the landscape of state and local funding dedicated to BH and found 207 different policies that illustrate the potential of earmarked taxes to generate sustainable funding for prevention. For example, California's millionaires' tax enacted in 2014 is used to support a range of BH programs, including in the state university and community college systems. The Washington State legislature enacted a law to allow counties to authorize and impose a sales and use tax of one-tenth of one percent "for chemical dependency or mental health treatment services or therapeutic courts."[9] Multiple counties have implemented such a tax. Surveys from California and Washington State have shown broad public support of the taxes, and respondents in California strongly agreed that the tax policy contributed to public awareness of BH and destigmatized the issue (Purtle et al., 2024).

Purtle and colleagues (2022) studied the potential of cannabis taxes and showed how a quarter of revenue in nine states with recreational cannabis excise taxes could be invested in MH, including in mobile psychiatric crisis unit and National Suicide Prevention Lifeline encounters.

As of August 2024, 21 states are collecting cannabis taxes: Alaska, Arizona, California, Colorado, Connecticut, Illinois, Maine, Maryland,

---

[9] Revised Code of Washington §82.14.46 *Sales a use tax for chemical dependency or mental health treatment services or therapeutic courts.* July 12, 2024.

Massachusetts, Michigan, Missouri, Montana, Nevada, New Jersey, New Mexico, New York, Ohio, Oregon, Rhode Island, Vermont, and Washington (Tax Policy Center, 2024). The revenues come from various types of taxation, including excise, sales, retail, and use taxes. In 2021, the first five states to legalize recreational cannabis (Colorado, Washington, Alaska, Oregon, and California) had collectively generated $2.78 billion in revenue from it. States are using the funds from cannabis taxes for traditional government programs, health care, substance abuse and drug education, law enforcement, education, other community needs determined by local jurisdictions (USAFacts, 2023). Purtle and colleagues (2022) noted the general consensus of the appropriateness of earmarking excise tax revenue for purposes that "offset externalities associated with the use of the good or engagement in the activity (i.e., when an individual's use of the good or engagement in the activity produces consequences for others or society)" (p. 1). More recently, Thom (2022) conducted a synthetic control analysis of CDC National Vital Statistics System data to examine how California's tax affected suicide deaths in the state and found beneficial effects on the death rate. Stadnick and colleagues (2024) surveyed officials from some of the 200 cities and counties that have implemented tax policies that earmark revenue for behavioral health services and found that most survey participants (82.7 percent, n = 225) agreed that the revenue provided by the tax increased funding for direct BH/social services and for improvements to BH/social services systems, but findings included concerns about "volatility of funding, inequities in the distribution of tax revenue, and, in some cases, administratively burdensome tax reporting." Purtle and colleagues (2024) compared tax policy implementers from Washington State and California and found broad support of the tax policies for the flexible resources they generated, some concern about design features that made reporting onerous and brought unwanted attention to the work, and also appreciation for other benefits of the tax policy, such as greater public awareness of behavioral health and decreased stigma.

Private-Sector Funding

Philanthropic funding has long played an important role in many aspects of public health and human services, and the philanthropic landscape for BH has grown and become more coordinated in recent years (KP, 2023; Sapatkin, 2024; Center for High Impact Philanthropy, 2020). The Well Being Trust and several partners helped to spark or intensify a movement for addressing the MH and SUD crises, and one of the movement's innovations was the creation of Mindful Philanthropy in 2020 to "catalyze impactful funding in mental health, addiction, and well-being" (Mindful Philanthropy, 2024).

There are numerous examples of the role of philanthropy in behavioral health, including as conveners and facilitators of collaboration. The Texas Behavioral Health Funders Collaborative brings together a variety of philanthropic organizations, including faith-based entities, to support a variety of collaborative efforts such as the South Texas Trauma-Informed Care Consortium, and in system transformation efforts with partners such as the Texas Association of Community Health Centers (MHM, 2020). The funders collaborative has also supported school districts in implementing peer-to-peer suicide prevention programming (CCC, 2023).

The Health Partners health system and community health plan in Minnesota supports school MH through its foundations. For example, the Park Nicollet Foundation has provided funding for grief support programming in 125 schools across 16 school districts and delivered tele-MH therapy to children who lack access to BH care, including teaching skills to manage negative feelings in three school districts (Park Nicollet Foundation, n.d.). Kaiser Permanente has been supporting educators and students in 10 Colorado school districts through its Thriving Schools Resilience in School Environments program to build resilience by integrating social and emotional wellness into the classroom. It provided more than $6 million in grants over the last 6 years and, in 2023, announced $3 million over the following 3 years (KP, 2023). The community-led programming supported by the grants has improved school climates and improved self-reported MH among teachers, staff, and students (KP, 2023).

MEETING THE NEED FOR SUFFICIENT AND SUSTAINABLE FUNDING

What does prevention funding support? In addition to supporting workforce and data components broadly, such as to help state governments implement their plans for prevention, funding is needed for the implementation costs of EBPs. Although it generally flows to the cost of programs or policies, there are associated costs that may not be sufficiently understood and addressed by decision makers. These include costs for initial deployment, the infrastructure to keep things going (implementation support, technical assistance), the workforce for specific programs, and updating the data infrastructure for specific community needs.

The cost of prevention programs, such as Family Check-up, can be a barrier to receiving or delivering services in community settings. Family Check-up costs $4,225 for an initial onsite 2-day training for one trainer and up to six trainees (e.g., a CBO that serves families with young children), and start-up costs are $4,400–6,500 (Blueprints for Healthy Youth Development, n.d.). Implementing the Good Behavior Game in classroom settings has an initial online training cost of $2,545 for up to 30 participants (or $200 each with a live instructor, or a self-paced training for $240 each). Teachers participating in the training must each obtain the Teacher Kit for $320–340. The initial in-person training costs $5,000 for up to 40 participants (IES, 2023).

Unlike with clinical preventive services, such as screening for alcohol or substance use, Medicaid does not reimburse EBPs such as these. That is the case with the vast majority of primary prevention services, whether they are training or other health-promoting interventions delivered to individuals or groups or population-based interventions, such as public health communication campaigns (Community Guide, n.d.).

Communities may receive some funding from SAMHSA through their state BH agency to, for example, support the work of a community coalition and a prevention specialist, but funding is often not available to finance data collection on community needs; the work of researching and selecting an EBP; and its implementation, evaluation, and sustainment. There are several potential ways to make the case for sustainable support for family and community-based primary prevention. Relatedly, payment considerations must include, in addition to the cost of the intervention, the cost of pre-implementation steps and the implementation process (Dopp et al., 2020).

OTHER, NONGOVERNMENTAL FUNDING OPPORTUNITIES

Health systems and hospitals that are tax exempt, which account for 58 percent of U.S. hospitals, are required by law to provide a community benefit commensurate with their tax exemptions (Godwin et al., 2023). These funds are used for a variety of purposes, including training and research, but the $28 billion in federal, state, and local tax exemptions in 2023, for example, did not contribute much to community health improvement efforts (DiGioia, 2022; Godwin et al., 2023). The Internal Revenue Service (IRS) provides guidance and enforces compliance with community benefit rules. Annual monitoring of community benefit spending is done through IRS Schedule H (Form 990). Hospitals failing to comply risk losing their tax-exempt status.

A critique of community benefit spending has been growing in the literature and in policy circles, along with a recognition that hospitals can serve as anchor institutions, such as investing in their local communities and playing an active role in workforce development and creating jobs, contributing to community development efforts (Koh et al., 2020; Healthcare Anchor Network, n.d.). Some hospitals have engaged in innovative and fruitful cross-sector partnerships to invest resources in programs and initiatives that address community conditions, such as building affordable housing (Affordable Housing Finance, 2018). Community benefit funding could serve as a potential resource for the promotion of MEB health directly by funding prevention and promotion programming in communities (which could, for example, yield dividends by reducing the need for hospitalization and costly treatment—a savings under value-based payment models). Community benefit funds could also benefit MEB health by being directed (and evaluated accordingly) to supporting the social determinants of BH and well-being (Carroll-Scott et al., 2017).

Under a provision of the ACA, tax-exempt hospitals are also required to conduct community health needs assessments, which can identify indicators of local risk and resilience (Carroll-Scott et al., 2017). By monitoring community needs assessments and encouraging partnership with public health officials, greater community linkage can be realized through existing mechanisms tied to protecting tax-exempt status with its associated tax breaks.

RECOMMENDATION 6-3: Congress should adopt and support the implementation of new or innovative funding mechanisms to generate sustainable and sufficient resources for promoting mental, emotional, and behavioral (MEB) health, and for prevention, particularly primary, of MEB disorders by

a. Offering incentives, such as tax credits, for large-scale social impact investing that supports universal prevention
b. Directing the Internal Revenue Service (IRS) to provide guidance on how tax-exempt hospitals can use community benefit funding to support MEB disorder prevention in communities where behavioral disorders are priority health needs within the mandated Community Health Needs Assessment. Specifically, the IRS should modify Lines 3, 6, 7, and 8 of Part II of IRS Schedule H (Form 990) that is used to monitor community benefit spending, to specifically include mental, emotional and behavioral disorder prevention. (see below; text in italics added to the text in Schedule H)

The changes to lines in IRS Schedule H (Form 990) are shown in italics.

- Line 3. "Community support" can include, but isn't limited to, childcare and mentoring programs for vulnerable populations or neighborhoods, neighborhood support groups, violence prevention programs, *mental, emotional and behavioral disorder prevention programs*, and disaster readiness and public health emergency activities, such as community disease surveillance or readiness training beyond what is required by accrediting bodies or government entities.
- Line 6. "Coalition building" includes, but isn't limited to, participation in community coalitions and other collaborative efforts with

the community to address *mental, emotional and behavioral health, and other* health and safety issues.
- Line 7. "Community health improvement advocacy" includes, but isn't limited to, efforts to support policies and programs to safeguard or improve public health, address *mental, emotional and behavioral health,* access to health care services, housing, the environment, and transportation.
- Line 8. "Workforce development" includes, but isn't limited to, *developing the prevention workforce for mental, emotional and behavioral health,* recruitment of physicians and other health professionals to medical shortage areas or other areas designated as underserved, and collaboration with educational institutions to train and recruit health professionals needed in the community (other than the health professions education activities entered on Part I, line 7f).

State, territorial, tribal, and local legislatures could consider different approaches to generate or maximize resources available to promote MEB health and well-being. The national opioid settlements have provided a much-needed, time-limited (e.g., 18 year) funding source for state opioid responses, but the funding is inadequate to meet all the specific costs of necessary services, and not all communities will receive it (Ban, 2024). State opioid settlement funding is variable, and while the settlements have expanded state coffers for addressing SUDs, it is unclear what proportion, if any, of the 70 percent required in the settlement agreement to be used for future opioid remediation (or abatement, term not defined by the settlement) is going to substance use prevention (Whaley, 2024). There are variations across settlements with different companies and differences in how the money is being paid out, and there is little public information about how states are investing it (Whaley, 2024). Several academic and research organizations have provided guidance on using the settlement funding, including for prevention, but more research is needed to inform the path forward (RAND, 2025; Johns Hopkins Bloomberg School of Public Health, 2025; Duke Margolis Institute for Health Policy, 2024; Faherty et al., 2020).

A variety of funding mechanisms are already in use in some states, such as California's 2004 tax on incomes over $1 million, which was established and continues to generate funding for MH services (Scheffler and Adams, 2005). These include excise taxes that account for the negative externalities—especially BH harms (e.g., of revenue streams from sales of alcohol, cannabis, and social media advertising[10])—and financial instruments, such as bonds, that allow states and municipalities to develop a funding source

---

[10] Refers to general advertising of any good or service on social media, as a potential funding source to account for negative externalities related to social media.

for an EBP or set of EBPs in anticipation of ROI (Chaloupka et al., 2019; Bloom et al., 2024; Lantz and Iovan, 2018; Raikov and Kalapchiev, 2023). Other options include mechanisms for coordinating and blending or layering funding sources from public and private entities with shared interests in improving the outcomes of a specific population, such as children (Weiner, 2022). Children's cabinets, for example, are an approach employed by many cities seeking to develop cradle-to-career pathways for supporting child and youth development and growth (Reville, 2020).

It is important for decision makers to weigh the evidence of benefits and challenges associated with each of these options for their specific context.

> **RECOMMENDATION 6-4:** State and territorial legislatures and tribal councils, respectively, should adopt and support the implementation of new or innovative funding mechanisms to generate sustainable and sufficient resources for promoting mental, emotional, and behavioral (MEB) health and prevention, particularly primary, of MEB disorders.

Such mechanisms could include the following:

- Enact new or revise current excise taxes to earmark funding to MEB health promotion programs.
    - New potential sources of funding include sales of recreational cannabis and social media advertising taxes.
    - Revise alcohol excise taxes to bring them up to inflation-adjusted levels.
- Establish prevention and wellness funds, which are pools of resources raised to support community prevention efforts (Local Wellness Funds, n.d.; TFAH, 2018).
- Establish children's cabinets and equivalent mechanisms to more effectively coordinate multiagency funding toward a shared mission.
- Use bonds, including social impact bonds (also known as pay for success financing), to support MEB prevention interventions (Segal et al., 2024).

Given the social, public health, and economic effects of BH disorders, promoting MEB health needs to be seen as a major national priority. The trajectories to these disorders begin early in life and as discussed in Chapters 2 and 7, are shaped by factors both distal (e.g., policies that affect poverty and economic mobility at a population level) and proximate to individuals (e.g., growing up in deep poverty and with caregivers who lack support and/or are experiencing BH disorders). Economic modeling that takes into consideration the multiplicity of causes and effects will be informative about the returns on investment in specific policies and major programs across different agencies.

There are several relevant bodies of work and entities. Yale University has a new Budget Lab that can inform policy making with a longer time horizon using a microsimulation tax model and open-source models. The Washington State Institute for Public Policy conducts cost–benefit analyses of policies and programs across multiple domains relevant to MEB health (e.g., education, adult and juvenile criminal legal, child welfare, health care, and MH) to guide policy making in Washington State (WSIPP, 2024b). But these are separate analyses for each intervention to inform policy makers about whether it is a good value. National Institutes of Health (NIH) has given increasing support to economic research relevant to MH and SUDs. A 2015 NIH Notice of Priorities for Health Economics Research signaled the agency's focus on the topic, and in 2023, National Institute of Mental Health and National Institute on Drug Abuse cohosted a conference on health economics. The NIH policy on funding health economics research calls for research that has "health outcomes and health-related behaviors as the primary focus, and the connection between the subject(s) of the study and improved understanding of health must be clear and explicit" (Humensky et al., 2024). None of these activities provide or are positioned to provide insights about the downstream effects on other federal agencies of investing in prevention in various domains and through various policies. That is a unique opportunity for HHS, which conducts economic impact analyses and modeling and simulation under the Assistant Secretary for Planning and Evaluation (often clinically oriented) and in 2012 prepared the report *A Review and Analysis of Economic Models of Prevention Benefits* (Miller et al., 2012).

> **RECOMMENDATION 6-5:** The Assistant Secretary for Planning and Evaluation should work with relevant experts to develop a comprehensive economic model that tests the downstream effects of investments in mental, emotional, and behavioral disorder (MEB) prevention. The model should include a range of inputs (e.g., quality early care and education), beneficiary federal agencies (e.g., Department of Health and Human Services/Centers for Medicare & Medicaid Services), and private-sector entities (employers/payers) that will reap the savings from enhancing mental, emotional, and behavioral health at a population level and eliminating MEB health disparities.

The Congressional Budget Office could refer to this model in informing the work of policy makers, in addition to their own work of scoring proposed prevention-oriented legislation.

The committee heard from several speakers at its information-gathering meetings about the burden of reporting and other requirements associated with SAMHSA and other funding sources (see Box 6-2). There are

> **BOX 6-2**
> **Insights on Funding from State, Local, and Federal Leaders**
>
> Speakers at the committee's information gathering meetings between January and April 2024 shared the following insights about funding for prevention services.
>
> New York State uses several funding sources for prevention programming in its Office of Addiction Services and Supports, including state aid funding and special revenue accounts (from the opioid settlement and cannabis tax) and federal resources from the SAMHSA Substance Use Prevention Treatment and Recovery Block Grant, American Rescue Plan Act (to be used by end of 2024), Coronavirus Response and Relief Supplemental Appropriations Act, Grant for Screening, Brief Intervention, Referral to Treatment, Partnership for Success Grant, and State Opioid Response Grant (Cunningham, 2024).
>
> Joe Neigel from Monroe County, Washington State, shared the funding sources for prevention efforts in his community and outlined several key needs. He suggested a consolidated application source, perhaps at the state level, to access funding, to reduce administrative burden; clear, common, and simple reporting expectations that will not overwhelm community coordinators; and consideration of the data entry burdens that he asserted keep communities like his from being able to scale programs (Neigel, 2024).
>
> The U.S. Department of Health and Human Services Administration for Community Living provides the policy framework of the Older Americans Act (1965) Title III, which includes supporting services and senior centers, disease prevention and health promotion, and the National Family Caregiver Support Program. Title III programs serve 11.4 million people, but in 2022, 29.4 percent of adults 65+ had incomes below 200 percent of poverty threshold, based on the official measure ($28,080 in 2022), and 42.2 percent of older adults, or 24.4 million people, based on the Supplemental Poverty Measure (Benson, 2024; Ochieng, 2024). Medicare provides some BH services but has gaps in coverage, and older adults struggle to get the care they need (Benson, 2024; McGinty, 2023). Although lay workers can be helpful, they cannot be reimbursed by Medicare or Medicaid, and paying for those services requires Title III funding.

numerous examples of innovative coordination and of flexibility in federal programs. Examples exist in the history of federal (and state) interagency cooperation of different agencies integrating data and reporting requirements to ease the difficulties of grantees and achieve both greater coordination and efficiency. The Sustainable Communities Initiative may offer a model for such coordination. This partnership among the Department of Housing and Urban Development, Environmental Protection Agency, and Department of Transportation offers a helpful example for several reasons: it facilitated coordination among the three different federal entities, promoted a holistic, cross-sectoral approach, and centered the needs and experience of communities and engaged them (Bates and Zapata, 2013). "Regional planning bodies like MPOs were to develop and extend their regional planning frameworks to integrate affordable housing and community and economic development into their land use and transportation plans" (Bates and Zapata, 2013, p. 15). In another compelling example, the Washington State Community Prevention & Wellness Initiative requires localities applying for funding to submit a single source application instead of several, one for each funding stream. See Box 6-3 for implementation considerations specifically related to funding MEB disorder prevention and health promotion programs.

BOX 6-3
Implementation Considerations in MEB Disorder Prevention Funding

Expanding Opportunities for MEB Health
- State-level distribution of resources:
  - Needs assessment—who is getting what
  - Transparency and accountability at the federal level
- Availability of technical assistance for applications for block and other grants for everyone
- Awareness among all communities of opportunities, and distribution of resources in a way that is commensurate with need
- Capacity building
- Funding for community engagement
- Pre-implementation (using maximally participatory community planning processes, such as Gathering of Native Americans)

Applying Implementation Science
- Bringing of all constituents to the table regarding funding decisions
- Exploration of how power is distributed
- Plan for implementation reflects community need
- Intentional de-implementation (and discontinuation of funding) of programs that cause harm
- Plan for sustained funding of effective programs
- Evaluation of cost effectiveness
- Allocation of funding for implementation support

REFERENCES

ACF (Administration for Children and Families). 2024. *FY 2024 justification of estimates for appropriations committees.* U.S. Department of Health and Human Services. https://www.acf.hhs.gov/sites/default/files/documents/olab/fy-2024-congressional-justification.pdf (accessed December 15, 2024).

Ackermann, R. T., E. A. Finch, E. Brizendine, H. Zhou, and D. G. Marrero. 2008. Translating the diabetes prevention program into the community: The DEPLOY pilot study. *American Journal of Preventive Medicine* 35(4):357–363. https://doi.org/10.1016/j.amepre.2008.06.035.

Afforable Housing Finance. 2018. *Kaiser Permanente announces $200 million affordable housing investment.* https://www.housingfinance.com/news/kaiser-permanente-announces-200-million-affordable-housing-investment_o (accessed December 16, 2024).

APHA (American Public Health Association). n.d. Prevention and public health fund: Dedicated to improving our nation's public health. https://www.apha.org/-/media/files/pdf/factsheets/200129_pphf_factsheet.pdf (accessed August 28, 2024).

ASTHO (The Association of State and Territorial Health Officials). 2021. Braiding and layering funding for adverse childhood experiences prevention. https://www.astho.org/globalassets/report/braiding-and-layering-funding-for-aces-prevention.pdf (accessed January 3, 2025).

Ban, C. 2024. *Opioid fight gets resources, faces pitfalls after settlement.* NACo. https://www.naco.org/news/opioid-fight-gets-resources-faces-pitfalls-after-settlement (accessed January 14, 2025).

Barna, M. 2024. States using Medicaid funds for firearm violence prevention. *The Nation's Health* 54(1):9–20. https://www.thenationshealth.org/content/54/1/9.1 (accessed January 3, 2025).

Bates, L. K., and M. A. Zapata. 2013. Revisiting equity: The HUD sustainable communities initiative. https://pdxscholar.library.pdx.edu/cgi/viewcontent.cgi?article=1083&context=usp_fac (accessed April 10, 2025).

BEA (Bureau of Economic Analysis). 2021. 2021 blended account release table rebate. https://www.bea.gov/sites/default/files/2023-12/2021-blended-account-release-table-rebate.xlsx (Accessed December 15, 2024).

Benson, K. 2024. National Aging Services Network: Infrastructure Supporting Prevention Among Older Adults, presented to the Committee on Blueprint for a National Prevention Infrastructure for Behavioral Health Disorders, Meeting 3. https://www.nationalacademies.org/event/42281_04-2024_blueprint-for-a-national-prevention-infrastructure-for-behavioral-health-disorders-meeting-3.

Bloom, D., A. Couffinhal, and C. Ozer. 2024. *Smart health taxes: A win for public health and the economy.* https://blogs.worldbank.org/en/health/Smart-health-taxes-A-win-for-public-health-and-the-economy (accessed October 20, 2024).

Blueprints for Healthy Youth Development. n.d. *Family check-up—toddler.* https://www.blueprintsprograms.org/programs/607999999/family-check-up-toddler/print/ (accessed December 15, 2024).

Brown, E., K. Conroy, and G. G. Kirby. 2019. *Aligning federal performance indicators accross programs promoting self-sufficiency: Local perspectives.* https://aspe.hhs.gov/sites/default/files/private/pdf/260606/EMPOWEREDPerfMeasuresLocal.pdf (accessed January 14, 2025).

Butler, S. 2018. How "wrong pockets" hurt health. *JAMA Forum Archive* A7(1). https://doi.org/10.1001/jamahealthforum.2018.0033.

Carroll-Scott, A., R. M. Henson, J. Kolker, and J. Purtle. 2017. The role of nonprofit hospitals in identifying and addressing health inequities in cities. *Health Affairs (Millwood)* 36(6):1102–1109. https://doi.org/10.1377/hlthaff.2017.0033.

CCC (Colorado County Citizen). 2023. RDF is painting the community red for mental health. https://www.coloradocountycitizen.com/article/178,rdf-is-painting-the-community-red-for-mental-health (accessed December 16, 2024).

The Center for High Impact Philanthropy. 2020. Health in mind. https://www.impact.upenn.edu/wp-content/uploads/2020/02/Heath-in-Mind-Mental-Health-and-Addiction.pdf (accessed December 16, 2024).

Chaloupka, F. J., L. M. Powell, and K. E. Warner. 2019. The use of excise taxes to reduce tobacco, alcohol, and sugary beverage consumption. *Annual Review of Public Health* 40:187–201. https://doi.org/10.1146/annurev-publhealth-040218-043816.

CHCS (Center for Health Care Strategies). 2023. *Gun violence prevention and Medicaid: State of the field*. https://www.chcs.org/resource/gun-violence-prevention-and-medicaid-state-of-the-field/ (accessed October 29, 2024).

CMS. n.d-a. *CMS behavioral health strategy*. https://www.cms.gov/cms-behavioral-health-strategy (accessed August 28, 2024).

CMS. n.d-b. *The Accountable Health Communities Health-Related Social Needs screening tool*. https://www.cms.gov/priorities/innovation/files/worksheets/ahcm-screeningtool.pdf (accessed January 3, 2025).

CMS (Centers for Medicare & Medicaid Services). 2023. *Coverage of services and supports to address health-related social needs in Medicaid and the Children's Health Insurance Program*. https://www.medicaid.gov/sites/default/files/2023-11/cib11162023.pdf (accessed December 12, 2024).

CMS. 2024a. *About the CMS innovation center*. https://www.cms.gov/priorities/innovation/about (accessed December 15, 2024).

CMS. 2024b. *Historical*. https://www.cms.gov/data-research/statistics-trends-and-reports/national-health-expenditure-data/historical (accessed. November 29, 2024).

CMS. 2024c. *Medicare payment*. https://www.cms.gov/cms-guide-medical-technology-companies-and-other-interested-parties/payment (accessed December 15, 2024).

Cohen Marill, M. 2022. Patients lift their voices to advance maternal health. *Health Affairs* 41(8). https://doi.org/10.1377/hlthaff.2022.00798.

The Community Guide. n.d. *Motor vehicle injury alcohol-impaired driving: Mass media campaigns*. https://www.thecommunityguide.org/findings/motor-vehicle-injury-alcohol-impaired-driving-mass-media-campaigns.html (accessed October 29, 2024).

The Community Guide. 2015. *School Based Health Centers*. https://www.thecommunityguide.org/media/pdf/SDOH-School-Based-Health-Centers-508.pdf (accessed October 8, 2024).

CRS (Congressional Research Service). 2024. Prevention and Public Health Fund: In Brief. https://crsreports.congress.gov/product/pdf/R/R47895 (accessed February 10. 2025).

CRS. 2023. The Centers for Disease Control and Prevention. https://crsreports.congress.gov/product/pdf/IF/IF12241 (accessed February, 10, 2025).

Cunningham, C. 2024. State-level infrastructure to support prevention, presented to the Committee on Blueprint for a National Prevention Infrastructure for Behavioral Health Disorders, Meeting 3. https://www.nationalacademies.org/event/42281_04-2024_blueprint-for-a-national-prevention-infrastructure-for-behavioral-health-disorders-meeting-3.

D'Alessandro, M., E. Higgins., S. Wilkniss. 2024. *Updates and FAQs: Developing and implementing a Medicaid state plan amendment to authorize community health worker reimbursement*. https://nashp.org/updates-and-faqs-developing-and-implementing-a-medicaid-state-plan-amendment-to-authorize-community-health-worker-reimbursement/ (accessed December 16, 2024).

DiGioia, K. 2022. *Hospital community benefit post-Affordable Care Act: An assessment of the effects of Medicaid expansion and 501 (r) on non-profit hospitals 2010–2018*: The George Washington University.

DiLorenzo, P., and J. Lukich. 2020. Perspective: The workforce crisis in child welfare might be the tip of an iceberg. *Children's Voice* 31(1).

DPC (Domestic Policy Council Office Of Science And Technology Policy). 2023. *The U.S. Playbook to address social determinants of health*.

Dopp, A. R., M. R. Narcisse, P. Mundey, J. F. Silovsky, A. B. Smith, D. Mandell, B. W. Funderburk, B. J. Powell, S. Schmidt, D. Edwards, D. Luke, and P. Mendel. 2020. A scoping review of strategies for financing the implementation of evidence-based practices in behavioral health systems: State of the literature and future directions. *Implementation Research and Practice* 1:2633489520939980. https://doi.org/10.1177/2633489520939980.

Duke Margolis Institute for Health Policy. 2024. *Leveraging opioid settlements to support sustainable community-based substance use disorder treatment and recovery infrastructure.* https://healthpolicy.duke.edu/opioidtools (accessed January 14, 2025).

Dunn, A., L. Rittmueller, and B. Whitmire. 2015. Introducing the new BEA health care satellite account. *Survey of Current Business* 95(1):1–21. https://citeseerx.ist.psu.edu/document?repid=rep1&type=pdf&doi=4fef84d36e4b54eab096548640b374796e167489 (accessed January 1, 2025).

ED (Department of Education). 2024. *Medicaid funding for school-based services.* https://www.ed.gov/sites/ed/files/about/offices/list/osers/docs/medicaid-funding-for-school-based-services-03-08-2024.pdf (accessed December 15, 2024).

Enomoto, K. 2023. *Harnessing mindful philanthropy to improve population health.* https://www.mckinsey.com/mhi/our-insights/harnessing-mindful-philanthropy-to-improve-population-health#/ (accessed October 29, 2024).

Fraser, M. R. 2019. A Brief History of the Prevention and Public Health Fund: Implications for Public Health Advocates. *Am J Public Health* Apr;109(4):572–577. https://doi.org/10.2105/AJPH.2018.304926.

Giliberti, M. 2023. *Fix the foundation: Unfair rate setting leads to inaccessible mental health care: Mental Health America.* https://mhanational.org/blog/fix-foundation-unfair-rate-setting-leads-inaccessible-mental-health-care (accessed December 31, 2024).

Godwin, J., Z. Levinson, and S. Hulver. 2023. *The estimated value of tax exemption for nonprofit hospitals was about $28 billion in 2020.* https://www.kff.org/health-costs/issue-brief/the-estimated-value-of-tax-exemption-for-nonprofit-hospitals-was-about-28-billion-in-2020/ (accessed October 29, 2024).

Haeder, S. F. 2021. As schools reopen, it's time to increase funding for school-based health centers. *Health Affairs Forefront.* https://doi.org/10.1377/hblog20210816.308933.

Harvard T.H. Chan School of Public Health. n.d. *South Carolina nurse-family partnership study.* https://www.hsph.harvard.edu/sc-nfp-study/ (accessed. October 29, 2024).

Healthcare Anchor Network. n.d. *Healthcare Anchor Network.* https://healthcareanchor.network/ (accessed October 24, 2024).

Heinrich, C. J., A. Colomer, and M. Hieronimus. 2023. Minding the gap: Evidence, implementation and funding gaps in mental health services delivery for school-aged children. *Children and Youth Services Review* 150:107023. https://doi.org/10.1016/j.childyouth.2023.107023.

Hinton, E. and A. Diana. 2024. *Medicaid authorities and options to address social determinants of health.* https://www.kff.org/medicaid/issue-brief/medicaid-authorities-and-options-to-address-social-determinants-of-health-sdoh/ (accessed November 19, 2024).

Hinton, E., R. Rudowitz, L. Stolyar, and N. Singer. 2020. *10 things to know about Medicaid managed care.* KFF. https://www.kff.org/medicaid/issue-brief/10-things-to-know-about-medicaid-managed-care/#:~:text=1.,case%20management%20(PCCM)%20programs.&text=As%20of%20July%202023%2C%2041,is%20both%20limited%20and%20mixed (accessed November 19, 2024).

HSCRC (Health Services Cost Review Commission). 2017. *Performance measurement work group meeting.* State of Maryland. https://hscrc.maryland.gov/Documents/Work%20Group%20Uploads/Performance%20Measurement/2017%20Meeting%20Materials/10-2017/2017-10-18%20FINAL%20PMWG%20Slides.pdf (accessed January 3, 2025).

Hsiung, H., K. Patel, H. Hundal, B. M. Baccouche, and K. W. Tsao. 2022. Preventing substance abuse in adolescents: A review of high-impact strategies. *Cureus* 14(7):e27361. https://doi.org/10.7759/cureus.27361.

Humensky, J. L., S. Q. Duffy, L. Cubillos, M. C. Freed, and A. Rupp. 2024. Perspective: Health economic interests at NIMH and NIDA to improve delivery of behavioral health services. *The Journal of Mental Health Policy and Economics* 27(1):33–39.

IES (Institute of Education Sciences). 2023. *Good behavior game.* https://ies.ed.gov/ncee/wwc/Docs/InterventionReports/WWC_GBG_IR-report.pdf (accessed December 15, 2024).

IOM (Institute of Medicine). 2012. *For the public's health: Investing in a healthier future.* Washington, DC: The National Academies Press. https://doi.org/10.17226/13268.

Johns Hopkins Bloomberg School of Public Health. 2025. *The principles for the use of funds from the opioid litigation.* https://opioidprinciples.jhsph.edu/ (accessed January 14, 2025).

Kaplan, R. M., M. Gold, S. Q. Duffy, N. Miller, J. R. Glassman, D. A. Chambers, T. G. Ganiats, S. Berndt, and D. K. Wilson. 2019. Economic analysis in behavioral health: Toward application of standardized methodologies. *Health Psychology* 38(8):672–679. https://doi.org/10.1037/hea0000769.

Kaufman, B. G., B. S. Spivack, S. C. Stearns, P. H. Song, and E. C. O'Brien. 2019. Impact of Accountable Care Organizations on utilization, care, and outcomes: A systematic review. *Medical Care Research and Review* 76(3):255–290. https://doi.org/10.1177/1077558717745916

KFF. 2021. Total Medicaid MCO Enrollment. https://www.kff.org/other/state-indicator/total-medicaid-mco-enrollment/?currentTimeframe=0&sortModel=%7B%22colId%22:%22Location%22,%22sort%22:%22asc%22%7D (accessed December 16, 2024).

KFF. 2024. Medicaid waiver tracker: Approved and pending section 1115 waivers by state. https://www.kff.org/medicaid/issue-brief/medicaid-waiver-tracker-approved-and-pending-section-1115-waivers-by-state/ (accessed January 3, 2025).

Koh, H. K., A. Bantham, A. C. Geller, M. A. Rukavina, K. M. Emmons, P. Yatsko, and R. Restuccia. 2020. Anchor institutions: Best practices to address social needs and social determinants of health. *American Journal of Public Health* 110(3):309–316. https://doi.org/10.2105/AJPH.2019.305472.

KP (Kaiser Permanente). 2023. *10 school districts receive next round of rise grants.* https://about.kaiserpermanente.org/commitments-and-impact/healthy-communities/news/ten-school-districts-receive-next-round-of-rise-grants (accessed December 15, 2024).

Lantz, P. M., and S. Iovan. 2018. Using pay-for-success financing for supportive housing interventions: Promise & challenges. *Behavioral Science & Policy* 4(1):39–49. https://doi.org/10.1177/237946151800400105.

LaVeist, T. A., E. J. Perez-Stable, P. Richard, A. Anderson, L. A. Isaac, R. Santiago, C. Okoh, N. Breen, T. Farhat, A. Assenov, and D. J. Gaskin. 2023. The economic burden of racial, ethnic, and educational health inequities in the US. *JAMA* 329(19):1682–1692. https://doi.org/10.1001/jama.2023.5965.

Le, L. K., A. C. Esturas, C. Mihalopoulos, O. Chiotelis, J. Bucholc, M. L. Chatterton, and L. Engel. 2021. Cost-effectiveness evidence of mental health prevention and promotion interventions: A systematic review of economic evaluations. *PLoS Med* 18(5):e1003606. https://doi.org/10.1371/journal.pmed.1003606.

Liu, Y., Y. Wang, Y. Wu, X. Chen, and J. Bai. 2021. Effectiveness of the Centering Pregnancy program on maternal and birth outcomes: A systematic review and meta-analysis. *International Journal of Nursing Studies* 120:103981. https://doi.org/10.1016/j.ijnurstu.2021.103981.

Local Wellness Funds. n.d. *What is a local wellness fund?* https://localwellnessfunds.org/local-wellness-funds/ (accessed October 9, 2024).

Loo, T. M., M. Altman, D. M. Bravata, and C. Whaley. 2024. Medical spending among US households with children with a mental health condition between 2017 and 2021. *JAMA Network Open* 7(3):e241860–e241860. https://doi.org/10.1001/jamanetworkopen.2024.1860.

MACPAC (Medicaid and CHIP Payment and Access Commission). 2021. *Medicaid's role in housing*. https://www.macpac.gov/wp-content/uploads/2021/06/Medicaids-Role-in-Housing-1.pdf (accessed December 15, 2024).

Martin, A. B., M. Hartman, J. Benson, and A. Catlin. 2023. National health care spending in 2021: Decline in federal spending outweighs greater use of health care. *Health Affairs (Millwood)* 42(1):6–17. https://doi.org/10.1377/hlthaff.2022.01397.

McDaid, D., A.-L. Park, and K. Wahlbeck. 2019. The economic case for the prevention of mental illness. *Annual Review of Public Health* 40(1):373–389. https://doi.org/10.1146/annurev-publhealth-040617-013629.

McGinty, B. 2023. *Medicare's mental health coverage: What's included, what's changed, and what gaps remain*. https://www.commonwealthfund.org/publications/explainer/2023/mar/medicare-mental-health-coverage-included-changed-gaps-remain (accessed July 30, 2024).

MHM (Methodist Healthcare Ministries). 2020. *Philanthropy to Support Trauma-Informed Care: Harnessing resilience to overcome adverse childhood experiences* https://www.mhm.org/philanthropy-to-support-trauma-informed-care-harnessing-resilience-to-overcome-adverse-childhood-experiences/ (accessed December 16, 2024).

Miller, J. E. 2012. *Too significant to fail: The importance of state behavioral health agencies in the daily lives of Americans with mental illness, for their families, and for their communities*. NASMHPD. https://www.nasmhpd.org/sites/default/files/Too%20Significant%20To%20Fail_0.pdf (accessed December 31, 2024).

Miller, W., D. Rein, M. O'Grady, J.-E. Yeung, J. Eichner, and M. McMahon. 2012. *Report on economic models of prevention benefits: A review and analysis of economic models of prevention benefits*. https://aspe.hhs.gov/sites/default/files/migrated_legacy_files//43986/rpt_EconomicModels.pdf (accessed June 7, 2012).

Mindful Philanthropy. 2024. *Our story*. https://www.mindfulphilanthropy.org/our-story (accessed October 29, 2024).

Mulvaney-Day, N., T. Marshall, K. Downey Piscopo, N. Korsen, S. Lynch, L. H. Karnell, G. E. Moran, A. S. Daniels, and S. S. Ghose. 2018. Screening for behavioral health conditions in primary care settings: A systematic review of the literature. *Journal of General Internal Medicine* 33:335–346. https://doi.org/10.1007/s11606-017-4181-0.

NASEM (National Academies of Sciences, Engineering, and Medicine). 2019. *Fostering healthy mental, emotional, and behavioral development in children and youth: A national agenda*. Washington, DC: The National Academies Press. https://doi.org/10.17226/25201.

NASEM. 2021. *Implementing high-quality primary care: Rebuilding the foundation of health care*. Washington, DC: The National Academies Press. https://doi.org/10.17226/25983.

NASHP (National Academy for State Health Policy). 2019. *50-state scan: How Medicaid agencies leverage their non-licensed substance use disorder workforce*. https://nashp.org/50-state-scan-how-medicaid-agencies-leverage-their-non-licensed-substance-use-disorder-workforce/ (accessed December 20, 2024).

NCCARE360. 2024. *Building connections for a healthier North Carolina*. https://nccare360.org/ (accessed December 16, 2024).

NCES (National Center for Education Statistics). 2024. *Over half of public schools report staffing and funding limit their efforts to effectively provide mental health services to students in need*. https://nces.ed.gov/whatsnew/press_releases/5_9_2024.asp (accessed December 16, 2024).

Neigel, J. 2024. Infrastructure supporting prevention among children and adolescents, presented to the Committee on Blueprint for a National Prevention Infrastructure for Behavioral Health Disorders, Meeting 3. https://www.nationalacademies.org/event/42281_04-2024_blueprint-for-a-national-prevention-infrastructure-for-behavioral-health-disorders-meeting-3.

Nichols, L., L. A. Taylor, P. Hughes-Cromwick, G. Miller, A. Turner, C. Rhyan, and R. Hamrick. 2020. Collaborative approach to public goods investments (CAPGI): Lessons learned from a feasibility study. *Health Affairs.* https://doi.org/10.1377/forefront.20200811.667525.

Niles, J., T. Litton, and R. Mechanic. 2019. An initial assessment of initiatives to improve care for high-need, high-cost individuals in accountable care organizations. *Health Affairs Forefront.* https://doi.org/10.1377/forefront.20190411.143015.

Ochieng, N., J. Cubanski, T. Neuman, and A. Damico. 2024. *How many older adults live in poverty?* https://www.kff.org/medicare/issue-brief/how-many-older-adults-live-in-poverty/ (accessed July 30, 2024).

ONDCP (Office of National Drug Control Policy). 2023. *National drug control budget: FY 2024 funding highlights.* https://www.whitehouse.gov/wp-content/uploads/2023/03/FY-2024-Budget-Highlights.pdf. (accessed December 16, 2024).

ONDCP. 2024. *National drug control strategy.* https://www.whitehouse.gov/wp-content/uploads/2024/05/2024-National-Drug-Control-Strategy.pdf (accessed January 3, 2025).

Panchal, N., and M. Guth. 2023. *Leveraging Medicaid for school-based behavioral health services: Findings from a survey of state Medicaid programs.* https://www.kff.org/mental-health/issue-brief/leveraging-medicaid-for-school-based-behavioral-health-services-findings-from-a-survey-of-state-medicaid-programs/ (accessed May 1, 2024).

Park Nicollet Foundation. n.d. *Children's mental health & well-being campaign.* https://fundraise.givesmart.com/e/JBHhyA?vid=18on1n (accessed October 29, 2024).

The Pew Charitable Trust. 2024. *Results First Initiative.* https://www.pewtrusts.org/en/projects/archived-projects/results-first-initiative (accessed December 26, 2024).

PTTC (Prevention Technology Transfer Center Network). 2024. *The return on investment of substance use prevention.* https://pttcnetwork.org/wp-content/uploads/2024/10/2024.09.27_PTTC_Return-on-Investment_FINAL.pdf (accessed December 9, 2024).

Purtle, J., K. Brinson, and N. A. Stadnick. 2022. Earmarking excise taxes on recreational cannabis for investments in mental health: An underused financing strategy. *JAMA Health Forum* 3(4):e220292. https://doi.org/10.1001/jamahealthforum.2022.0292.

Purtle, J., N. A. Stadnick, M. Wynecoop, S. C. Walker, E. J. Bruns, and G. A. Aarons. 2024. A tale of two taxes: Implementation of earmarked taxes for behavioral health services in California and Washington state. *Psychiatric Services* 75(5):410–418. https://doi.org/10.1176/appi.ps.20230257.

Purtle, J., M. Wynecoop, M. E. Crane, and N. A. Stadnick. 2023. Earmarked taxes for mental health services in the United States: A local and state legal mapping study. *Milbank Quarterly* 101(2):457–485. https://doi.org/10.1111/1468-0009.

Quality Improvement Center for Workforce Development. 2022. The child welfare workforce crisis—what we're hearing from the field. https://www.qic-wd.org/blog/child-welfare-workforce-crisis-%E2%80%93-what-we%E2%80%99re-hearing-field (accessed February 4, 2025).

Raikov, M., and M. Kalapchiev. 2023. *Differentiated taxation of products with harmful externalities.* https://www.ey.com/en_bg/tax/differentiated-taxation-of-products-with-harmful-externalities (accessed October 20, 2024).

RAND. 2025. *Strategies for effectively allocation opioid settlement funds.* https://www.rand.org/health-care/centers/optic/tools/fund-allocation.html (accessed January 14, 2025).

Reville, P. 2020. *The urgent need for children's cabinets.* https://www.gse.harvard.edu/ideas/usable-knowledge/20/03/urgent-need-childrens-cabinets (accessed December 26, 2024).

Rising, S. S. 1998. Centering pregnancy. An interdisciplinary model of empowerment. *Journal Nurse Midwifery* 43(1):46–54. https://doi.org/10.1016/s0091-2182(97)00117-1.

Rosenthal, M., S. Alidina, H. Ding, and A. Kumar. 2023. *Realizing the potential of accountable care in Medicaid. The Commonwealth Fund.* https://www.commonwealthfund.org/publications/issue-briefs/2023/apr/realizing-potential-accountable-care-medicaid (accessed October 29, 2024).

SAMHSA (Substance Abuse and Mental Health Services Administration). 2019. Behavioral Health Spending & Use Accounts 2006–2015. HHS Pub. No. (SMA) 19-5095. Rockville, MD: Substance Abuse and Mental Health Services Administration.

Sapatkin, D. 2024. *Philanthropy's 'uneasy journey' to supporting behavioral health.* MindSiteNews. https://mindsitenews.org/newsletter/philanthropys-uneasy-journey-to-supporting-behavioral-health/ (accessed January 14, 2025).

Scheffler, R. M., and N. Adams. 2005. Millionaires and mental health: Proposition 63 in California. *Health Affairs (Millwood)* Suppl Web Exclusives:W5-212-W215-224. https://doi.org/10.1377/hlthaff.w5.212.

Schlenker, T., and C. A. Huber. 2015. A unique funding opportunity for public health in Texas. *Journal of Public Health Management & Practice* 21(Suppl 1):S81–86. https://doi.org/10.1097/PHH.0000000000000131.

Segal, J., R. Khare., L. Cornell, I. Brewer, E. Carpenter, R. Levy, and N. Summerall. 2024. *Pay for success issue brief series.* https://socialfinance.org/insight/pay-for-success-issue-brief-series/ (accessed October 29, 2024).

Stadnick, N. A., C. Geremia, A. I. Mauri, K. Swanson, M. Wynecoop, and J. Purtle. 2024. A mixed-methods exploration of the implementation of policies that earmarked taxes for behavioral health. *The Milbank Quarterly.* https://doi.org/10.1111/1468-0009.12715.

Stelmach, R., E. L. Kocher, I. Katarina, A. M. Jackson-Morris, S. Saxena, and R. Nugent. 2022. The global return on investment from preventing and treating adolescent mental health disorders and suicide: A modelling study. *BMJ Global Health* 7(6):e007759. https://doi.org/10.1136/bmjgh-2021-007759.

Tax Policy Center. 2024. *How do state and local cannabis (marijuana) taxes work?* https://taxpolicycenter.org/briefing-book/how-do-state-and-local-cannabis-marijuana-taxes-work (accessed October 29, 2024).

Taylor, L. A., and L. M. Nichols. 2024. Insights from implementation of a community-based model for collaborative public good investing. *Health Affairs (Millwood)* 43(1):72–79.

TFAH. n.d. *Sustainable funding for healthy communities: Local health trusts: Structures to support local coordination of funds.* https://www.tfah.org/wp-content/uploads/2018/01/Local-Health-Trusts-Convening-Summary.pdf (accessed January 3, 2025).

TFAH (Trust for America's Health). 2017. *The value of prevention.* https://www.tfah.org/wp-content/uploads/2018/02/The-Value-of-Prevention.pdf (accessed October 10, 2024).

TFAH. 2018. *Local health trusts: Structures to support local coordination of funds.* https://www.tfah.org/wp-content/uploads/2018/01/Local-Health-Trusts-Convening-Summary.pdf (accessed January 14, 2025).

TFAH. 2024. *The impact of chronic underfunding on america's public health system 2024: Trends, risks, and recommendations.* https://www.tfah.org/report-details/funding-2024/ (accessed October 10, 2024).

Thau, S. 2024. Perspectives on Community Based Prevention to Address Substance Use and Misuse, presented to the Committee on Blueprint for a National Prevention Infrastructure for Behavioral Health Disorders, Meeting 2. https://www.nationalacademies.org/event/41980_02-2024_blueprint-for-a-national-prevention-infrastructure-for-behavioral-health-disorders-meeting-2.

Thom, M. 2022. Can additional funding improve mental health outcomes? Evidence from a synthetic control analysis of California's millionaire tax. *PLoS One* 17(7):e0271063. https://doi.org/10.1371/journal.pone.0271063.

Tsega, M., C. Lewis, D. McCarthy, T. Shah, and K. Coutts. 2019. Review of evidence for health-related social needs interventions. *Journal of Preventive Medicine* 53, no. 5 (2017): 719–729.

USAFacts. 2023. *How much revenue do states make from marijuana taxes?* https://usafacts.org/articles/how-much-revenue-do-states-make-from-marijuana-taxes/ (accessed October 29, 2024).

USPSTF (U.S. Preventive Services Task Force). 2024. *A & B recommendations.* https://www.uspreventiveservicestaskforce.org/uspstf/recommendation-topics/uspstf-a-and-b-recommendations (accessed December 12, 2024).

Weiner, R. 2022. *How children's cabinets can meet the needs of families and youth.* https://www.ecs.org/how-childrens-cabinets-can-meet-the-needs-of-families-and-youth/ (accessed December 16, 2024).

Whaley, S. 2024. Maximizing the impact of opioid settlement funds, presented to the Committee on Blueprint for a National Prevention Infrastructure for Behavioral Health Disorders, Meeting 3. https://www.nationalacademies.org/event/42281_04-2024_blueprint-for-a-national-prevention-infrastructure-for-behavioral-health-disorders-meeting-3 (accessed January 14, 2025).

WSIPP (Washington State Institute for Public Policy). 2024a. *Good Behavior Game: Public health & prevention: School-based.* https://www.wsipp.wa.gov/benefitcost/program/82 (accessed December 16, 2024).

WSIPP. 2024b. *Overview of WSIPP's Benefit-Cost Model: A brief guide.* https://www.wsipp.wa.gov/TechnicalDocumentation/Overview%20of%20WSIPPs%20Benefit-Cost%20Model.pdf (accessed December 16, 2024).

7

The Evidence Base on Policies

As discussed in Chapter 1, the national infrastructure to prevent mental, emotional, and behavioral (MEB) disorders requires multilevel approaches that include adopting and expanding the set of evidence-based programs (see Chapter 2) and policies (Akers et al., 2022; Alegría et al., 2022). This chapter responds to study sponsors' request that the committee consider policy as an intervention. Policy is critical infrastructure because it can function as universal prevention—with broad reach to large portions of the population. Policies can positively or negatively affect population MEB health and therefore represent critical infrastructure both indirectly and directly. First, policies indirectly influence the upstream factors that promote MEB well-being, such as economic stability, health care and education quality and accessibility, as well as neighborhood and social context. Second, policies can directly affect MEB health by promoting protective factors and reducing risk factors. Ultimately, all types of policies can shape individual behavior—for example, policies that discourage alcohol use through taxation and other strategies lead to lower rates of excessive alcohol use (CDC, 2024b), and policies that expanded Medicaid and improved health care access led to reduced symptoms of depression (Baicker et al., 2013). Policies are necessary to promote MEB health and well-being, but they need to be enforced and implemented effectively. Policies also can be part of multilevel interventions that incorporate programs (Moore et al., 2024).

This chapter briefly highlights U.S. social, economic, and environmental policies that have been shown to have positive effects on MEB health in National Academies of Sciences, Engineering, and Medicine (National Academies) reports (see simple chapter "map" in Table 7-1). For example,

TABLE 7-1 A Map to the Chapter Contents

Policies with robust evidence of effects on MEB health and described in past National Academies work	• Economic policies • Social policies • Environmental policies
Policies with robust but more recently amassed evidence of effects on MEB health, not the focus of recent National Academies work	• Incarceration policies • Firearms and community safety policies
Policies with a somewhat recent history, some evidence of effects on MEB health available, more research needed to shed light	• Policies that affect lesbian, gay, bisexual, transgender, queer (or questioning), and other sexual identities (LGBTQ+) people • Social media policies

Fostering Healthy Mental, Emotional, and Behavioral Development in Children and Youth: A National Agenda stated that "policies influence the distribution of wealth, employment and the health care, education, welfare, and juvenile justice system—all of which have implications for MEB development and health" (NASEM, 2019a, p. 188). In addition to discussing indirect effects on MEB health, the report also briefly examined policies that are known to directly influence MEB health outcomes, many of which have been evaluated in previous National Academies reports. The list includes health care access and affordability; Maternal, Infant, and Early Childhood Home Visiting; Mental Health Parity Act; Special Supplemental Nutrition for Women Infants and Children (WIC), Supplemental Nutrition Assistance Program (SNAP), and the National School Lunch Program (NSLP).

The 2019 report also reviewed the effects on MEB outcomes of minimum wage laws, paid family leave, Earned Income Tax Credit (EITC), child care subsidies, and Temporary Assistance for Needy Families (TANF). The report further discussed policies that impact access to alcohol and tobacco, regulate lead exposure, require seatbelts and bicycle helmets, and promote firearm and community safety, as well as education policies including Every Student Succeeds Act (ESSA), Individuals with Disabilities Education Act (IDEA), and state policies on socioemotional learning. This chapter briefly highlights many of the economic, social, and environmental policies examined in the 2019 report. It also discusses in much greater detail two topics very briefly addressed in the 2019 report (and not substantively explored in other recent National Academies work) and for which the evidence base has grown considerably in recent years: mass incarceration and firearm violence. The committee points to their role as important indirect and direct factors in MEB health, especially for low-income and minoritized communities, veterans, and children. Firearm injuries are the leading cause of death for young people, involved in 30 percent of suicides in youth, and also a major cause of psychiatric disorders in youth who are survivors of firearm violence (McKie et al., 2024; Song et al., 2023). Incarceration has clear and explicit links to poor MEB outcomes, pointing to key opportunities for prevention (Mendel, 2023b). A final section briefly discusses two areas of evolving policy at the national and state levels, where additional research is needed: the effects of social media on MEB health and well-being, and the effects on LGBTQ+ youth of policies that limit what they can do and the care they can receive.

ECONOMIC POLICIES AND MEB HEALTH

Income Support, Earnings Replacement, and Employment Support

Income support policies, such as the EITC and Child Tax Credit, have shown positive effects on MEB health. Both policies function to alleviate poverty, which places stress on families. Further, evidence shows that reducing poverty can improve educational outcomes, reduce interactions with the criminal legal system, and improve access to health care (NASEM, 2017; NASEM, 2019d). According to the *Reducing Intergenerational Poverty* report, "interventions such as the EITC that promote employment and increase income improve children's long-run outcomes; interventions that promote employment in the absence of increased income do not appear to improve child outcomes; and evidence on whether income supplementation alone improves long-term child outcomes is inconclusive, with some studies showing positive effects and others showing no improvement" (NASEM, 2024b, pp. 157–58).

The EITC has been consistently shown to increase employment for single parents and, in 2018, lifted about 5.6 million people above the poverty line, including nearly 3 million children, based on the Supplemental Poverty Measure (SPM) (CBPP, 2023). It has been associated with improvements in infant and maternal health and educational attainment (see review by Hoynes and colleagues [2015]). The EITC is associated with fewer depressive symptoms and reduction in deaths by suicide, and recent research on the effects of the temporary expansion of the Child Tax Credit (from $2,000 to $3,600 and covering a larger subset of low-income families) showed positive effects on the mental health (MH) and well-being of adults in affected families (Batra et al., 2023; Boyd-Swan et al., 2015; Dow et al., 2020).

Employment support includes paid leave and child care subsidies. Paid maternity leave is associated with improved maternal MH (Heshmati et al., 2023). Mothers who received some paid leave had lower levels of depressive symptoms than those who did not. Longer leave has also been associated with lower levels of depressive symptoms (Heshmati et al., 2023). A study found increases in exercise and improved stress management among women who took paid parental leave compared to those who took no or unpaid leave (Jou et al., 2018). Paid family leave is also associated with improved MEB health. A 2021 study found that levels of emotional distress statistically decreased among adults with paid family leave policies (Irish et al., 2021). Direct cash transfers have shown positive (though sometimes temporary) effects—one recent randomized trial showed reductions in emergency room visits for MH disorders, and another showed modest and time-limited improvements in subjective well-being (Agarwal et al., 2024; McKay et al., 2023).

Research has shown that the expanded Child Tax Credit was associated with a reduction in anxiety symptoms for recipients (Batra et al., 2023; Cha et al., 2023; Nam and Kwon, 2024), with some noting significantly more pronounced effects for Black and Hispanic adults with children (Batra et al., 2023; Cha et al., 2023) and women (Cha et al., 2023) compared with non-Hispanic White adults (Batra et al., 2023; Cha et al., 2023). Batra and colleagues (2023) also found reduced depressive symptoms among low-income adults.

Social Security Income (SSI) benefits have also been shown to reduce depressive symptoms among older adults. Golberstein (2015) exploited the "notch" in SSI that led certain cohorts of beneficiaries to receive payments doubly indexed for inflation. These increases in payments were especially large for women, given their lower overall income, and the study reports that $1,000 of SSI led to an improvement of 0.541 points (27 percent) on the Center for Epidemiologic Studies Depression Scale, CES-D (Golberstein, 2015).

In-Kind Support: Housing, Health Insurance, and Nutrition

Housing

Housing is a basic human need with direct linkage to MEB health. Research comparing families randomly assigned to a permanent housing subsidy, community-based rapid rehousing, project-based transitional housing, or "usual care" (any services that are not an immediate referral to other interventions) over 3 years found the families who received the permanent subsidy experienced reduced psychological distress, signs of substance and alcohol use issues, and intimate partner violence incidence (by half) compared with families receiving usual care (Gubits et al., 2015). In children, research shows reduced behavioral challenges and more prosocial behavior when provided improved housing conditions (Gubits et al., 2015; Sard et al., 2018). In addition, the quality of neighborhoods matters: the Moving to Opportunity experiment found that living in a low-poverty neighborhood had positive impacts on adults' mental and physical health, including decreased rates of depression, and on the MH of female children (Chetty et al., 2016). As the frequency and severity of natural disasters increases due to climate change, the consequences, including destruction of housing and displacement, pose additional risks for MEB disorders (SAMHSA, 2024a,b).

Health Insurance

The ability to pay for health care is included in the Global Social Development Innovation's definition of economic security (GSDI, 2021). Expanding Medicaid and the State Children's Health Insurance Program in 1997–2002 was associated with improved MH for teenagers, with boys specifically experiencing a significant increase in the likelihood of the highest level of MH. It also created spillover effects for parents, who experienced slightly better MH (Hamersma and Ye, 2021). Expanding Medicaid in Oregon via lottery also improved adult MH; some effects could be due to reduced financial precarity, as medical bills are a leading cause of household debt (Baicker et al., 2013; Kluender et al., 2021; Maas, 2016).

Nutrition

Food insecurity is a well-documented source of stress, undermining the psychological well-being of adults and children (Pourmotabbed et al., 2020; Wolfson et al., 2021). A patchwork of federal programs provides food assistance to specific groups considered particularly vulnerable: WIC, NSLP, and SNAP. NSLP was expanded during COVID-19 to include all students—though federal support stopped in June 2022, several states have decided to continue free school meals because they are destigmatizing. Evidence has shown free school meals improved psychosocial functioning, anxiety, and depression symptoms in children (Murphy et al., 1998). WIC recipients who are more food insecure have been shown to have more depressive symptoms (Herman et al., 2024). Moreover, preschool children whose mothers participated in WIC were less likely to be diagnosed with attention-deficit/hyperactivity disorder (Carlson and Neuberger, 2021). Research suggests that states that removed asset tests for SNAP benefits, resulting in program expansions, experienced reduced suicidality and depressive symptoms at the population level (Austin et al., 2023).

SOCIAL POLICIES THAT PROMOTE MEB HEALTH

Infancy and Early Childhood

The 2019 National Academies report *Vibrant and Healthy Kids* found that home visiting during pregnancy and early childhood by a nurse, social worker, or early educator "improves a wide range of child and family outcomes, including promotion of maternal and child health, prevention of child abuse and neglect, positive parenting, child development, and school readiness" and recommended expanding evidence-based home visiting programs (NASEM, 2019c, p. 10). Estimates from U.S. Census Bureau data indicate that approximately five million pregnant women and families with children under 6 live in poverty (NHVRC, 2018); home-visiting programs reach only about 15 percent of them due to funding constraints (Zaid et al., 2022). Expanding funding for home visiting would need to be paired with training additional nurses, social workers, and early educators to deliver evidence-based interventions in families.

Early Childhood Care and Education and K–12 Education

The Administration for Children and Families, part of the Department of Health and Human Services, Head Start, and Early Head Start programs, reports that enrolled children have improved social, emotional, and behavioral development and fewer child welfare encounters related to sexual or physical abuse (ACF, 2024). As they mature, they are more likely to graduate from high school, attend college, and feel better prepared to be parents themselves compared with children who are not enrolled (ACF, 2024). However, similar to home-visiting programs, Head Start and Early Head Start services serve only 30 percent of 3- to 5-year-old children and 9 percent of infants and toddlers living in poverty, according to 2020–2021 data (First Five Years Fund, 2022). The need greatly outpaces the available resources. Although all children at or below 100 percent of the federal poverty level qualify for Head Start and Early Head Start, less than half of them receive the services (First Five Years Fund, 2022). Quality early childhood care and education is associated with improved MEB development, can mediate risk factors such as trauma and inadequate parental support (NASEM, 2019c; Penney et al., 2019), and may promote MH "through developmentally supportive learning opportunities and secure caregiving relationships" (Hutchins et al., 2023, p. 2).

National Academies reports have underscored how opportunities for educational attainment contribute to improved health, health equity, and well-being (IOM, 2013; NASEM, 2019b,c, 2023). But schools also contribute to MH directly, by implementing trauma-informed practices, providing MH services and curricula and teaching resources that center social and emotional learning, and creating safe and supportive learning environments (CASEL, n.d.; NASEM, 2019b). Federal policies, such as the No Child Left Behind Act, Every Student Succeeds Act, and IDEA, inform state education programming and set national standards and guidelines, including for implementing multitier systems of supports. Chapter 2 discusses school-based programs and other interventions in more detail.

Safety and Belonging

The 2023 National Academies report *Federal Policy to Advance Racial, Ethnic, and Tribal Health Equity* discussed the history of discriminatory federal policies including those that have harmed and traumatized specific communities, including people with disabilities, immigrants, people from certain racial and ethnic groups, and LGBTQ+ people.

Schools are an important setting for creating safe and supporting environments for youth development. *The Promise of Adolescence* recommended that to "[p]rotect the overall health and well-being of each student . . . school districts should enact policies and practices that promote supportive school climates and ensure safety for all students" (NASEM, 2019b, p. 199). For example, research shows that LGBTQ+ youth face greater risk of substance use, bullying, isolation, rejection, anxiety, depression, and suicide (Hafeez et al., 2017; Levengood and Hadland, 2024). Youth who are LGBTQ+ and are also Native American/Indigenous, Black, Latina/Latino, or multiracial, are more likely to have attempted suicide compared to their White LGBTQ+ peers (TTP, 2021). Seventy-two percent of LGBTQ+ youth reported symptoms of generalized anxiety disorder, and 62 percent reported symptoms of major depressive disorder in the past 2 weeks (TTP, 2021).

Since 2016, multiple states have enacted policies intended to enforce traditional gender norms that reflect binary sex at birth, from banning the use of bathrooms consistent with one's gender identity to prohibiting classroom discussion about sexual orientation or gender identity. In 2023, 20 states enacted legislation limiting what LGBTQ+ people can do and the care they can receive (ACLU, 2024b). While it is still early to draw definitive conclusions about the effects of such policies, a 2023 national survey conducted by the Trevor Project reported that nearly one in three LGBTQ+ young people reported their mental health was poor most of the time or always due to anti-LGBTQ+ policies and legislation. Additionally, almost two in three LGBTQ+ youth said that hearing about potential state or local laws banning discussions about people like them in schools worsened their mental health (TTP, 2023).

An adverse policy environment can affect all LGBTQ+ communities, but young people are more vulnerable due to their dependence on the presence or absence of supports at school and at home (Hatzenbuehler, 2009). The literature also indicates that the social environment of sexual and gender diverse youth affects their behavioral health outcomes (Newcomb et al., 2019; Hatzenbuehler, 2011). For example, lower depression, suicidal ideation, and suicidal behaviors in gender diverse youth are associated with greater number of contexts where youth are referred to by their chosen name (Russell et al., 2018). There is also a growing body of work that illustrates that distal stressors such as structural stigma and discrimination at different levels of government also influence the health outcomes of LGBTQ+ youth (Hatzenbuehler 2014, 2017; Hatzenbuehler and Link, 2014).

Ramos and colleagues (2023) found that:

> Over 2 decades of rigorous scientific inquiry indicates that mental health among LGBTQ+ youth is directly and indirectly affected by laws pertaining to their civil rights. For example, in states that legalized same-sex marriage before the U.S. Supreme Court required it, the rate of suicide attempts among sexual minority high school students—and high school students overall—declined (Raifman et al., 2017). Legal developments affecting civil rights often garner significant media exposure and spark discussion about perceptions of LGBTQ+ populations more generally. Youth in those populations may experience such developments both practically (e.g., by gaining the right to marry the partner of their choice) and psychologically (e.g., by internalizing messages that they are worthy of rights). Legal changes amounting to an expression of public affirmation and support for LGBTQ+ rights and identity may promote a more positive self-image and a sense of safety among LGBTQ+ youth, while publicity regarding the restriction or loss of civil rights may contribute to feelings of stigma, hopelessness, internalized homophobia, and poor self-image. (Bauermeister, 2014; Woodford et al., 2015)

New findings from the 2023 Behavioral Risk Factor Surveillance System (BRFSS) indicate that 25.3 percent of transgender and 26.4 percent of questioning students, compared to 8.5 percent of cisgender male students, missed school because they felt unsafe (Suarez, 2024). Of the 3.3 percent of U.S. high school students who identify as transgender, 72 percent reported feeling sad or hopeless (Suarez, 2024).

Research is needed to assess the effects on MEB health of recent state anti-LGBTQ+ policies on the MEB health of LGBTQ+ individuals, especially young people. State education and school district policies, in particular, appear to influence school climate, contributing to an environment that feels unsafe, unwelcoming, and even threatening. This stands in stark contrast to research highlighting the positive impact of social and emotional learning approaches in K–12 educational settings and the important relationship between schools and their communities (CASEL, n.d.; NASEM, 2019b, 2023).

Social Media Policies

The 2023 National Academies report *Social Media and Adolescent Health* examined the effects of social media on the mental and physical health of U.S. adolescents and made recommendations intended to "maximize the benefits and minimize the harms" of social media (NASEM, 2024c, p. 2). The report highlighted, and the present committee endorses, the research needs discussed in that report, especially identifying what laws and regulations are needed to curb potential harms of exposure to unregulated violent or otherwise harmful content conveyed through social media (NASEM, 2024c).

In May 2023, the U.S. Surgeon General issued the *Advisory on Social Media and Youth Mental Health*, which called on policy makers, social media companies, researchers, youth, and their families to better understand the full impact of social media on MH, and maximize benefits and minimize harms (OSG, 2023). The advisory concluded that greater exposure to social media (more than 3 hours per day) is associated with twice the risk of poor MEB outcomes, such as depression and anxiety. Additionally, social media exposure can act as a mediator for other pathways to poor MEB outcomes, such as inadequate sleep.

In the last 5 years, Congress has introduced at least five legislative proposals related to further research and protecting user safety (NASEM, 2024c). In July 2024, the Senate passed the Kids Online Safety and Privacy Act[1] (which includes the Children and Teens' Online Privacy Protection Act 2.0). As demonstrated in the proposed legislation, this topic warrants additional research to ascertain what guardrails may be necessary to mitigate potential harms of social media to the MEB health and well-being of youth.

As briefly discussed above, there are several domains where the relationship between MEB disorders and policies is clear, and others, such as social media, where there is a need for more evidence of effects on MEB health and well-being. Basing public policy on the best available knowledge is essential to enhancing protective factors and mitigating risk factors. As noted in Chapter 1, MEB disorders present major social and economic costs. It is crucial to identify, understand, and carefully consider the implications of policies on this public health issue.

RECOMMENDATION 7-1: In keeping with the Foundations for Evidence-Based Policymaking Act of 2018, federal and state policy makers should use the best available evidence to sustain, restore, develop, or de-implement social and economic policies, considering the direct or indirect effects of such policies on mental, emotional, and behavioral health and population well-being.

Policy makers have tools they can use to inform this work, including health impact assessments and a range of modeling approaches, including economic models as discussed in Chapter 5 (NASEM, 2016; NRC, 2011).

---

[1] https://www.congress.gov/bill/118th-congress/senate-bill/1409 (accessed January 3, 2025).

Incarceration

Scale and Scope of Mass Incarceration

Mass incarceration is both a response to and risk factor for the disproportionately high rates of MEB disorders and substance use disorders (SUDs). The year 2023 marked 50 years of mass incarceration in the United States, defined by a period of unprecedented legal and policy decisions that have led to massive expansion of the use of incarceration as punishment, especially for drug use and crimes related to MEB disorders, and restrictions on the rights of people with criminal records, including limited access to publicly funded social services. Tens of millions of adults, especially those with low incomes and those from populations historically marginalized on the basis of their race or ethnicity, have been incarcerated, and almost 80 million have a criminal record (NCSL, 2023; Sawyer and Wagner, 2024). At any point in time, 60,000 children are incarcerated in juvenile facilities, and 5 million have parents who have been or are currently incarcerated (ACLU, 2024a; The Annie E. Casey Foundation, 2016). People released from incarceration face its "collateral consequences" of 42,000 laws and policies that create additional barriers for those with a criminal record, especially drug felonies, including to securing housing, transportation, health insurance, and employment (CSI, 2024). The effects of incarceration and stigma of a criminal record have lasting effects and spill over to the health of family members, and this risk is not shared equally across the population. Black men and women have an imprisonment rate six and two times more than their White counterparts, respectively (The Pew Charitable Trusts, 2023), leading to disproportionate effects on Black families (Lee, 2014). Almost 25 percent of Black individuals have three or more immediate family members who have been incarcerated, compared with 5 percent of White individuals (Sundaresh et al., 2021).

The Effect of Incarceration on MEB Health

Imprisonment and exposure to the conditions of confinement create new risks for MEB well-being. Furthermore, the overcrowding and exposure to violence that are commonplace in carceral facilities and the continued use of solitary confinement for punishment lead to severe psychological distress and MEB disorders, including anxiety, depression, and posttraumatic stress disorder (PTSD) (Edgemon and Clay-Warner, 2019; Huey and McNulty, 2005; Solitary Watch and the Unlock the Box Campaign, 2023). Incarceration is a broad structural pathway that exposes individuals to intersecting risks, including peer antisocial behavior, disruption of community connections, limited ability to practice prosocial behavior, and increased likelihood of aggressive behavior due to the violent nature of prisons (Teplin et al., 2013, Tisdale, 2020). The lack of prevention programs and services, substance use treatment, and MH care within carceral facilities means that trauma exposure goes unaddressed, while substance use and MH problems worsen (Volkow, 2021). Studies of adults who have been incarcerated have shown robust and long-lasting relationships with certain disorders, including major depressive disorder, PTSD, and bipolar disorder; those who were incarcerated as children or with longer sentences had worse outcomes (Barnert et al., 2017). Upon release, "relapse to drug use can be fatal due to loss of opioid tolerance," underscoring an opportunity and need for secondary prevention (Volkow, 2021, p. 2048).

For youth, having a criminal record diminishes one's opportunities for protective factors for MEB health. It decreases educational attainment, residential independence, gainful activity, desistance from criminal activity and substance use, and impairs interpersonal functioning and parenting responsibility (Abram et al., 2017). The excess burden of felony drug convictions and imprisonment has radiating impacts on the children and families who are disproportionately incarcerated, such as Black, Latino, and Native American children and families. In 2021, Volkow writes, "Parents who are arrested can lose custody of their children, entering the latter into the child welfare system. According to . . . analysis by the Pew Charitable Trusts, 1 in 9 African American children (11.4 percent) and 1 in 28 Hispanic children (3.5 percent) have an incarcerated parent, compared to 1 in 57 White children (1.8 percent), (The Pew Charitable Trust, 2010)," (Volkow, 2021). Among American Indian and Alaska Native children in 2019–2020, 16 percent had a parent who was in jail or had served time when they were born (Casey Family Programs, 2023). Having a partner incarcerated is associated with symptoms consistent with major depressive disorder, higher levels of life dissatisfaction, and high rates of substance use and addiction (Wildeman et al., 2012). Children with incarcerated parents have been found to be more depressed; as young adults, they suffer from worse MEB outcomes compared to those whose parents have not been incarcerated (Geller et al., 2012).

Several states and jurisdictions have passed laws or instituted new policies to decarcerate, which have been rigorously studied, including addressing youth lawbreaking outside the criminal legal system; halting the use of confinement in response to probation violations and low-level drug offenses; and reinvesting dollars earmarked for youth incarceration to community alternatives to build community supports and prevention infrastructure (Mendel, 2023a; The Annie E. Casey Foundation, 2022). For example, to divert youth away from arrest and criminal charges, Florida passed a law to implement a civil citation program for juveniles (TJCHC, 2024). Civil citations are a civil alternative to arrest (DSCYF, n.d.). The U.S. Department of Justice (DOJ) evaluated the program, comparing those who were eligible for civil citation but arrested with those given a civil citation. It concluded that civil citation reduced the likelihood of rearrest within the study's 3-year follow-up period (Bales et al., 2019). Ohio passed a statute in 1993 to use a variety of strategies to decrease its juvenile incarceration rate, including the RECLAIM program, which gave jurisdictions choice in allocating dollars for adjudicated youth to either incarceration or community programming, allowing money to be kept locally and spent on developing supportive infrastructure in the community (Latessa et al., 2014; Lux et al., 2015; OJJDP, 1997). Low- and moderate-risk youth were much less likely to return to prison systems, and high-risk youth were also less likely to recidivate and be incarcerated after being supported by community programming compared with imprisonment. California passed Proposition 47 (2014),[2] which reduced penalties for certain lower-level drug and property crimes and showed modest but significant reductions in rearrest and reconvictions and no evidence that violent crime increased but some evidence that property crime did (NIJ, 2021). The state reallocated funds from incarceration to community-based treatment initiatives, such as MH and substance use disorder treatment, funds to K–12 schools, and victim services.

Most states have passed statutes to create problem-solving courts, also called "drug," "treatment," or "mental health" courts, that divert people with hazardous drug and alcohol use and MEB disorders from the carceral system (OJP, 2020). A recent study assessed the effect of a problem-solving court in the county on county-level overdose deaths and researchers found a significant effect in reducing county overdose mortality (Lindenfeld et al., 2022). Several studies have also found that providing medications for opioid use disorder for people in carceral facilities has shown reductions in overdose mortality (Lindenfeld et al., 2022). Twelve states, including New Mexico and New York, have passed legislation to mandate medications for opioid use disorder in carceral facilities (Weizman et al., 2021).

The Juvenile Detention Alternative Initiative (JDAI) is an example of a multisite implementation network of counties and states that has worked to reduce exposure to incarceration as a risk factor for MEB health by applying evidence-based laws, policies, and programs. Launched in the early 1990s, it was adopted by 300 counties across 39 states. It uses a variety of approaches to reduce youth incarceration, including passing laws that expand diversionary opportunities and reduce detention for probation violations, promoting cross-sector collaboration, implementing objective admissions criteria, and identifying policies that may have a harsher effect on racial or ethnic minority youth. The JDAI network is multisectoral, engages in community partnership, involves and consults those with lived

---

[2] In November 2024, California voters passed proposition 36, which repealed some parts of Proposition 47 (Duara, 2024).

experience, and attends to and measures inequitable impact of policies on racial and ethnic minorities. Participating jurisdictions have seen reductions in detention among youth and state custody populations of more than 40 percent and more than 50 percent, respectively. These and other such efforts have achieved a 75 percent reduction in youth incarceration between 2000 and 2022; in 2022, 27,587 youths were held in juvenile justice facilities, down from 108,800 in 2000 (Rovner, 2024).

Policies exist in many jurisdictions that layer additional challenges to current and formerly incarcerated individuals, including denying access to protective factors, such as education and health care. A 2023 National Academies report examined the effects of federal policy on health disparities, with exclusions faced by previously incarcerated individuals as one specific example of policies that could be harmful to health and well-being. The report noted that although incarcerated people had been excluded from Pell Grant eligibility since 1994, Pell Grant access for people enrolled in qualifying prison education programs was reinstated in 2020. This, the report noted, is a promising example of how removing barriers to access to federal programs for specific populations can even the playing field in terms of the broad factors known to affect health (NASEM, 2023). The report also recommended a review of policies, such as those pertaining to Medicaid coverage, that exclude incarcerated people and other specific populations, for their effects on health outcomes (see Appendix F).

CONCLUSION 7-1: *Evidence shows that incarceration has a detrimental impact on the mental, emotional, and behavioral health of millions of children and adults in the United States.*

RECOMMENDATION 7-2: Federal, state, tribal, and county officials should enact evidence-based policies to divert from the criminal legal system and reduce reliance on incarceration where appropriate, while simultaneously building a robust community prevention infrastructure, thus enabling protective factors that support mental, emotional, and behavioral health.

As noted above, there are many opportunities to intervene before incarceration, such as civil court, drug courts, and community programming for youth, overseen by the criminal legal juvenile system.

Community prevention infrastructure refers to a range of investments and interventions that create protective factors and help reduce exposure to risk factors. For youth, school-based evidence-based programs, for example, may reduce problem behavior, strengthen coping skills and behavioral regulation, lessen aggressive behavior, and over the long-term lead to other positive outcomes, such as lower criminal legal system involvement (WSIPP, 2023).

ENVIRONMENTAL POLICIES THAT PROMOTE MEB HEALTH

Environmental policies represent a heterogenous set of interventions, but they share in common modifications to the environment to decrease or mitigate risk factors for MEB disorders, with causal pathways that generally include exposure to violence and trauma. Two protective factors discussed—mandating seat belt use and reducing lead exposure—are among the 10 greatest public health achievements of the 20th century (CDC, 2011).

Motor Vehicle Crashes

Research shows that policies can mitigate risk factors related to tobacco and alcohol. Policies setting age limits for sales, raising taxes, and limiting availability and advertising are among some of the approaches that states and localities have used to lower rates of drinking among teens and adults and thus reduce the public health effects (deaths and disease associated with alcohol, and also injuries from alcohol). The MEB disorders related to alcohol impairment are evident in motor vehicle crashes associated with driving while intoxicated—which is a major cause of PTSD, affecting an estimated 2.5–7 million U.S. people (Blanchard and Hickling, 2004). Each day, 37 people die in alcohol-impaired driving crashes, or one death every 39 minutes (NHTSA, n.d.). A range of evidence-based policy strategies can reduce driving while intoxicated and its social harms, but one of the most effective, taxation (which is inversely associated with binge drinking), has been eroded by inflation over the past 3 decades (Naimi et al., 2018). The 2018 NASEM report on alcohol-impaired driving called for increasing alcohol taxes and indexing them to inflation (this can generate funding for MEB promotion—see Chapter 5) and adopting universal primary seatbelt laws (i.e., a motorist can be stopped for not wearing a seat belt) to reduce motor vehicle accident fatalities.

Firearm Violence

Firearm violence—the intentional and unintentional injuries, deaths, and attendant physical and emotional trauma caused by exposure to firearm use—is a major contributor to poor MEB outcomes. The U.S. Surgeon General has highlighted the cascading harms to survivors and communities, including much higher rates of depression and psychiatric disorders (OSG, 2024). Although mental illness is frequently blamed for incidents of firearm violence, research indicates that it accounts for only 4 percent of violent acts (with or without firearms), and most people with mental illness are never violent (Swanson et al., 2015). In 2020 and 2021, more children and adolescents 1–17 years old died from injury by firearms (homicides, not suicide) than any other cause (Cabral et al., 2024; McGough et al., 2023;

Rossin-Slater et al., 2020). More than half of all suicide deaths are with a firearm, and 85 to 90 percent of all suicide attempts that involve a firearm are fatal (Drexler, 2016). Veterans and members of the military tragically experience elevated risk of suicide (Dempsey et al., 2019). Suicide rates are 57.3 percent higher among the veteran than among the age- and sex-adjusted non-veteran U.S. population, and 72.2 percent of veteran suicides are by firearm compared to 52.2 percent of non-veterans (OMHSP, 2022, 2023).

As noted in the 2024 Surgeon General's Advisory, "beyond the profound consequences of surviving a firearm-related injury, those who do not experience direct bodily harm often grapple with MEB consequences related to firearm violence exposure, including community members, children and adolescents, and families" (OSG, 2024, p. 14). In her presentation to the committee, Therese Richmond of the University of Pennsylvania echoed this finding, describing firearm-related harms as a pyramid, with deaths at the top, morbidity in the middle, and myriad effects on the MEB health of individuals and families and well-being of communities at the base (Richmond, 2024). The morbidities among survivors include MEB issues (such as PTSD and depression), and those indirectly exposed to firearm violence are more likely to receive a MH diagnosis or report symptoms of depression and drug and alcohol use (Magee et al., 2023; Rheingold et al., 2012). Smith and colleagues (2020b) found that 24 percent of participants in the Survey of Police-Public Encounters across four urban areas reported exposure to firearm violence fatality and those exposed had "significantly higher levels of psychological distress, depression, suicidal ideation, and/or psychotic experiences compared to those not exposed" (p. 1).

Richmond made some key points about how the relationship between MEB health and firearm violence needs to inform the infrastructure to prevent MEB disorders. She underscored that the induction period for firearm violence is not a split second (the finger on the trigger) but can be quite long, allowing consideration of a prevention infrastructure that addresses joint risks for both firearm violence and MEB disorders. She also noted that the prevention infrastructure for MEB disorders needs to be maximally accessible to youth, families, and communities at risk for firearm violence (Richmond, 2024).

There is ample evidence that firearm violence contributes to MH disorders for children and adolescents. Repeated exposure to firearm violence, particularly in neighborhoods with high crime rates, can lead to chronic PTSD, affecting a child's functioning in school and social settings (Collins and Swoveland, 2014; Panchal, 2024). In addition, Song and colleagues (2023) analyzed data from 2007–2021 to assess the impacts of firearm injuries on 2,052 child and adolescent survivors and their families, finding increases in pain disorders (117 percent), psychiatric disorders (68 percent), and SUDs (144 percent) among survivors. Health care spending surged by $34,884 per survivor in the first year (Song et al., 2023).

Turning to indirect effects, firearm violence affects not only the direct victims but also their families and communities, creating cycles of trauma and worsening MEB outcomes. Families of victims often experience profound psychological distress, including grief, anxiety, and depression (Panchal, 2024). Among rural youth ages 13–18 interviewed at Iowa's FFA (formerly Future Farmers of America) leadership conference, more than one-third said "they knew someone who had been killed or injured by a firearm," more than "two-thirds knew of someone who had died or was injured unintentionally" by a firearm, and 30 percent "knew of someone killed or injured intentionally" by a firearm (Jennissen et al., 2021, p. 1). Song and colleagues (2023) found that firearm injuries among children and young adults had harmful effects on their family members. Mothers in particular faced increased MEB challenges, with a 30 percent rise in psychiatric disorders for parents and a 75 percent increase in MH visits for mothers (Washburn, 2024). Box 7-1 outlines a community coalition's multi-faceted work to address community violence as a cause of

---

BOX 7-1
Community-Led Prevention to Reduce Violence on Chicago's South Side

Beginning in 2015, a coalition of 70 community partners from the Bronzeville community on the South Side of Chicago collaborated on data-driven development, implementation, and evaluation of the Greater Bronzeville Community Action Plan (BSCO, 2018). Supported by the Centers for Disease Control and Prevention-funded Chicago Center for Youth Violence Prevention at the University of Chicago, the Bronzeville community coalition used the Communities That Care (CTC) framework to structure and guide the development and implementation of its community action plan. Rates of violent crime were also among the highest in Chicago, with consequences for the mental, emotional, and behavioral health of residents. The community's assessment showed that approximately one in three students between 6th and 12th grade experienced depressive symptoms and a majority of students felt worried for the safety of friends and family members. The Community Action Plan stated that among Chicago's 15- and 17-year-olds "nearly all had been exposed to some form of violence. Thirty-two percent had a close friend or family member murdered. Eighteen percent—nearly 1 child in 5—had witnessed a shooting that resulted in death" (BSCO, 2018, p.2). The Plan noted that "[v]iolence hurts a wide circle—victims, families, witnesses, and perpetrators. The physical and emotional consequences can last a lifetime, cause deep pain, and trigger other serious problems, including depression, posttraumatic stress

poor MH and provides an illustration of programming that could be paired with municipal or state-level policies that promote safety.

Community violence is not randomly distributed but is highest in communities that experienced discriminatory banking practices on the basis of race and ethnicity under the Home Owners' Loan Corporation in the mid-20th century (Poulson et al., 2021). Firearm violence disproportionately affects Black children and adolescents, with higher rates of exposure to assaults, police shootings, and community violence. Black individuals are nearly 14 times more likely to die from firearm homicide than White individuals, and inpatient admission rates for firearm-related injuries are 9 times higher among Black patients (Schnippel et al., 2021; Semenza et al., 2024). Bor and colleagues (2018) used data from the 2013–2015 BRFSS and Mapping Police Violence databases to examine the MEB impacts of police killings of unarmed Black individuals on other Black adults, finding that each additional police killing in the respondent's state of residence was associated with 0.14 additional poor MH days.

---

disorder (PTSD), aggression and violence, substance abuse, suicide, and poor academic achievement, among other disorders" (BSCO, 2018, p. 2). Given the role of such factors as economic disinvestment and municipal neglect in the community's high rates of violence, the coalition focused not only on preventing violence through evidence-based interventions but also on adapting the CTC framework to address Bronzeville's social and economic health more holistically.

The ensuing action plan had four components: (1) violence prevention through positive youth, family, and community development; (2) supporting schools and school leaders to level the playing field for all schools in the community; (3) faith-led trauma support services for people affected by violence; and (4) employment and placement services for residents. Programs implemented by the community partners included the evidence-based Check and Connect school-based intervention (University of Chicago, 2021) that has been shown to "have positive effects on staying in school" and "potentially positive effects on progressing in school" (IES, 2015).

The coalition's evaluation compared trends in violent crime from 2010-2020 in Bronzeville and similar communities in Chicago. Findings included statistically significant reductions in aggravated assaults and robberies in Bronzeville beginning in 2018, about 3 years after the coalition began its work.

SOURCES: Garthe et al., 2024; Gorman-Smith et al., 2024.

Although mass shootings do not account for the majority of incidents of firearm violence, they have a profound psychological impact on both the individuals directly involved and the broader community. Rossin-Slater and colleagues (2020) examined the impact of local exposure to school shootings on youth antidepressant use. The results showed a 21.4 percent increase in antidepressant use among youth within 2 years of fatal shootings.

A range of interventions have been established as promising at preventing one or more negative health outcomes, including suicide: one 2024 systematic review found that laws requiring secure storage of firearms and preventing child access can reduce rates of suicide, unintentional injury and death, and violent crime (Smart et al., 2024). Emerging evidence indicates that these programs could be implemented at scale (Beidas et al., 2024). Anderson and colleagues (2021) found that child access prevention laws reduced juvenile firearm-related homicides by up to 17 percent. Grossman and colleagues (2005) demonstrated that secure storage was also associated with reductions in youth firearm-related suicide and accidents, which reduces exposure to trauma, preventing the onset of aforementioned MEB issues, such as PTSD.

Smart and colleagues' (2024) systematic review also found that minimum age requirements for purchasing a firearm reduce suicides among young adults. Anestis and Anestis (2015) found that four policies (waiting periods, background checks, gun locks, and open carry permits) were all associated with a lower rate of suicide overall and by firearms specifically; conversely, repeal of such laws led to an associated increase. Researchers in Washington state found that requirements for a permit to purchase assault rifles reduced firearm violence incidents, including those with an assault weapon for individuals under 21 (Bhullar et al., 2024).

Research indicates that red flag laws, also called "Extreme Risk Protection Orders" (ERPOs), civil court orders that temporarily prevent the purchase or possession of firearms, are effective in preventing suicides and homicides or mass shootings (Swanson, 2019; Wintemute et al., 2019; Zeoli et al., 2019). The 2022 Bipartisan Safer Communities Act included $750 million in incentives for states to implement ERPOs and other crisis intervention approaches (Geller, 2023). In March 2024, DOJ launched a National ERPO Resource Center to assist in implementation (OPA, 2024). A composite measure of state-level firearm legislation for 1991–2017 found that states with a higher number of safety policies experienced a lower rate of suicides and homicides (Gunn et al., 2022). Research shows that firearm violence can be heavily concentrated in low-income communities and communities or subpopulations marginalized on the basis of race and ethnicity, and lead to a cycle of violence that leads to trauma and jeopardizes MEB health. Community violence intervention (CVI) uses "evidence-informed strategies to reduce violence through tailored community-centered initiatives" and has been recently supported through a historic federal investment launched by DOJ in FY 2022 (CGVS, n.d.; OJP, n.d.). These approaches are community driven and multisectoral. In 2021, the City of Baltimore released its first Community Violence Prevention Plan, which included support of the CVI ecosystem, including Safe Streets, a violence interrupter program that uses trusted messengers to serve as intermediaries and de-escalate violent situations. The evaluation showed that Safe Streets decreased homicides and nonfatal shootings (Webster et al., 2023). A recent randomized trial of another CVI, Rapid Employment and Development Initiative Chicago, which includes cognitive behavioral therapy and access to social services, found a 65 percent decrease in shootings and homicide arrests (Bhatt et al., 2023).

According to the Department of Veterans Affairs, lethal means safety counseling (LMSC) "is a patient-centered counseling strategy that aims to promote safety behaviors by aligning evidence-based recommendations with patients' preferences and values." It is a health care–centered approach that involves asking if a person at risk of injury or death has access to lethal means and working to reduce that access until the risk subsides (U.S. Department of Veterans Affairs, n.d.; EFSGV, n.d.). A recent review found that LMSC changed behaviors in 14 out of 19 studies, although the quality of these studies varied (Spitzer et al., 2024). A 2021 randomized trial of LMSC coupled with cable locks, however, did find an increase in protective behaviors (Anestis et al., 2021).

CONCLUSION 7-2: *Evidence shows that firearm violence erodes mental, emotional, and behavioral (MEB) health, directly contributing to poor MEB outcomes, including suicide, depression, and anxiety, especially for youth and heavily affected communities.*

RECOMMENDATION 7-3: Federal, state and local policy makers should implement evidence-based policies to prevent firearm violence—a risk factor for mental, emotional, and behavioral disorders—including but not limited to safe and secure gun storage, community violence interventions, and lethal means safety counseling.

Lead Poisoning Prevention

Lead poisoning prevention is a major component of public health programming at the federal, state, and local levels. Because high blood lead levels cause neurological harm, they are associated with lower levels of educational attainment, more behavioral problems (e.g., in school), and other risk factors for poor health and social outcomes, including juvenile detention (NASEM, 2019a, 2024b). Childhood lead exposure is also linked with mental disorders in adulthood (Reuben et al., 2019). Despite the decrease in lead exposure owing to federal regulations and related environmental changes (removing lead from gasoline), approximately 500,000 U.S. children ages 1–5 years have blood lead levels at or above the CDC blood lead reference value of 5 µg/dL (Dignam et al., 2019). Those most at risk for lead exposure are from low-income and minoritized communities (Yeter et al., 2020). The effective interventions needed to address lead hazards are well documented, and National Academies and other reports have called for such interventions, ranging from removing lead water service lines to increasing the enforcement of the Environmental Protection Agency rule that "requires lead-safe renovation, repair, and painting" (NASEM, 2019c, p. 425).

Neighborhood Factors

The quality of neighborhoods matters for MEB health. Policies can support healthy neighborhoods and built environments. One well-known example is the federal Moving to Opportunity experiment, which demonstrated the impact of neighborhood on adult well-being. Researchers found that living in a low-poverty neighborhood had positive impacts on adults' mental and physical health, including decreased rates of depression. Evidence indicates that neighborhood characteristics have considerable effects on MH, well-being, and safety (South et al., 2018; Tach et al., 2016). For example, Branas and colleagues (2016) found that blight remediation measures significantly reduced firearm violence and provided "taxpayer and societal returns on investment for the prevention of firearm violence" of "$5 and $79 for every dollar spent on abandoned building remediation and $26 and $333 for every dollar spent on vacant lot remediation" (p. 2158). Enhancing green spaces, such as greening vacant lots and building parks, is associated with multiple positive outcomes, including enhanced community safety and greater well-being/lower levels of stress (Ashcraft et al., 2024; Hunter et al., 2019).

INCLUDING MEB HEALTH OUTCOMES IN POLICY RESEARCH

Research from various federal agencies has demonstrated that policies can positively impact MEB health and resilience (Purtle, 2016). Examples include housing vouchers, rental assistance, urban green spaces, and the Medicaid Early and Periodic Screening, Diagnostic and Treatment benefit (Ashcraft et al., 2024; Branas et al., 2011; Hunter et al., 2019; PD&R, n.d.; Rosenbaum, 2016). However, MEB health outcomes are not consistently included as a policy target, which represents a missed opportunity to learn whether and to what extent policies are effective at preventing MEB disorders.

RECOMMENDATION 7-4: The Department of Health and Human Services (through the National Institutes of Health, Centers for Disease

Control and Prevention, and Centers for Medicare & Medicaid Services), and the relevant research entities in the Departments of Defense, Education, Housing and Urban Development, Justice, and Veterans Affairs should direct more targeted funding to research that assesses mental, emotional, and behavioral health and population well-being outcomes related to specific policies directed at social, economic, and environmental factors. Studies should include direction and strength of associations, as well as an assessment of causality.

In closing, the overview of implementation considerations for policy provided in Box 7-2 restates the earlier description of the steps for program implementation.

BOX 7-2
8 Steps to Support Implementation of Policies for Mental, Emotional, and Behavioral (MEB) Disorder Prevention

As noted in Chapter 1, these steps toward implementation that benefits all communities are not strictly sequential; many can and should be taken concurrently.

1. **Identify the Need:** To address a problem, policy makers and other constituents will need to take steps to clearly identify it. This can be achieved through needs assessments, such as a community health assessment or community health improvement plan (CDC, 2024a).
2. **Select the Intervention:** Social, economic, and environmental policies that would mitigate risk factors and promote protective factors to prevent MEB disorders.
3. **Map the Constituents:** Community members and leaders, policy makers, and others invested in addressing the need identified in Step 1 need to be engaged to ensure buy-in from all those potentially affected by the policy and to assess whether the policy effectively addresses the need.
4. **Assess Barriers and Facilitators and Understand Context:** Barriers and facilitators, or "determinants," are factors that enable or hinder the adoption, implementation, and sustainment of interventions. These may include costs, workforce availability, and political or collective will to address the issue. Constituents will need to be able to rapidly assess them. Many tools exist to support this assessment, such as a pragmatic context assessment tool (Robinson and Damschroder, 2023).

(continued)

BOX 7-2 Continued

5. **Create a Logic Model:** Once Steps 1–4 are completed, constituents can create a road map for implementation. There is no single correct approach; what matters is that the plan is intentional, forward-looking, and clearly documents the identified need or problem, proposed intervention, required resources, target outcomes, and data and evaluation plans. The Implementation Research Logic Model may be a helpful starting point (Smith et al., 2020a).
6. **Evaluate:** As outlined in the logic model, constituents will need to engage in ongoing evaluation of the intervention to assess its effectiveness and identify whether adjustments are needed.
7. **Adapt:** Early evaluations may indicate that an intervention is on the right track but needs to be adapted to better suit the community's needs. Adaptation is necessary to ensure the interventions success and its alignment with the community to context (Chambers, 2023; Geng et al., 2023; Wiltsey Stirman et al., 2019).
8. **Sustain:** Sustainment is a key focus throughout the entire process. In addition to tools like Designing for Dissemination and Sustainability,[3] emerging evidence on various sustainment strategies may provide valuable insights for communities (Wolfenden et al., 2024).

NOTE: "Constituents" is used to describe any parties with an investment in a policy and its outcomes and not exclusively individuals whom a legislator has been elected to represent.

REFERENCES

Abram, K. M., N. M. Azores-Gococo, K. M. Emanuel, D. A. Aaby, L. J. Welty, J. A. Hershfield, M. S. Rosenbaum, and L. A. Teplin. 2017. Sex and racial/ethnic differences in positive outcomes in delinquent youth after detention: A 12-year longitudinal study. *JAMA Pediatrics* 171(2):123–132. https://doi.org/10.1001/jamapediatrics.2016.3260.

ACF (Administration for Children and Families). 2024. *Head Start services*. https://www.acf.hhs.gov/ohs/about/head-start (accessed December 12, 2024).

ACLU (American Civil Liberties Union). 2024a. *Juvenile justice*. https://www.aclu.org/issues/juvenile-justice (accessed December 16, 2024).

ACLU. 2024b. *Mapping attacks on LGBTQ rights in U.S. state legislatures in 2023*. https://www.aclu.org/legislative-attacks-on-lgbtq-rights-2023 (accessed December 13, 2024).

Agarwal, S. D., B. Lê Cook, and J. B. Liebman. 2024. Effect of cash benefits on health care utilization and health: A randomized study. *JAMA* 332(17):1455–1463. https://doi.org/10.1001/jama.2024.13004.

---

[3] https://implementationresearch.wustl.edu/support-your-research/di-methods-tool-2/ (accessed January 16, 2025).

Akers, L., J. Tippins, S. Hauan, and M. Lynch-Smith. 2022. *Advancing primary prevention in human services: Convening findings.* https://aspe.hhs.gov/sites/default/files/documents/8228e700f6e369df9382ac8e0d3976c1/primary-prevention-convening-brief.pdf (accessed December 16, 2024).

Alegría, M., J. Zhen-Duan, I. S. O'Malley, and K. DiMarzio. 2022. A new agenda for optimizing investments in community mental health and reducing disparities. *American Journal of Psychiatry* 179(6):402–416. https://doi.org/10.1176/appi.ajp.21100970.

Anderson, D. M., J. J. Sabia, and E. Tekin. 2021. Child access prevention laws and juvenile firearm-related homicides. *Journal of Urban Economics* 126:103387. https://doi.org/10.1016/j.jue.2021.103387.

Anestis, M. D., and J. C. Anestis. 2015. Suicide rates and state laws regulating access and exposure to handguns. *American Journal of Public Health* 105(10):2049–2058. https://doi.org/10.2105/ajph.2015.302753.

Anestis, M. D., C. J. Bryan, D. W. Capron, and A. O. Bryan. 2021. Lethal means counseling, distribution of cable locks, and safe firearm storage practices among the Mississippi National Guard: A factorial randomized controlled trial, 2018-2020. *American Journal of Public Health* 111(2):309–317. https://doi.org/10.2105/AJPH.2020.306019.

Ashcraft, L. E., K. I. Cabrera, M. B. Lane-Fall, and E. C. South. 2024. Leveraging implementation science to advance environmental justice research and achieve health equity through neighborhood and policy interventions. *Annual Review of Public Health* 45(1):89–108. https://doi.org/10.1146/annurev-publhealth-060222-033003.

Austin, A. E., M. Frank, M. E. Shanahan, H. L. M. Reyes, G. Corbie, and R. B. Naumann. 2023. Association of state supplemental nutrition assistance program eligibility policies with adult mental health and suicidality. *JAMA Network Open* 6(4):e238415. https://doi.org/10.1001/jamanetworkopen.2023.8415.

Baicker, K., S. L. Taubman, H. L. Allen, M. Bernstein, J. H. Gruber, J. P. Newhouse, E. C. Schneider, B. J. Wright, A. M. Zaslavsky, and A. N. Finkelstein; Oregon Health Study Group. 2013. The Oregon experiment — effects of Medicaid on clinical outcomes. *New England Journal of Medicine* 368(18):1713–1722. https://doi.org/10.1056/NEJMsa1212321.

Bales, W., M. Nadel, and G. Pesta. 2019. Research project #1 an assessment of the effectiveness of civil citation as an alternative to arrest among youth apprehended by law enforcement.

Barnert, E. S., R. Dudovitz, B. B. Nelson, T. R. Coker, C. Biely, N. Li, and P. J. Chung. 2017. How does incarcerating young people affect their adult health outcomes? *Pediatrics* 139(2). https://doi.org/10.1542/peds.2016-2624.

Batra, A., K. Jackson, and R. Hamad. 2023. Effects of the 2021 expanded child tax credit on adults' mental health: A quasi-experimental study. *Health Affairs* 42(1):74–82. https://doi.org/10.1377/hlthaff.2022.00733.

Bauermeister, J. A. 2014. How statewide LGB policies go from "under our skin" to "into our hearts": Fatherhood aspirations and psychological well-being among emerging adult sexual minority men. *Journal of Youth and Adolescence* 43:1295–1305. https://doi.org/10.1007/s10964-013-0059-6.

Beidas, R. S., K. A. Linn, J. M. Boggs, S. C. Marcus, K. Hoskins, S. Jager-Hyman, C. Johnson, M. Maye, L. Quintana, C. B. Wolk, L. Wright, C. Pappas, A. Beck, K. Bedjeti, A. M. Buttenheim, M. F. Daley, M. Elias, J. Lyons, M. L. Martin, B. McArdle, D. P. Ritzwoller, D. S. Small, N. J. Williams, S. Zhang, and B. K. Ahmedani. 2024. Implementation of a secure firearm storage program in pediatric primary care: A cluster randomized trial. *JAMA Pediatrics*. https://doi.org/10.1001/jamapediatrics.2024.3274.

Bhatt, M. P., S. B. Heller, M. Kapustin, M. Bertrand, and C. Blattman. 2023. Predicting and preventing gun violence: An experimental evaluation of READI Chicago. *The Quarterly Journal of Economics* 139(1):1–56. https://doi.org/10.1093/qje/qjad031.

Bhullar, A., J. Shipley, L. Alaniz, A. Grigorian, S. Burruss, L. Swentek, C. Kuza, and J. Nahmias. 2024. Washington State assault weapon firearm violence before and after firearm legislation reform. *The American Journal of Surgery* 90(10):2384–2388. https://doi.org/10.1177/00031348241244644.

Blanchard, E. B., and E. J. Hickling. 2004. After the crash: Psychological assessment and treatment of survivors of motor vehicle accidents: American Psychological Association.

Bor, J., A. S. Venkataramani, D. R. Williams, and A. C. Tsai. 2018. Police killings and their spillover effects on the mental health of black Americans: A population-based, quasi-experimental study. *Lancet* 392(10144):302–310. https://doi.org/10.1016/ S0140-6736(18)31130-9.

Boyd-Swan, C., C. M. Herbert, J. Ifcher, and H. Zarghamee. 2015. The earned income tax credit, mental health, and happiness. *Journal of Economic Behavior & Organization* 126:18–38. https://doi.org/10.1016/j.jebo.2015.11.004.

Branas, C. C., R. A. Cheney, J. M. MacDonald, V. W. Tam, T. D. Jackson, and T. R. Ten Have. 2011. A difference-in-differences analysis of health, safety, and greening vacant urban space. *American Journal of Epidemiology* 174(11):1296–1306. https://doi.org/10.1093/aje/kwr273.

Branas, C. C., M. C. Kondo, S. M. Murphy, E. C. South, D. Polsky, and J. M. MacDonald. 2016. Urban blight remediation as a cost-beneficial solution to firearm violence. *American Journal of Public Health* 106(12):2158–2164. https://doi.org/10.2105/ajph.2016.303434.

BSCO (Bright Star Community Outreach). 2018. Greater Bronzeville community action plan. https://cpb-us-w2.wpmucdn.com/voices.uchicago.edu/dist/6/954/files/2018/06/community_action_plan_working_document-19517ps.pdf (accessed December 16, 2024).

Cabral, M., B. Kim, M. Rossin-Slater, M. Schnell, and H. Schwandt. 2024. Trauma at school: The impacts of shootings on students' human capital and economic outcomes. National Bureau of Economic Research Working Paper Series, No. 28311. http://www.nber.org/papers/w28311 (accessed January 2, 2025).

Carlson, S., and Z. Neuberger. 2021. *WIC works: Addressing the nutrition and health needs of low-income families for more than four decades.* Center on Budget and Policy Priorities. https://www.cbpp.org/research/food-assistance/wic-works-addressing-the-nutrition-and-health-needs-of-low-income-families (accessed January 2, 2025).

CASEL (Collaborative for Academic, Social, and Emotional Learning). n.d. *SEL and mental health.* https://casel.org/fundamentals-of-sel/how-does-sel-support-your-priorities/sel-and-mental-health/ (accessed October 20, 2024).

Casey Family Programs. 2023. *What should child protection agencies consider when working with children whose parent or primary caregiver is incarcerated?* https://www.casey.org/parental-incarceration-issue (accessed January 2, 2025).

CBPP (Center on Budget and Policy Priorities). 2023. *Policy basics: The earned income tax credit.* https://www.cbpp.org/research/policy-basics-the-earned-income-tax-credit (accessed December 13, 2024).

CDC (Centers for Disease Control and Prevention). 2011. Ten great public health achievements—United States, 2001–2010. *Morbidity and Mortality Weekly Reoport* 60(19);619–623. https://www.cdc.gov/mmwr/preview/mmwrhtml/mm6019a5.htm (accessed January 2, 2024).

CDC. 2024a. *Community planning for health assessment: CHA & CHIP.* https://www.cdc.gov/public-health-gateway/php/public-health-strategy/public-health-strategies-for-community-health-assessment-health-improvement-planning.html (accessed November 11, 2024).

CDC. 2024b. *Excessive Alcohol Use in the United States.* https://www.cdc.gov/alcohol/fact-sheets/states/excessive-alcohol-use-united-states.html

CGVS (Johns Hopkins Bloomberg School of Public Health Center for Gun Violence Solutions). n.d. *Community violence intervention.* https://publichealth.jhu.edu/center-for-gun-violence-solutions/solutions/community-violence-intervention (accessed October 28, 2024).

Cha, E., J. Lee, and S. Tao. 2023. Impact of the expanded child tax credit and its expiration on adult psychological well-being. *Social Science and Medicine* 332:116101. https://doi.org/10.1016/j.socscimed.2023.116101.
Chambers, D. A. 2023. Advancing adaptation of evidence-based interventions through implementation science: Progress and opportunities. *Frontiers in Health Services* 3:1204138. https://doi.org/10.3389/frhs.2023.1204138.
Chetty, R., N. Hendren, and L. F. Katz. 2016. The effects of exposure to better neighborhoods on children: New evidence from the moving to opportunity experiment. *American Economic Review* 106(4):855–902. https://doi.org/10.1257/aer.20150572.
Collins, J., and E. Swoveland. 2014. The impact of gun violence on children, families, & communities. *Children's VOICE* 23(1):10–13. https://www.cwla.org/the-impact-of-gun-violence-on-children-families-communities/ (accessed November 20, 2024).
CSI (Clean Slate Initiative). 2024. *Barriers and restrictions*. https://www.cleanslateinitiative.org/maryland (accessed December 16, 2024).
Delpin-Rittmon, M. E. 2023. *Lethal means safety for suicide prevention*. https://www.samhsa.gov/blog/lethal-means-safety-suicide-prevention (accessed October 29, 2024).
Dempsey, C. L., D. M. Benedek, K. L. Zuromski, C. Riggs-Donovan, T. H. H. Ng, M. K. Nock, R. C. Kessler, and R. J. Ursano. 2019. Association of firearm ownership, use, accessibility, and storage practices with suicide risk among us army soldiers. *JAMA Network Open* 2(6):e195383–e195383. https://doi.org/10.1001/jamanetworkopen.2019.5383.
Dexler, M. 2016. *Guns & suicide*. Harvard Public Health. https://hsph.harvard.edu/news/guns-suicide/ (accessed December 16, 2024).
Dignam, T., R. B. Kaufmann, L. LeStourgeon, and M. J. Brown. 2019. Control of lead sources in the United States, 1970–2017: Public health progress and current challenges to eliminating lead exposure. *Journal of Public Health Management and Practice* 25(Suppl 1):S13–S22. https://doi.org/10.1097/PHH.0000000000000889.
Dow, W. H., A. Godoy, C. Lowenstein, and M. Reich. 2020. Can labor market policies reduce deaths of despair? *Journal of Health Economics* 74:102372. https://doi.org/10.1016/j.jhealeco.2020.102372.
Drexler, Madeline. 2016. *Guns & Suicide*. Harvard T. H. Chan School of Public Health. https://hsph.harvard.edu/news/guns-suicide/ (accessed January 14, 2025).
DSCYF (Delaware Department of Services for Children, Youth, & Their Families). n.d. *Juvenile civil citation*. https://kids.delaware.gov/youth-rehabilitative-services/juvenile-civil-citation/ (accessed November 18, 2024).
Duara, K. 2024. *California voters get tough on crime, pass Prop 36*. Cal Matters. https://calmatters.org/politics/elections/2024/11/prop-36-california-election-result/ (accessed December 12, 2024).
Edgemon, T. G., and J. Clay-Warner. 2019. Inmate mental health and the pains of imprisonment. *Society and Mental Health* 9(1):33–50. https://doi.org/10.1177/2156869318785424.
EFSGV (The Educational Fund to Stop Gun Violence). n.d. *Lethal means safety counseling*. https://efsgv.org/learn/policies/lethal-means-safety-counseling/ (accessed November 14, 2024).
First Five Years Fund. 2022. *Report demonstrates inequitable access to head start services*. https://www.ffyf.org/resources/2022/12/report-inequitable-access-to-head-start-services/ (accessed September 11, 2024).
Garthe, R. C., D. Gorman-Smith, S. Kim, S. Yoon, S. Mwima, and F. N. Cosey-Gay. 2024. Promotive Factors Within Neighborhood, Family, and School Contexts for Adolescents Living in an Urban, High-Burden Community. Youth & Society, 0044118X241282348.
Geller, A., C. E. Cooper, I. Garfinkel, O. Schwartz-Soicher, and R. B. Mincy. 2012. Beyond absenteeism: Father incarceration and child development. *Demography* 49:49–76. https://doi.org/10.1007/s13524-011-0081-9.
Geller, L., and S. Cantrell. 2023. *A critical opportunity for extreme risk protection order implementation*. https://rockinst.org/blog/a-critical-opportunity-for-extreme-risk-protection-order-implementation/ (accessed October 19, 2024).

Geng, E. H., A. Mody, and B. J. Powell. 2023. On-the-go adaptation of implementation approaches and strategies in health: Emerging perspectives and research opportunities. *Annual Review of Public Health* 44(1):21–36. https://doi.org/10.1146/annurev-publhealth-051920-124515.

Golberstein, E. 2015. The effects of income on mental health: Evidence from the Social Security notch. *Journal of Mental Health Policy and Economics* 18(1):27–37. https://pubmed.ncbi.nlm.nih.gov/25862202/ (accessed January 3, 2025).

Golden, L., and J. Kim. 2020. *The involuntary part-time work and underemployment problem in the U.S.* Center for Law and Social Policy. https://www.clasp.org/sites/default/files/publications/2020/08/GWC2029_Center%20For%20Law.pdf (accessed January 3, 2024).

Gorman-Smith, D., R. C. Garthe, M. E. Schoeny, F. N. Cosey-Gay, C. Harris Sr., C. H. Brown, and J. A. Villamar. 2024. The impact of the Communities that Care approach in reducing violence and crime within an urban, high-burden community. *Prevention Science*, 25(6):863–877. https://doi.org/10.1007/s11121-024-01707-5.

Grossman, D. C., B. A. Mueller, C. Riedy, M. D. Dowd, A. Villaveces, J. Prodzinski, J. Nakagawara, J. Howard, N. Thiersch, and R. Harruff. 2005. Gun storage practices and risk of youth suicide and unintentional firearm injuries. *JAMA* 293(6):707–714. https://doi.org/10.1001/jama.293.6.707.

GSDI (Global Spatial Data Infrastructure Association). 2021. *Economic security*. https://gsdi.unc.edu/our-work/economic-security/ (accessed December 13, 2024).

Gubits, D. M. S., B. Bell, M. Wood, S. R. Dastrup, C. Solari, S. Brown, S. Brown, L. Dunton, W. Lin, D. McInnis, J. Rodriguez, G. Savidge, and B. Spellman,. 2015. *Family options study: Short-term impacts of housing and services interventions for homeless families*. U.S. Department of Housing and Urban Development. https://papers.ssrn.com/sol3/papers.cfm?abstract_id=3055272 (accessed January 3, 2025).

Gunn, J. F., P. Boxer, T. Andrews, M. Ostermann, S. L. Bonne, M. Gusmano, E. Sloan-Power, and B. Hohl. 2022. The impact of firearm legislation on firearm deaths, 1991–2017. *Journal of Public Health* 44(3):614–624. https://doi.org/10.1093/pubmed/fdab047.

Hafeez, H., M. Zeshan, M. A. Tahir, N. Jahan, and S. Naveed. 2017. Health care disparities among lesbian, gay, bisexual, and transgender youth: A literature review. *Cureus* 9(4):e1184. https://doi.org/10.7759/cureus.1184.

Hamersma, S., and J. Ye. 2021. The effect of public health insurance expansions on the mental and behavioral health of girls and boys. *Social Science and Medicine* 280:113998. https://doi.org/10.1016/j.socscimed.2021.113998.

Hatzenbuehler, M. L. 2009. How does sexual minority stigma "get under the skin"? A psychological mediation framework. *Psychological Bulletin* 135(5):707. https://doi.org/10.1037/a0016441.

Hatzenbuehler, M. L. 2011. The social environment and suicide attempts in lesbian, gay, and bisexual youth. *Pediatrics* 127(5):896–903. https://doi.org/10.1542/peds.2010-3020.

Hatzenbuehler, M. L. 2014. Structural stigma and the health of lesbian, gay, and bisexual populations. *Current Directions in Psychological Science* 23(2):127–132. https://doi.org/10.1177/0963721414523775.

Hatzenbuehler, M. L. 2017. Advancing research on structural stigma and sexual orientation disparities in mental health among youth. *Journal of Clinical Child & Adolescent Psychology* 46(3):463–475. https://doi.org/10.1080/15374416.2016.1247360.

Hatzenbuehler, M. L., and B. G. Link. 2014. Introduction to the special issue on structural stigma and health: Elsevier. https://doi.org/10.1016/j.socscimed.2013.12.017.

Herman, D. R., M. Westfall, M. Bashir, and P. Afulani. 2024. Food insecurity and mental distress among WIC-eligible women in the United States: A cross-sectional study. *Journal of the Academy of Nutrition and Dietetics* 124(1):65–79. https://doi.org/10.1016/j.jand.2023.09.006.

Heshmati, A., H. Honkaniemi, and S. P. Juarez. 2023. The effect of parental leave on parents' mental health: A systematic review. *Lancet Public Health* 8(1):e57–e75. https://doi.org/10.1016/S2468-2667(22)00311-5.

HHS (Department of Health and Human Services). n.d. *Mental health*. https://eclkc.ohs.acf.hhs.gov/mental-health (accessed December 13, 2024).

Hoynes, H., D. Miller, and D. Simon. 2015. Income, the earned income tax credit, and infant health. *American Economic Journal: Economic Policy* 7(1):172–211. https://doi.org/10.1257/pol.20120179.

Huey, M. P., and T. L. McNulty. 2005. Institutional conditions and prison suicide: Conditional effects of deprivation and overcrowding. *The Prison Journal* 85(4):490–514. https://doi.org/10.1177/0032885505282258.

Hunter, R. F., C. Cleland, A. Cleary, M. Droomers, B. W. Wheeler, D. Sinnett, M. J. Nieuwenhuijsen, and M. Braubach. 2019. Environmental, health, wellbeing, social and equity effects of urban green space interventions: A meta-narrative evidence synthesis. *Environment International* 130:104923. https://doi.org/10.1016/j.envint.2019.104923/.

Hutchins, H., J. Abercrombie, and C. Lipton. 2023. Promotion of early childhood development and mental health in quality rating and improvement systems for early care and education: A review of state quality indicators. *Early Childhood Research Quarterly* 64:229–241. https://doi.org/10.1016/j.ecresq.2023.03.006.

IES (Institute of Education Sciences). 2015. WWC intervention report: Check & connect. https://ies.ed.gov/ncee/WWC/Docs/InterventionReports/wwc_checkconnect_050515.pdf (accessed December 16, 2024).

IOM (Institute of Medicine). 2013. *U.S. Health in international perspective: Shorter lives, poorer health*. Washington, DC: The National Academies Press. https://doi.org/10.17226/13497.

Irish, A. M., J. S. White, S. Modrek, and R. Hamad. 2021. Paid family leave and mental health in the US: A quasi-experimental study of state policies. *American Journal of Preventive Medicine* 61(2):182–191. https://doi.org/10.1016/j.amepre.2021.03.018.

Jennissen, C. A., R. P. King, K. M. Wetjen, G. M. Denning, C. C. Wymore, N. R. Stange, P. J. Hoogerwerf, J. Liao, and K. E. Wood. 2021. Rural youth's exposure to firearm violence and their attitudes regarding firearm safety measures. *Injury Epidemiol* 8(Suppl 1):29. https://doi.org/10.1186/s40621-021-00317-x.

Johnson, M. 2022. The dangerous consequences of Florida's "Don't Say Gay" bill on LGBTQ+ youth in Florida. *The Georgetown Journal of Gender and Law* XXIII(3). https://www.law.georgetown.edu/gender-journal/online/volume-xxiii-online/the-dangerous-consequences-of-floridas-dont-say-gay-bill-on-lgbtq-youth-in-florida/ (accessed December 13, 2024).

Jou, J., K. B. Kozhimannil, J. M. Abraham, L. A. Blewett, and P. M. McGovern. 2018. Paid maternity leave in the United States: Associations with maternal and infant health. *Maternal and Child Health Journal*, 22(2):216–225.

Kluender, R., N. Mahoney, F. Wong, and W. Yin. 2021. Medical debt in the US, 2009–2020. *JAMA* 326(3):250–256. https://doi.org/10.1001/jama.2021.8694.

Latessa, E. J., B. Lovins, and J. Lux. 2014. Evaluation of Ohio's reclaim programs. *Center for Criminal Justice Research: Cincinnati*. https://ojjdp.ojp.gov/sites/g/files/xyckuh176/files/pubs/reform2/ch3_d.html#340 (accessed January 3, 2025).

Lee, H., C. Wildeman, E. A. Wang, N. Matusko, and J. S. Jackson. 2014. A heavy burden: The cardiovascular health consequences of having a family member incarcerated. *American Journal of Public Health* 104(3):421–7. https://doi.org/10.2105/AJPH.2013.301504.

Levengood, T. W., and S. E. Hadland. 2023. Hostile laws and hospitalization: Why anti-lgbtq+ legislation threatens adolescent lives. *Journal of Hospital Medicine* 18(5):449. https://doi.org/10.1002/jhm.13038.

Lindenfeld, Z., S. Kim, and J. E. Chang. 2022. Assessing the effectiveness of problem-solving courts on the reduction of overdose deaths in the United States: A difference-in-difference study. *Drug and Alcohol Dependence Reports* 4:100088. https://doi.org/10.1016/j.dadr.2022.100088.

Lux, J. L., M. Schweitzer, and C. Chouhy. 2015. Downsizing juvenile institutions in Ohio: Five innovations. *Victims & Offenders* 10(4):379–400. https://doi.org/10.1080/15564886.2015.1078181.

Maas, S. 2016. *Financial impacts of medicaid expansion under the ACA.* https://www.nber.org/digest/aug16/financial-impacts-medicaid-expansion-under-aca (accessed September 21, 2024).

Magee, L. A., D. Semenza, S. Gharbi, and S. E. Wiehe. 2023. Addressing mental health needs of secondary homicide survivors through a social determinants of health framework. *Homicide Studies* 27(4):435–453. https://doi.org/10.1177/10887679231163099.

McGough, M., K. Amin, N. Panchal, and C. Cox. 2023. *Child and teen firearm mortality in the U.S. and peer countries.* https://www.kff.org/mental-health/issue-brief/child-and-teen-firearm-mortality-in-the-u-s-and-peer-countries/ (accessed December 12, 2024).

McKay, F. H., R. Bennett, and M. Dunn. 2023. How, why and for whom does a basic income contribute to health and wellbeing: A systematic review. *Health Promotion International* 38(5):daad119. https://doi.org/10.1093/heapro/daad119.

McKie, K. A., R. C. Bell, and L. K. Lee. 2024. Variations by state in firearm suicide among US children and young adults, 2016–2021. *JAMA Pediatrics* 178(7):722–25. https://doi.org/10.1001/jamapediatrics.2024.1128.

Mendel, R. 2023a. *System reforms to reduce youth incarceration: Why we must explore every option before removing any young person from home.* The Sentencing Project. https://www.sentencingproject.org/reports/system-reforms-to-reduce-youth-incarceration-why-we-must-explore-every-option-before-removing-any-young-person-from-home/ (accessed December 16, 2024).

Mendel, R. 2023b. *Why youth incarceration fails: An updated review of the evidence.* The Sentencing Project. https://www.sentencingproject.org/reports/why-youth-incarceration-fails-an-updated-review-of-the-evidence/ (accessed December 16, 2024).

Moore, S. A., J. M. Cooper, J. Malloy, and A. R. Lyon. 2024. Core components and implementation determinants of multilevel service delivery frameworks across child mental health service settings. *Administration and Policy in Mental Health* 51(2):172–195. https://doi.org/10.1007/s10488-023-01320-8.

Murphy, J. M., M. E. Pagano, J. Nachmani, P. Sperling, S. Kane, and R. E. Kleinman. 1998. The relationship of school breakfast to psychosocial and academic functioning: Cross-sectional and longitudinal observations in an inner-city school sample. *Archives of Pediatrics & Adolescent Medicine* 152(9):899–907. https://doi.org/10.1001/archpedi.152.9.899.

Naimi, T. S., J. G. Blanchette, Z. Xuan, and F. J. Chaloupka. 2018. Erosion of state alcohol excise taxes in the United States. *Journal of Studies on Alcohol and Drugs* 79(1):43–48. https://doi.org/10.15288/jsad.2018.79.43.

Nam, J., and S. J. Kwon. 2024. Expansion of child tax credits and mental health of parents with low income in 2021. *JAMA Network Open* 7(2):e2356419. https://doi.org/10.1001/jamanetworkopen.2023.56419.

NASEM (National Academies of Sciences, Engineering, and Medicine). 2016. *How Modeling Can Inform Strategies to Improve Population Health: Workshop Summary.* Washington, DC: The National Academies Press. https://doi.org/10.17226/21807.

NASEM. 2017. *Communities in Action: Pathways to Health Equity.* Washington, DC: The National Academies Press. https://doi.org/10.17226/24624.

NASEM. 2018. *Getting to zero alcohol-impaired driving fatalities: A comprehensive approach to a persistent problem.* Washington, DC: The National Academies Press. https://doi.org/10.17226/24951.

NASEM. 2019a. *Fostering healthy mental, emotional, and behavioral development in children and youth: A national agenda.* Washington, DC: The National Academies Press. https://doi.org/10.17226/25201.
NASEM. 2019b. *The promise of adolescence: Realizing opportunity for all youth.* Washington, DC: The National Academies Press. https://doi.org/10.17226/25388.
NASEM. 2019c. *Vibrant and healthy kids: Aligning science, practice, and policy to advance health equity.* Washington, DC: The National Academies Press. https://doi.org/10.17226/25466.
NASEM. 2019d. *A Roadmap to Reducing Child Poverty.* Washington, DC: The National Academies Press. https://doi.org/10.17226/25246.
NASEM. 2023. *Federal policy to advance racial, ethnic, and tribal health equity.* Washington, DC: National Academies Press. https://doi.org/10.17226/26834.
NASEM. 2024b. *Reducing intergenerational poverty.* Washington, DC: The National Academies Press. https://doi.org/10.17226/27058.
NASEM. 2024c. *Social media and adolescent health.* Washington, DC: The National Academies Press. https://doi.org/10.17226/27396.
NCSL (National Conference of State Legislatures). 2023. Criminal record and reentry toolkit. https://www.ncsl.org/civil-and-criminal-justice/criminal-records-and-reentry-toolkit (accessed January 3, 2025).
Newcomb, M. E., M. C. LaSala, A. Bouris, B. Mustanski, G. Prado, S. M. Schrager, and D. M. Huebner. 2019. The influence of families on LGBTQ youth health: A call to action for innovation in research and intervention development. *LGBT Health* 6(4):139–145. https://doi.org/10.1089/lgbt.2018.0157.
NHTSA (National Highway Traffic Safety Administration). n.d. *Drunk driving.* https://www.nhtsa.gov/risky-driving/drunk-driving (accessed January 14, 2025).
NHVRC (National Home Visiting Resource Center). 2018. *Home visiting yearbook.* https://www.nhvrc.org/wp-content/uploads/NHVRC_Yearbook_2018_FINAL.pdf (accessed January 3, 2025).
NIJ (National Institute of Justice). 2021. *Impact of California's Proposition 47 (The Reduced Penalties for Some Crimes Initiative) on recidivism.* https://crimesolutions.ojp.gov/ratedprograms/impact-californias-proposition-47-reduced-penalties-some-crimes-initiative-recidivism (accessed January 2, 2025).
NRC (National Research Council). 2011. *Improving Health in the United States: The Role of Health Impact Assessment.* Washington, DC: The National Academies Press. https://doi.org/10.17226/13229.
OJJDP (DOJ Office of Juvenile Justice and Delinquency Prevention). 1997. Juvenile justice reform initiatives in the States 1994–1996: Ohio: Sharing responsibility for administration of juvenile justice. https://www.ojp.gov/pdffiles/reform.pdf (accessed November 20, 2024).
OJP (Department of Justice Office of Justice Programs). n.d. *Community violence intervention.* https://www.ojp.gov/topics/community-violence-intervention (accessed October 28, 2024).
OJP. 2020. *Treatment courts.* https://www.ojp.gov/feature/treatment-courts/overview (accessed October 29, 2024).
OMHSP (U.S. Department of Veterans Affairs, Office of Mental Health and Suicide Prevention). 2022. *National Veteran Suicide Prevention Annual Report 2022.* https://www.mentalhealth.va.gov/docs/data-sheets/2022/2022-National-Veteran-Suicide-Prevention-Annual-Report-FINAL-508.pdf (accessed December 16, 2024).
OMHSP. 2023. *National Veteran Suicide Prevention Annual Report 2023.* https://www.mentalhealth.va.gov/docs/data-sheets/2023/2023-National-Veteran-Suicide-Prevention-Annual-Report-FINAL-508.pdf (accessed December 12, 2024).
OPA (DOJ Office of Public Affairs). 2024. Justice department launches the national extreme risk protection order resource center. https://www.justice.gov/opa/pr/justice-department-launches-national-extreme-risk-protection-order-resource-center (accessed October 21, 2024).

OSG (Office of the Surgeon General). 2023. *Social media and youth mental health.* https://www.hhs.gov/sites/default/files/sg-youth-mental-health-social-media-advisory.pdf (accessed January 3, 2025).

OSG. 2024. *Firearm violence in America.* https://www.hhs.gov/sites/default/files/firearm-violence-advisory.pdf (accessed November 20, 2024).

Panchal, N. 2024. *The impact of gun violence on children and adolescents.* https://www.kff.org/mental-health/issue-brief/the-impact-of-gun-violence-on-children-and-adolescents/ (accessed September 11, 2024).

Parrish, K. 2012. Dempsey: Military must persevere to solve suicide issue. *American Forces Press Service.* https://www.army.mil/article/80940/dempsey_military_must_persevere_to_solve_suicide_issue (accessed January 3, 2025).

PD&R (Housing and Urban Development Office of Policy Development and Research). n.d. *Moving to Opportunity (MTO).* https://www.huduser.gov/portal/mto.html (accessed November 20, 2024).

Penney, S. C., G. Young, E. Butler, K. Maich, and D. F. Philpott. 2019. The role of quality ECE in facilitating mental health and well-being in children. *Exceptionality Education International* 29(3):57–76. https://doi.org/10.5206/eei.v29i3.9387.

Poulson, M., M. Y. Neufeld, T. Dechert, L. Allee, and K. M. Kenzik. 2021. Historic redlining, structural racism, and firearm violence: A structural equation modeling approach. *The Lancet Regional Health–Americas* 3. https://doi.org/10.1016/j.lana.2021.10 0 052.

Pourmotabbed, A., S. Moradi, A. Babaei, A. Ghavami, H. Mohammadi, C. Jalili, M. E. Symonds, and M. Miraghajani. 2020. Food insecurity and mental health: A systematic review and meta-analysis. *Public Health Nutrition* 23(10):1778–1790. https://doi.org/10.1017/S136898001900435X.

Purtle, J., R. Peters, R. C. Brownson. 2016. A review of policy dissemination and implementation research funded by the national institutes of health, 2007–2014. *Implementation Science* 11(1):1. https://doi.org/10.1186/s13012-015-0367-1.

Raifman, J., E. Moscoe, S. B. Austin, and M. McConnell. 2017. Difference-in-differences analysis of the association between state same-sex marriage policies and adolescent suicide attempts. *JAMA Pediatrics* 171(4):350–356. https://doi.org/10.1001/jamapediatrics.2016.4529.

Ramos, N., A. Burgess, and E. Ollen. 2023. The current status of sociopolitical and legal issues faced by lesbian, gay, bisexual, transgender, queer, and questioning youth. *Adolescent Psychiatry* 12, no. 3 (2022): 180-195. https://doi.org/10.2174/2210676611666211105120645.

RAND. 2024. *Gun policy research review.* https://www.rand.org/research/gun-policy/analysis.html#modalDialog (accessed October 28, 2024).

Reuben, A., J. D. Schaefer, T. E. Moffitt, J. Broadbent, H. Harrington, R. M. Houts, S. Ramrakha, R. Poulton, and A. Caspi. 2019. Association of childhood lead exposure with adult personality traits and lifelong mental health. *JAMA Psychiatry* 76(4):418–425. https://doi.org/10.1001/jamapsychiatry.2018.4192.

Rheingold, A. A., H. Zinzow, A. Hawkins, B. E. Saunders, and D. G. Kilpatrick. 2012. Prevalence and mental health outcomes of homicide survivors in a representative US sample of adolescents: Data from the 2005 national survey of adolescents. *Journal of Child Psychology and Psychiatry* 53(6):687–694. https://doi.org/10.1111/j.1469-7610.2011.02491.x.

Richmond, T. 2024. The bidirectional relationship between firearm violence and behavioral health. Presented on February 22, 2024, at Meeting 2 of the Committee on a Blueprint for a National Prevention Infrastructure for Behavioral Health Ddisorders. https://www.nationalacademies.org/event/41980_02-2024_blueprint-for-a-national-prevention-infrastructure-for-behavioral-health-disorders-meeting-2 (accessed October 5, 2024).

Robinson, C. H., and L. J. Damschroder. 2023. A Pragmatic Context Assessment Tool (pCAT): Using a think aloud method to develop an assessment of contextual barriers to change. *Implementation Science Communications* 4(1):3. https://doi.org/10.1186/s43058-022-00380-5.

Rosenbaum, S. 2016. When old is new: Medicaid's EPSDT benefit at fifty, and the future of child health policy. *The Milbank Quarterly* 94(4):716. https://www.milbank.org/quarterly/articles/old-new-medicaids-epsdt-benefit-fifty-future-child-health-policy/ (accessed January 3, 2025).

Rossin-Slater, M., M. Schnell, H. Schwandt, S. Trejo, and L. Uniat. 2020. Local exposure to school shootings and youth antidepressant use. *Proceedings of the National Academy of Science* 117(38):23484–23489. https://doi.org/10.1073/pnas.2000804117.

Rovner, J. 2024. *Youth justice by the numbers.* https://www.sentencingproject.org/app/uploads/2024/08/Youth-Justice-By-The-Numbers.pdf (accessed January 3, 2025).

Russell, S. T., A. M. Pollitt, G. Li, and A. H. Grossman. 2018. Chosen name use is linked to reduced depressive symptoms, suicidal ideation, and suicidal behavior among transgender youth. *Journal of adolescent Health* 63(4):503–505. https://doi.org/10.1016/j.jadohealth.2018.02.003.

SAMHSA (Substance Abuse and Mental Health Services Administration). 2024a. *Climate change and health equity.* https://www.samhsa.gov/find-help/disasters/climate-change-health-equity (accessed October 20, 2024).

SAMHSA. 2024b. *Disaster technical assistance center supplemental research bulletin: Climate change and behavioral health.* https://www.samhsa.gov/sites/default/files/dtac-climate-change-behavioral-health.pdf (accessed January 2, 2025).

Sard, B., M. Cunningham, and R. Greenstein. 2018. *Helping young children move out of poverty by creating a new type of rental voucher.* https://www.mobilitypartnership.org/file/1218671/JOe-i15a.pdf (accessed December 13, 2024).

Sawyer, W., and P. Wagner. 2024. *Mass incarceration: The whole pie 2024.* Prison Policy Initiative. https://www.prisonpolicy.org/reports/pie2024.html (accessed December 16, 2024).

Schnippel, K., S. Burd-Sharps, T. R. Miller, B. A. Lawrence, and D. I. Swedler. 2021. Nonfatal firearm injuries by intent in the United States: 2016–2018 hospital discharge records from the healthcare cost and utilization project. *Western Journal of Emergency Medicine* 22(3):462. https://doi.org/10.5811/westjem.2021.3.51925.

Semenza, D. C., S. Daruwala, J. R. B. Stephens, and M. D. Anestis. 2024. Gun violence exposure and suicide among black adults. *JAMA Network Open* 7(2):e2354953–e2354953. https://doi.org/10.1001/jamanetworkopen.2023.54953.

Smart, R., A. R. Morral, J. P. Murphy, R. Jose, A. Charbonneau, and S. Smucker. 2024. *The science of gun policy: A critical synthesis of research evidence on the effects of gun policies in the United States, fourth edition.* Santa Monica, CA: RAND Corporation. https://www.rand.org/pubs/research_reports/RRA243-9.html (accessed January 3, 2024).

Smith, J. D., D. H. Li, and M. R. Rafferty. 2020a. The implementation research logic model: A method for planning, executing, reporting, and synthesizing implementation projects. *Implementation Science* 15:1–12. https://doi.org/10.1186/s13012-020-01041-8.

Smith, M. E., T. L. Sharpe, J. Richardson, R. Pahwa, D. Smith, and J. DeVylder. 2020b. The impact of exposure to gun violence fatality on mental health outcomes in four urban U.S. settings. *Social Science & Medicine* 246:112587. https://doi.org/.org/10.1016/j.socscimed.2019.112587.

Solitary Watch and the Unlock the Box Campaign. 2023. *Calculating torture.* https://solitarywatch.org/wp-content/uploads/2023/05/Calculating-Torture-Report-May-2023-R2.pdf (accessed January 3, 2024).

Song, Z., J. R. Zubizarreta, M. Giuriato, K. A. Koh, and C. A. Sacks. 2023. Firearm injuries in children and adolescents: Health and economic consequences among survivors and family members: Study examines firearm injuries in children and adolescents and the health and economic consequences among survivors and family members. *Health Affairs* 42(11):1541–1550. https://doi.org/10.1377/hlthaff.2023.00587.

South, E. C., B. C. Hohl, M. C. Kondo, J. M. MacDonald, and C. C. Branas. 2018. Effect of greening vacant land on mental health of community-dwelling adults: A cluster randomized trial. *JAMA Network Open* 1(3):e180298. https://doi.org/10.1001/jamanetworkopen.2018.0298.

Spitzer, E. G., K. A. Stearns-Yoder, A. S. Hoffberg, H. M. Bailey, C. J. Miller, and J. A. Simonetti. 2024. A systematic review of lethal means safety counseling interventions: Impacts on safety behaviors and self-directed violence. *Epidemiologic Reviews* 46(1):1–22. https://doi.org/10.1093/epirev/mxae001.

Suarez, N. A. 2024. Disparities in school connectedness, unstable housing, experiences of violence, mental health, and suicidal thoughts and behaviors among transgender and cisgender high school students—youth risk behavior survey, United States, 2023. *Morbidity and Mortality Weekly Report Supplements* 73. https://www.cdc.gov/mmwr/volumes/73/su/su7304a6.htm (accessed January 3, 2025).

Sundaresh, R., Y. Yi, T. D. Harvey, B. Roy, C. Riley, H. Lee, C. Wildeman, and E. A. Wang. 2021. Exposure to family member incarceration and adult well-being in the United States. *JAMA Network Open* 4(5):e2111821–e2111821. https://doi.org/10.1001/jamanetworkopen.2021.11821.

Swanson, J. W. 2019. Understanding the research on extreme risk protection orders: Varying results, same message. *Psychiatric Services* 70(10):953–954. https://doi.org/10.1176/appi.ps.201900291.

Swanson, J. W., E. E. McGinty, S. Fazel, and V. M. Mays. 2015. Mental illness and reduction of gun violence and suicide: Bringing epidemiologic research to policy. *Annals of Epidemiology* 25(5):366–376. https://doi.org/10.1016/j.annepidem.2014.03.004.

Tach, L., S. Jacoby, D. J. Wiebe, T. Guerra, and T. S. Richmond. 2016. The effect of microneighborhood conditions on adult educational attainment in a subsidized housing intervention. *Housing Policy Debate* 26(2):380–397. https://doi.org/10.1080/10511482.2015.1107118.

Teplin, L. A., K. M. Abram, J. J. Washburn, L. J. Welty, J. A. Hershfield, and M. K. Dulcan. 2013. *Northwestern juvenile project: Overview.* U.S. Department of Justice, Office of Justice Programs, Office of Juvenile Justice and Delinquency Prevention. https://ojjdp.ojp.gov/sites/g/files/xyckuh176/files/pubs/234522.pdf (accessed December 16, 2024).

The Annie E. Casey Foundation. 2016. A shared sentence: The devastating toll of parental incarceration on kids, families, and communities. https://assets.aecf.org/m/resourcedoc/aecf-asharedsentence-2016.pdf (accessed January 3, 2025).

The Annie E. Casey Foundation. 2022. Maryland enacts sweeping youth justice reforms. https://www.aecf.org/blog/maryland-enacts-sweeping-youth-justice-reforms (accessed January 3, 2025).

The Pew Charitable Trusts. 2010. *Collateral costs: Incarceration's effect on economic mobility.* https://www.pewtrusts.org/~/media/legacy/uploadedfiles/pcs_assets/2010/collateralcosts1pdf.pdf (accessed January 3, 2025).

The Pew Charitable Trusts. 2023. *Racial disparities persist in many U.S. jails.* https://www.pewtrusts.org/en/research-and-analysis/issue-briefs/2023/05/racial-disparities-persist-in-many-us-jails (accessed January 3, 2025).

The University of Chicago. 2021. *Chicago Center for Youth Violence Prevention collaborates with the Great Bronzeville community to reduce violence and address critical needs elevated through community planning process.* Crown Family School News. https://crownschool.uchicago.edu/news-events/all-news/chicago-center-youth-violence-prevention-collaborates-greater-bronzeville (accessed January 17, 2025).

Tiberii, J. 2016. N.C.'s "bathroom law" energizes voters on both sides of the issue. *NPR.* https://www.npr.org/2016/05/09/477301444/n-c-s-bathroom-law-energizes-voters-on-both-sides-of-the-issue (accessed December 13, 2024).

Tisdale, A. 2020. Youth, interrupted: Encouraging a holistic approach to juvenile incarceration policy. *Modern Psychological Studies* 25(2). https://scholar.utc.edu/mps/vol25/iss2/1 (accessed January 3, 2025).

TJCHC (Thirteenth Judicial Circuit Hillsborough County). 2024. *Juvenile Arrest Avoidance program (civil citation).* https://www.fljud13.org/CourtPrograms/JuvenileDiversionPrograms/JuvenileArrestAvoidanceProgram.aspx#:~:text=Civil%20Citation%20is%20an%20alternative,citation%20in%20lieu%20of%20arrest (accessed November 18, 2024).

TTP (The Trevor Project). 2021. *National survey on LGBTQ youth mental health.* https://www.thetrevorproject.org/wp-content/uploads/2021/05/The-Trevor-Project-National-Survey-Results-2021.pdf (accessed January 3, 2025).

TTP. 2023. *2023 U.S. national survey on the mental health of LGBTQ+ young people.* https://www.thetrevorproject.org/survey-2023/ (accessed January 14, 2025).

U.S. Department of Veterans Affairs. n.d. *What is lethal means safety counseling?* https://www.mirecc.va.gov/visn19/lethalmeanssafety/counseling/ (accessed November 14, 2024).

Ursano, R. J., C. S. Fullerton, R. S. Epstein, B. Crowley, T.-C. Kao, K. Vance, K. J. Craig, A. L. Dougall, and A. Baum. 1999. Acute and chronic posttraumatic stress disorder in motor vehicle accident victims. *American Journal of Psychiatry* 156(4):589–595. https://doi.org/10.1176/ajp.156.4.589.

Volkow, N. D. 2021. Addiction should be treated, not penalized. *Neuropsychopharmacology* 46(12):2048–2050. https://doi.org/10.1038/s41386-021-01087-2.

Washburn, K. 2024. *Gun violence increases physical, mental health disorders among children, survivors and families, study says.* https://healthjournalism.org/blog/2024/01/gun-violence-increases-physical-mental-health-disorders-among-children-survivors-and-families-study-says/ (accessed November 14, 2024).

Webster, D. W., J. M. Whitehill, J. S. Vernick, and F. C. Curriero. 2023. Effects of Baltimore's Safe Streets program on gun violence: A replication of Chicago's ceasefire program. *Journal of Urban Health* 90(1):27–40. https://doi.org/10.1007/s11524-012-9731-5.

Weizman, S., J. Perez, I. Manoff, M. Baney, and T. El-Sabawi. 2021. *National snapshot: Access to medications for opioid use disorder in U.S. jails and prisons.* https://oneill.law.georgetown.edu/wp-content/uploads/2021/07/National-Snapshot-Access-to-Medications-for-Opioid-Use-Disorder-in-U.S.-Jails-and-Prisons.pdf (accessed January 3, 2025).

Wildeman, C., J. Schnittker, and K. Turney. 2012. Despair by association? The mental health of mothers with children by recently incarcerated fathers. *American Sociological Review* 77(2):216–243. https://doi.org/10.1177/0003122411436234.

Wiltsey Stirman, S., A. A. Baumann, and C. J. Miller. 2019. The frame: An expanded framework for reporting adaptations and modifications to evidence-based interventions. *Implementation Science* 14:1–10. https://doi.org/10.1186/s13012-019-0898-y.

Wintemute, G. J., V. A. Pear, J. P. Schleimer, R. Pallin, S. Sohl, N. Kravitz-Wirtz, and E. A. Tomsich. 2019. Extreme risk protection orders intended to prevent mass shootings: A case series. *Annals of Internal Medicine* 171(9):655–658. https://doi.org/10.7326/M19-2162.

WSIPP (Washington State Institute for Public Policy). 2023. *Primary care in behavioral health settings (community-based settings) adult mental health: Serious mental illness.* https://www.wsipp.wa.gov/BenefitCost/ProgramPdf/334/Primary-care-in-behavioral-health-settings-community-based-settings (accessed November 7, 2024).

Wolfenden, L., A. Shoesmith, A. Hall, A. Bauman, and N. Nathan. 2024. An initial typology of approaches used by policy and practice agencies to achieve sustained implementation of interventions to improve health. *Implementation Science Communications* 5(1):21. https://doi.org/10.1186/s43058-024-00555-2.

Wolfson, J. A., T. Garcia, and C. W. Leung. 2021. Food insecurity is associated with depression, anxiety, and stress: Evidence from the early days of the Covid-19 pandemic in the United States. *Health Equity* 5(1):64–71. https://doi.org/10.1089/heq.2020.0059.

Woodford, M. R., M. S. Paceley, A. Kulick, and J. S. Hong. 2015. The LGBQ social climate matters: Policies, protests, and placards and psychological well-being among LGBQ emerging adults. *Journal of Gay & Lesbian Social Services* 27(1):116–141. https://doi.org/10.1080/10538720.2015.990334.

Yeter, D., E. C. Banks, and M. Aschner. 2020. Disparity in risk factor severity for early childhood blood lead among predominantly African American Black children: The 1999 to 2010 US NHANES. *International Journal of Environmental Research and Public Health*. Feb 28;17(5):1552. https://doi.org/10.3390/ijerph17051552.

Zaid, S., K. McCombs-Thornton, K. Faucetta, L. Childress, P. Cachat, and J. Filene. 2022. *Family Level Assessment and State of Home Visiting outreach and recruitment study report* (OPRE Report No. 2022-110). Office of Planning, Research, and Evaluation; Administration for Children and Families; U.S. Department of Health and Human Services. https://www.acf.hhs.gov/sites/default/files/documents/opre/FLASHVOutreachRecruitment_508_v2_0.pdf (accessed January 6, 2025).

Zeoli, A. M., S. Frattaroli, K. Roskam, and A. K. Herrera. 2019. Removing firearms from those prohibited from possession by domestic violence restraining orders: A survey and analysis of state laws. *Trauma, Violence, & Abuse* 20(1):114–125. https://doi.org/10.1177/1524838017692384.

Appendix A

Committee and Staff Biosketches

COMMITTEE MEMBERS

Marcella Alsan, M.D., Ph.D., M.P.H. (*CoChair*), is Angelopulos Professor of Public Policy at Harvard Kennedy School. Dr. Alsan received a B.A. from Harvard University (1999), an M.P.H. from Harvard School of Public Health (2005), an M.D. from Loyola University (2005), and a Ph.D. in economics from Harvard (2012). She trained at Brigham and Women's Hospital Hiatt Global Health Equity Residency Fellowship and combined her Ph.D. with an infectious disease fellowship at Massachusetts General Hospital (2013). Before returning to Harvard, she was on faculty at Stanford University. She is an applied microeconomist studying health inequality. Some of her recent papers include "Does Diversity Matter for Health: Experimental Evidence from Oakland" and "Tuskegee and the Health of Black Men," published in the *American Economic Review* and *Quarterly Journal of Economics*, respectively. These papers have been cited in the *New York Times* and other major media outlets, and findings have been presented to the Association of American Medical Colleges and the Centers for Disease Control and Prevention. She is on the board of editors for *Science Magazine*, coeditor of the *Journal of Health Economics*, and cochair of the Health Care Delivery Initiative of Poverty Action Lab based out of Massachusetts Institute of Technology. She is the corecipient of the 2019 Arrow Award for Best Paper in Health Economics. She served as a member on the National Academies of Sciences, Engineering, and Medicine (the National Academies) consensus study team that authored *Improving Representation in Clinical Trials and Research: Building Research*

Equity for Women and Underrepresented Groups and is an elected member of the National Academy of Medicine.

Marthe R. Gold, M.D., M.P.H. (*CoChair*), is a senior scholar at the New York Academy of Medicine and the Logan Professor Emeritus in the Department of Community Health and Social Medicine at the City University of New York Medical School. A graduate of the Tufts University School of Medicine and Columbia School of Public Health, she received her clinical training in family medicine. Dr. Gold has been a primary care provider in urban and rural underserved settings. She served as senior policy advisor in the Office of the Assistant Secretary for Health in the U.S. Department of Health and Human Services 1990–1996, where her focus was on financing of clinical preventive services, the economics and outcomes of public health programs, and health care reform. She directed the work of the expert Panel on Cost-Effectiveness in Health and Medicine, whose report remains an influential guide to cost-effectiveness methodology for academic and policy uses. Her work focuses on patient, public, and decision maker views on using economic and comparative effectiveness information to inform health policy. Dr. Gold served as chair of the National Academies of Sciences, Engineering, and Medicine consensus study team that authored *For the Public's Health: The Role of Measurement in Action and Accountability*, *For the Public's Health: Revitalizing Law and Policy to Meet New Challenges*, and *For the Public's Health: Investing in a Healthier Future* and a member of the Roundtable on Population Health Improvement between 2013 and 2018. She is an elected member of the National Academy of Medicine.

Rinad S. Beidas, Ph.D., is chair and Ralph Seal Paffenbarger Professor of Medical Social Sciences at the Feinberg School of Medicine at Northwestern University. Dr. Beidas is an internationally recognized implementation scientist leading a department that is ranked first in the nation for public health in medical schools. Using innovative methods from implementation science to advocate and amplify the needs of various communities in pursuit of achieving population health and social justice at scale, she has done work to close the research-to-practice gap in firearm injury prevention, mental health (MH), cancer care, HIV, and cardiovascular disease. Her work with the MH system in Philadelphia directly informed how the Department of Behavioral Health supports implementing evidence-based practice. She is at the forefront of integrating approaches from behavioral economics and IS, has published more than 300 peer-reviewed publications, and has led to two National Institutes of Health (NIH) center grants. She is an associate editor for *Implementation Science* and has served on numerous scientific advisory boards. She is on the NIH National Advisory Mental Health Council. She earned the Association for Behavioral and Cognitive Therapies President's

New Researcher Award, American Psychological Foundation Diane J. Willis Early Career Award, and Acenda Institute Research Pioneer Award. Dr. Beidas holds a B.A. in psychology from Colgate University and a Ph.D. in psychology from Temple University. She served on the Optum Behavioral Health Clinical and Scientific Advisory Board and is completing a consultation for Optum Behavioral Health. She is a senior advisor to the University of Pennsylvania Center for Health Incentives and Behavioral Economics and an advisory board member for the Certified Community Behavioral Health Clinic-Expansion Evaluation Advisory Panel, ETUDES NIMH P50 Center (University of Pittsburgh), and NCHATS NIMH P50 Center (Michigan State University). She is an active researcher in the field.

Camille C. Cioffi, Ph.D., is a research assistant professor at the University of Oregon and research scientist at Oregon Research Institute and Influents Innovations. Her research focuses on supporting families impacted by substance use disorders (SUDs) to improve health outcomes and prevent the intergenerational transmission of SUDs. She is particularly interested in identifying evidence-based programs developed by communities most impacted by disparities in substance use and preventing harms associated with substance use among individuals at risk for overdose. Dr. Cioffi is a member of the College on Problems of Drug Dependence and Society for Implementation Research Collaboration and has provided overall and domain-specific leadership on more than 10 National Institutes of Health grants. She received her Ph.D. from the University of Oregon in prevention science in 2020 and has experience as a K–12 administrator and educator.

Joseph P. Gone, Ph.D., M.A., is faculty director of the Harvard University Native American Program, professor of anthropology in the Faculty of Arts and Sciences, and professor of global health and social medicine in the Faculty of Medicine at Harvard. He taught at the University of Michigan in Ann Arbor for 16 years, where he directed the Native American Studies program before joining the faculty at Harvard. An enrolled member of the Aaniiih-Gros Ventre Tribal Nation of Montana, he also served briefly as the chief administrative officer for the Fort Belknap Indian reservation. An international expert in the psychology and mental health of American Indians and other Indigenous peoples, Dr. Gone has collaborated with tribal communities for nearly 30 years to re-envision conventional mental health services for advancing Indigenous well-being. As a clinical-community psychologist and action researcher, he has published more than 100 scientific articles. Honored with more than 20 fellowships and career awards, including a Guggenheim Fellowship, he was the recipient of the 2021 American Psychological Association Award for Distinguished Professional Contributions to Applied Research, and 2023 American Psychological Foundation

Gold Medal Award for Impact in Psychology. He is a graduate of Harvard College and the University of Illinois, and he also trained at Dartmouth College and McLean Hospital/Harvard Medical School. Dr. Gone is an elected member of the National Academy of Medicine.

Kyle Lynn Grazier, Dr.P.H., M.P.H., M.S., is Richard Carl Jelinek Professor in the School of Public Health at the University of Michigan (UM), professor of psychiatry at the Medical School, and recent director of the UM Behavioral Health Workforce Research Center. Prior academic positions include Cornell University (J. Thomas Clark Chair in Entrepreneurship and Personal Enterprise), University of California (UC)—Berkeley (King Sweesy and Robert Womack Chair in Medical Research and Public Health), and Yale University. Dr. Grazier received a Dr.P.H. and M.P.H. from UC Berkeley, an M.S. in engineering from the University of Notre Dame, and a B.S. from Valparaiso University. Her research seeks to understand and improve access to behavioral health care services by vulnerable populations. She conducts research on systems approaches to equitable, high-quality, culturally appropriate services through alternative models of delivery, payment, and workforce. Dr. Grazier studies and tests strategies for structural changes, coordination and integration with primary care, housing, and support services and estimates the costs of processes and outcomes. She has conducted international research in Croatia as a Fulbright Scholar and nationally with support from National Institutes of Health, Health Resources and Services Administration, Substance Abuse and Mental Health Services Administration, and Robert Wood Johnson Foundation. She has served on grant reviews committees for National Institute of Mental Health, National Institute on Drug Abuse, National Institute on Alcohol Abuse and Alcoholism, Agency for Healthcare Research and Quality, John A. Hartford Foundation, Robert Wood Johnson Foundation, the Nuffield Trust, Centers for Medicare & Medicaid Services, and California, New York, and Michigan. Dr. Grazier is on the board of directors for the Indiana University Health System. She is an active researcher in the field.

Jeffrey Hom, M.D., M.P.H., M.S.H.P., is the director of population behavioral health in the Behavioral Health Services division of the San Francisco Department of Public Health, which uses population-level and equity-driven approaches to advance the well-being of San Franciscans. A board-certified internist, Dr. Hom oversees the Office of Overdose Prevention, focusing on reducing overdoses and the harms associated with substance use. He most recently served as the medical director of the Division of Substance Use Prevention and Harm Reduction in the Philadelphia Department of Public Health, where he helped lead the city's response to addiction and overdose.

He was also a board member of Mental Health Partnerships and faculty member at the University of Pennsylvania and Jefferson College of Population Health. He has been selected as a Zuckerman Fellow at Harvard's Center for Public Leadership and a fellow of the College of Physicians of Philadelphia, received an AcademyHealth Presidential Scholarship, and awarded the Common Good Award by Bowdoin College's Board of Trustees. Dr. Hom received his M.D. from Harvard Medical School and M.P.H. from the Harvard School of Public Health. He completed his internal medicine residency at University of California, San Francisco and his fellowship as a Robert Wood Johnson Foundation Clinical Scholar at the University of Pennsylvania, where he obtained his M.S. in health policy research. He is pursuing a Dr.P.H. as a Bloomberg Fellow at the Johns Hopkins Bloomberg School of Public Health.

Margaret Kuklinski, Ph.D., is the director of the Social Development Research Group (SDRG), acting director of the Center for Communities That Care (CTC), and endowed associate professor of prevention in social work in the School of Social Work, University of Washington. At SDRG and CTC, she oversees multidisciplinary staff dedicated to promoting healthy development and preventing substance misuse and other problem behaviors in young people through rigorous prevention science and dissemination of effective preventive interventions. Dr. Kuklinski is a prevention scientist and health economist whose National Institutes of Health– and foundation-funded research focuses on demonstrating the long-term impact of effective family-focused and community-based preventive interventions; partnering with communities, agencies, and services systems to implement and scale them; and building policy support for them by demonstrating their benefits and costs. She is a member of the Board on Children Youth and Families in the Health and Medicine Division of the National Academies and former member of the board of the Society for Prevention Research. She received a Ph.D. in psychology from the University of California—Berkeley and an A.B. in economics from Harvard University.

David S. Mandell, Sc.D., is the Kenneth E. Appel Professor of Psychiatry at the University of Pennsylvania Perelman School of Medicine. He is trained as a psychiatric epidemiologist and mental health services researcher. The goal of his research is to improve the quality of care that individuals with and at risk for psychiatric and developmental disabilities receive in their communities. Dr. Mandell's research is of two types: the first examines, at the state and national level, the effects of different strategies to organize, finance, and deliver services on service use patterns and outcomes. The second consists of experimental studies designed to determine the best strategies to successfully implement proven-efficacious practices in community settings. Dr. Mandell holds a B.A. in psychology from Columbia University and an Sc.D. from the Johns Hopkins School of Hygiene and Public Health.

Velma McBride Murry, Ph.D., is the Lois Autrey Betts Endowed Chair and associate provost, Office of Research and Innovation and University Distinguished Professor in the Departments of Health Policy at Vanderbilt School of Medicine and Human and Organizational Development at Peabody College in Nashville, Tennessee. Her research focuses on examining the significance of context to everyday life experiences of African American families and youth with specific consideration to processes through which racism, and other social structural stressors, cascade through families to influence parenting and family functioning, quality of life, and youth developmental outcomes and adjustment, including mental and physical health. She is associate director of the Institute for Clinical and Translational Research, Community Engagement Research Core, Vanderbilt University Medical Center, past president of the Society for Research on Adolescence, and president of the International Consortium of Developmental Science Societies. She was a member of the Board on Children, Youth, and Families and serves on numerous other boards and governing councils, including the National Academy of Medicine (NAM)'s Culture of Health, Foundation for Child Development, and Society for Research in Child Development. She earned her Ph.D. in human development and family studies from the University of Missouri–Columbia and was appointed by the Department of Health and Human Services to serve a 4-year term to the National Institutes of Health National Advisory Mental Health Council. Dr. McBride Murry is an elected member of NAM.

Anand Parekh, M.D., M.P.H., is chief medical advisor at the Bipartisan Policy Center (BPC), where he provides clinical and public health expertise across the organization, including on behavioral health issues. His health care expertise has been recognized by *The Washingtonian* in its listing of Washington, DC's 500 Most Influential People. Before BPC, he completed a decade of service at the Department of Health and Human Services (HHS). As an HHS Deputy Assistant Secretary for Health in the Senior Executive Service (2008–2015), he developed and implemented national initiatives focused on prevention, wellness, and care management. Specifically, he played instrumental roles in implementing the Recovery Act's Prevention and Wellness Fund, Affordable Care Act's prevention initiatives, and HHS' Multiple Chronic Conditions Initiative. He received the Surgeon General's Outstanding Service Award for his efforts. Dr. Parekh is a board-certified internal medicine physician, a fellow of the American College of Physicians, and an adjunct professor of health management and policy at the University of Michigan (UM) School of Public Health. He serves on the National Academies Board of Population Health and Public Health Practice. His book *Prevention First: Policymaking for a Healthier America* argues that prevention must be our nation's top health policy priority. A native of Michigan, he received a B.A. in political science and an M.D. and M.P.H. in health management and policy from UM.

Lisa Saldana, Ph.D., M.A., is a senior research scientist and associate director of the Chestnut Health Systems, Lighthouse Institute. She has expertise in measuring implementation process and resource use and has collaborated to operationalize the implementation process of more than 85 prevention and intervention programs in more than 2,500 sites. This repository of data has generated knowledge regarding optimal implementation of evidence-based practice. Dr. Saldana also is an intervention developer and has produced an evidence-based integrated behavioral preventive program for parental opioid/methamphetamine use, parenting deficits, mental health symptoms, and identified social determinants of health needs. Combined with her implementation expertise, she has worked with state and Medicaid systems to create sustainable funding models to support implementation of the program in her own and other dually licensed behavioral health clinics. Dr. Saldana has been fully funded by National Institute on Drug Abuse and/or National Institute of Mental Health since 2002 and, in 2023, received the National Institutes of Health Helping to End Addiction Long-term Initiative Director's Award for Excellence in Research for her prevention program for families involved in the child welfare and self-sufficiency systems. She is a clinical psychologist by training and received her doctorate from the University of Missouri—Columbia. She was a 2011–2012 Implementation Research Institute fellow and now serves as core faculty. Dr. Saldana co-owns a small consulting LLC, Western Implementation Research and Evaluation.

Paula Smith, Ph.D., M.A., is an associate professor in the Department of Educational Leadership & Policy at the University of Utah. She is a developmental psychologist with expertise in school-based prevention in middle and high schools. Her primary research interests lie at the intersection of schools and juvenile justice systems—the school-to-prison pipeline, juvenile justice, restorative justice, and access to mental health resources. Her currently funded research projects are concerned with maximizing youth potential via evidence-based research. She is the evaluator of a 5-year suicide prevention intervention in three Utah school districts, and her most recently funded research project is a collaborative effort to develop student-led coalitions on Utah's public institutions of higher education to improve mental health and decrease substance misuse among college students. She is a board member for the National Prevention Science Coalition and served two terms on the board of directors for the Society for Prevention Research, of which she is a member. Dr. Smith received her Ph.D. from the University of Illinois at Chicago, where she was a National Institute of Mental Health predoctoral fellow and National Institute on Drugs and Addiction postdoctoral fellow.

Lonnie Snowden, Ph.D., M.A.,[1] was professor of the Graduate School in the Health Policy and Management Division in the School of Public Health, University of California (UC), Berkeley. He held affiliated appointments in Berkeley's Psychology Department and the UC, Berkeley–UC, San Francisco Joint Medical Program. Past appointments included Berkeley's Institute for Personality and Social Research, at the Brown School, Washington University, St. Louis and at RAND. His research focused on mental health and other health care disparities approached from treatment systems and health policy perspectives. Dr. Snowden published more than 200 papers in peer-reviewed research literature. He served as principal investigator on seven National Institute of Mental Health grants and coinvestigator on many others. His awards included the American Psychological Association Award for Distinguished Contributions to Research in Public Policy, Division 27 Award for Outstanding Contributions to Theory and Research in Community Psychology, and Presidential Citation; American Public Health Association Carl Taube Award for Lifetime Contributions to Mental Health Services Research and Steve Banks Mentoring Award; Surgeon General's Exemplary Service Award; and Berkeley Citation.

Emily Wang, M.D., M.A.S., is a professor in the Yale School of Medicine and School of Public Health and directs the new SEICHE Center for Health and Justice, a collaboration between the Yale School of Medicine and Yale Law School working to stimulate community transformation by identifying the legal, policy, and practice levers that can improve the health of individuals and communities impacted by mass incarceration. Dr. Wang leads the Health Justice Lab research program, which receives National Institutes of Health funding to investigate how incarceration influences chronic health conditions, including cardiovascular disease, cancer, and opioid use disorder, and uses a participatory approach to study interventions that mitigate the impacts of incarceration. As an internist, she has cared for thousands of individuals with a history of incarceration and is cofounder

---

[1] Deceased January 25, 2025.

of the Transitions Clinic Network, a consortium of 45 community health centers nationwide dedicated to caring for individuals recently released from correctional facilities by employing community health workers with histories of incarceration. Dr. Wang served as cochair of the National Academies of Sciences, Engineering, and Medicine (the National Academies) consensus study team that authored *Decarcerating Correctional Facilities During COVID-19* and the planning committee for a National Academies workshop on improving the collection of indicators of criminal justice system involvement in population health data programs and has presented at National Academies workshops on health and incarceration and the means of violence. Her work been published in *Lancet*, *JAMA*, *American Journal of Public Health*, and *Health Affairs* and showcased in national outlets, such as the *New York Times*, NPR, and CNN. She has an A.B. from Harvard University, an M.D. from Duke University, and an M.A.S. from the University of California—San Francisco. Dr. Wang is an elected member of National Academy of Medicine.

Donald Warne, M.D., M.P.H., is an acclaimed physician, one of the world's preeminent scholars in Indigenous health, health education, policy, and equity, and a member of the Oglala Lakota tribe from Pine Ridge, South Dakota. He is the codirector of the Johns Hopkins Center for Indigenous Health and Johns Hopkins Provost Fellow for Indigenous Health Policy. He is an educational leader who created the first Indigenous health–focused M.P.H. and Ph.D. programs in the United States or Canada at the North Dakota State University and the University of North Dakota, respectively. Dr. Warne served at the University of North Dakota as professor of Family and Community Medicine and associate dean of diversity, equity, and inclusion, and director of the Indians Into Medicine and Public Health programs at the School of Medicine and Health Sciences. He served the Pima Indian population in Arizona as a primary care physician and later worked as a staff clinician with the National Institutes of Health. He has also been the health policy research director for the Inter-Tribal Council of Arizona, executive director of the Great Plains Tribal Chairmen's Health Board, and faculty member at the Indian Legal Program of the Sandra Day O'Connor College of Law at Arizona State University. Dr. Warne has received many awards recognizing his research accomplishments, educational leadership, and service work, including the American Public Health Association Helen Rodríguez-Trías Award for Social Justice and the Explorer's Club 50 People Changing the World. He received a B.S. from Arizona State University, M.D. from Stanford University's School of Medicine, and an M.P.H. from the Harvard T.H. Chan School of Public Health.

NAM FELLOWS AND EMERGING LEADERS

NAM Emerging Leaders in Health and Medicine Scholar

Lucinda Leung, M.D., Ph.D., M.P.H., is an assistant professor of medicine and psychiatry at University of California, Los Angeles (UCLA) David Geffen School of Medicine. She is a general internal medicine physician at VA Greater Los Angeles Healthcare System who teaches medical students and residents and cares for hospitalized and clinic patients. Dr. Leung was a first-generation college student who earned her A.B. at Dartmouth College, M.D. at Brown Medical School, M.P.H. at Harvard School of Public Health, and Ph.D. at UCLA School of Public Health. She completed fellowship through the Robert Wood Johnson Foundation VA Clinical Scholars Program and was selected chief fellow for UCLA's Specialty Training and Advanced Research Program. Dr. Leung is a board-certified clinical informatics subspecialist.

NAM Puffer/American Board of Family Medicine Fellow

Sebastian Tong, M.D., M.P.H., is a family physician, addiction medicine specialist, and primary care researcher. He is an assistant professor of family medicine at the University of Washington in Seattle, where he also serves as the codirector of the Washington, Wyoming, Alaska, Montana, and Idaho region Practice and Research Network. He practices both primary care and addiction medicine at an outpatient safety-net clinic in Seattle and conducts research in substance use, loneliness, and chronic pain. He is one of the NAM 2023–2025 James C. Puffer/American Board of Family Medicine Fellows. Dr. Tong completed medical school at Boston University School of Medicine, received an M.P.H. from the Harvard School of Public Health, and finished his residency training in family medicine at the Greater Lawrence Family Health Center in Lawrence, MA.

STUDY STAFF

Alina B. Baciu, Ph.D., M.P.H., is a senior program officer in the Health and Medicine Division Board on Population Health and Public Health Practice (BPH). She has directed the activities of the Roundtable on Population Health Improvement since 2013. After joining the National Academies of Sciences, Engineering, and Medicine in 2001, Dr. Baciu staffed or directed several consensus study teams, including those that produced *Leading Health Indicators 2030: Advancing Health, Equity, and Well-Being* (2020) and the *For the Public's Health* series of reports on measurement, law, and funding. She worked at the Orange County (California) Health Care Agency as a program evaluation specialist (1997–2000) and later at the Public Health Agency as a health educator in maternal, child, and adolescent health. After earning her M.P.H. (international health) in 1996 from Loma Linda University School of Public Health, Dr. Baciu spent 1 year as training coordinator on a USAID-funded maternal and child health project in Zambia. In 2010, she received a Ph.D. in human sciences (an interdisciplinary program in language, culture, and society) from George Washington University.

Alexis Wojtowicz, M.P.H., is a program officer for Board on Population Health and Public Health Practice. She has worked on several consensus studies and roundtables at the National Academies of Sciences, Engineering, and Medicine (the National Academies) on topics including improving clinical prevention research; promoting health literacy; preventing gun violence; building an infrastructure to improve wastewater-based disease surveillance; and the health effects of e-cigarettes, PFAS exposure, and social media use. Before the National Academies, Ms. Wojtowicz managed intake for a culinary job training program at DC Central Kitchen and coordinated an AmeriCorps VISTA summer associate program for Hunger-Free America. She earned a B.A. in art history from the University of Maryland and an M.P.H. from Johns Hopkins Bloomberg School of Public Health, where she was a Bloomberg American Health Initiative Fellow with a focus on adolescent health.

Madeleine Deye, B.A., is a research associate for Board on Population Health and Public Health Practice (BPH). Before BPH, she served as the editorial projects coordinator for the National Academy of Medicine, where she developed and edited discussion papers on a variety of public health topics, including systems thinking in public health, accountable communities for health, and women's health research. She received a B.A. in English literature from Boston College, where her thesis on disability representation in adaptations of Samuel Beckett's plays won the 2021 Doherty Honors Project Award. She is pursuing an M.Sc. in public health from the London School of Hygiene and Tropical Medicine.

Ella Castanier, B.A., is a senior program assistant for Board on Population Health and Public Health Practice. She currently supports a study on women's health in addition to this project. She received a B.A. in history from Georgetown University with a minor in medical humanities and completed an honors thesis on the intellectual history of Black psychiatry during the civil rights period. She has previously interned at Georgetown University Press on the acquisitions editorial and publicity teams and volunteered for the Georgetown-Howard Center for Medical Humanities and Health Justice, assisting with early planning for the center and reviewing inaugural fellowship applications.

Rose Marie Martinez, Sc.D., has served as senior director of the Health and Medicine Division (formerly the Institute of Medicine) Board on Population Health and Public Health Practice since 1999. Dr. Martinez was a senior health researcher at Mathematica Policy Research, where she conducted research on the impact of health system change on the public health infrastructure, access to care for vulnerable populations, managed care, and the health care workforce. She is a former assistant director for Health Financing and Policy with the Government Accountability Office and served for 6 years directing research studies for the Regional Health Ministry of Madrid, Spain.

Y. Crysti Park is a program coordinator for Board on Population Health and Public Health Practice. Before the National Academies of Sciences, Engineering, and Medicine, she worked in marketing and sales management for more than 15 years, creating catalogs, merchandising, and production in the garment industry. She attended the Fashion Institute of Technology and Cornell University.

Appendix B

Clearinghouses of Preventive Interventions

This appendix offers a sample, not exhaustive or comprehensive, of some of the major evidence clearinghouses that collate programs and interventions for mental, emotional, and behavioral disorder prevention.

Name (evaluative Y/N)	Link	Topics
Blueprints for Healthy Youth Development (Y)	https://www.blueprintsprograms.org/	Children, child development, risk factors
Boston University Mental Health Clearinghouse	URL N/A	mental health
California Evidence-Based Clearinghouse for Child Welfare (Y)	https://www.cebc4cw.org/	children, welfare, state
Canadian Best Practices Portal	https://cbpp-pcpe.phac-aspc.gc.ca/	children, violence, equity, disability, CA
ChildTrends/What Works	https://www.childtrends.org/what-works	children, families, poverty, Indigenous, Hispanic, LGBTQ, education
Clearinghouse for Military Family Readiness	https://militaryfamilies.psu.edu/	families, military, children, mental health, substance use disorder (SUD)

continued

Name (evaluative Y/N)	Link	Topics
Collaborative for Academic, Social, and Emotional Learning	https://casel.org/	education, children
Compendium of Evidence-Based Interventions and Best Practices for HIV Prevention	https://www.cdc.gov/hiv/research/interventionresearch/compendium/rr/complete.html	HIV, prevention
Connecticut Clearinghouse	https://www.ctclearinghouse.org/	children, education, SUD, harm reduction, LGBTQ
CrimeSolutions.gov	https://crimesolutions.ojp.gov/	crime, prevention
Diffusion of Effective Behavioral Interventions for HIV	https://www.denverptc.org/debi.html	HIV, prevention
Early intervention Foundation Guidebook	https://guidebook.eif.org.uk/	children, SUD, crime, violence, mental health
Effective Child Therapy	https://effectivechildtherapy.org/	mental health, children
EPIS Center (Y)	https://epis.psu.edu/	prevention, children, families, crime
European Platform for Investing in Children	https://ec.europa.eu/social/main.jsp?catId=1246&langId=en	children, economics, financing, disability
Friends National Resource Center	https://friendsnrc.org/	children, families, outcomes, abuse, prevention
Home Visiting Evidence of Effectiveness	https://homvee.acf.hhs.gov/	children, implementation
JBI Evidence-Based Practices Database	https://jbi.global/ebp	implementation, synthesis
National Child Traumatic Stress Network	https://www.nctsn.org/	mental health, children, trauma
National Gang Center Strategic Planning Tool	https://nationalgangcenter.ojp.gov/about/strategic-planning-tool	crime, prevention
National Governor's Association Center for Best Practices	https://www.nga.org/bestpractices/	behavioral health, mental health, SUD
National Registry of Evidence-Based Programs and Practices	URL N/A	mental health, SUD, behavioral health
OJJDP Model Programs Guide (Y)	https://ojjdp.ojp.gov/model-programs-guide/home	children, crime, prevention

APPENDIX B

Name (evaluative Y/N)	Link	Topics
PracticeWise	https://www.practicewise.com/	children, mental health
Prevention Services Clearinghouse	https://preventionservices.acf.hhs.gov/program	mental health, SUD, prevention, children
Promising Practices Network	Yhttp://www.promisingpractices.net/	policy
Resource Center for Adolescent Pregnancy Prevention	https://www.etr.org/ebi/programs/	pregnancy prevention
Results First Clearinghouse Database	https://evidence2impact.psu.edu/what-we-do/research-translation-platform/results-first-resources/clearing-house-database/	crime, SUD, mental health, education, pregnancy prevention
SAMHSA Evidence-Based Practices Resource Center	https://www.samhsa.gov/resource-search/ebp	SUD, mental health, communities, clinicians
Social Programs That Work	https://evidencebasedprograms.org/programs/	education, children, employment, welfare, housing, finance, pregnancy prevention
Society for Clinical Psychology	https://div12.org/psychological-treatments/	mental health, treatments
Suicide Prevention Resource Center	https://www.sprc.org/	mental health, prevention
Teen Pregnancy Prevention Evidence Review	https://tppevidencereview.youth.gov/	pregnancy prevention, finance
University of Washington Addictions, Drug, and Alcohol Institute	http://adaiclearinghouse.net/	SUD
Washington State Institute for Public Policy Inventory	https://www.wsipp.wa.gov/Publications	SUD, mental health, crime, education, foster care, state level
What Works Clearinghouse	https://ies.ed.gov/ncee/WWC	education, children
What Works for Children's Social Care Evidence Store	https://whatworks-csc.org.uk/evidence-store/	SUD, mental health, children, violence, family (UK)
What Works in Reentry Clearinghouse	https://whatworks.csgjusticecenter.org/	mental health, crime, SUD, housing, education, employment
Youth.Gov	https://youth.gov/	mental health, children, implementation

NOTE: Y/N = yes/no.

Appendix C

Mental Health and Substance Use Disorder Prevention Financing Landscape Analysis

Tami L. Mark, Ph.D., M.B.A.
RTI International
TMark@RTI.org
July 30, 2024

TABLE OF CONTENTS

MENTAL HEALTH AND SUBSTANCE USE DISORDER PREVENTION FINANCING LANDSCAPE ANALYSIS	267
Table of Contents	267
INTRODUCTION	**270**
Background	270
Purpose of the paper	271
Methods	271
FEDERAL SPENDING ON BH PREVENTION	**274**
Federal Spending Overview	274
Discretionary Versus Mandatory Funding	275
Prevention and Public Health Fund	276
Total Federal Spending on Prevention	277
Total Federal Spending on SuD Prevention	277
Total Federal Spending on MH Disorder Prevention	279
Total Federal Spending on BH (MH/SUD) Prevention	279

Medicaid	282
Medicare	286
SAMHSA	287
CDC	290
ACF	296
HRSA	298
ACL	299
Department of Education	300

STATE SPENDING BH PREVENTION	300
State Financing Overview	300
State Spending on BH Prevention	301
Expanding State Spending on BH Prevention Through Earmarked Taxes	302
Expanding State Spending on BH Prevention Through Settlement Funds	303

PRIVATE SPENDING ON BH PREVENTION	303
Charitable/Nonprofit Organizations	303
Private Insurance	304
Employers	304

CONCLUSIONS	304
REFERENCES	305

TABLES

TABLE 1	Federal government total outlays, fiscal year 2023	274
TABLE 2	Federal Agency's Total Outlays, FY 2023 (millions)	275
TABLE 3	Federal substance use disorder prevention funding, fiscal year 2023 (millions)	278
TABLE 4	Federal mental health disorder prevention funding, fiscal year 2023 (millions)	279
TABLE 5	Federal substance use and mental health disorder prevention funding, fiscal year 2023 (millions)	280
TABLE 6	Department of Health and Human Services total outlays, fiscal year 2023 (millions)	281
TABLE 7	SAMHSA substance use disorder prevention funding, fiscal year 2023 (millions)	287
TABLE 8	SAMHSA total mental health funding and mental health disorder prevention funding, fiscal year 2023 (millions)	289

TABLE 9	Description of SAMHSA's major mental health programs (treatment and prevention focused)	291
TABLE 10	CDC total funding and mental health/substance use disorder prevention funding, fiscal year 2023 (millions)	294
TABLE 11	CDC substance use prevention funding, fiscal year 2023 (millions)	295
TABLE 12	CDC budget for mental health disorder prevention funding, fiscal year 2023 (millions)	296
TABLE 13	Administration on Children and Families mental health prevention funding, fiscal year 2023 (millions)	297
TABLE 14	HRSA substance use disorder prevention funding, fiscal year 2023 (millions)	299
TABLE 15	HRSA mental health disorder prevention funding, fiscal year 2023 (millions)	299
TABLE 16	State primary substance use disorder prevention spending, 2023 (millions)	301
TABLE 17	State mental health disorder prevention spending, 2023 (millions)	302

Introduction

BACKGROUND

Mental health and substance use disorders (MH/SUDs) are disabling conditions that drive a sizable proportion of morbidity and mortality in the United States and worldwide. By many indications, MH/SUD in United States have worsened over the past 2 decades:

- Deaths from suicide increased from 10.4 per 100,000 in 2000 to 13.5 in 2020 (Ehlman et al., 2022).
- Drug overdose deaths increased from 6.1 per 100,000 in 1999 to 28.3 in 2020 (Hedegaard, Miniño, and Warner, 2020).
- Alcohol-related deaths increased from 7.9 per 100,000 in 2012 to 13.5 in 2022 (Saunders and Rudowitz, 2024).

The increase in deaths from suicide, drugs, and alcohol is one of key drivers of the U.S. decline in life expectancy in recent years (Arias et al., 2022).

The prevalence of MH/SUD is high and has increased for some conditions and populations:

- In 2022, 48.7 million people aged 12 or older (17.3 percent) had an SUD in the past year, including 29.5 million who had an alcohol use disorder (AUD), 27.2 million who had a drug use disorder, and 8.0 million who had both (SAMHSA, 2023a).
- Among adults aged 18 years and older, 15.4 million (6 percent) had a serious mental illness (SMI) in 2022.
- The percent of adolescents reporting ever getting drunk was 26.4 in 2020 (Johnston et al., 2021).
- The percent of adolescents reporting using illicit drugs was 34.7 in 2020 (Johnston et al., 2021).
- Major depression among adolescents increased from 8.1 percent in 2009 to 15.8 percent in 2019 (Daly, 2022).
- Anxiety among adults increased from 5.1 percent in 2008 to 6.6 percent in 2018 (Goodwin et al., 2020).

Spending on MH/SUD treatment more than tripled, from $40 billion in 2000 to $140 billion in 2021, driven by a combination of increased prevalence, use, and cost of care (BEA, n.d.).

These trends require a new examination of the nation's MH/SUD prevention infrastructure and financing.

PURPOSE OF THE PAPER

This paper scans the funding landscape for MH/SUD prevention, also referred to collectively as "prevention of behavioral health (BH) disorders." It describes the amount of funding for BH prevention activities at the federal, state, and local levels and through private insurance, charitable/not for profit organizations, and employers. The paper also discusses options to generate sustained and adequate funding for the prevention infrastructure.

METHODS

Defining MH/SUD

This paper relies on the definitions and criteria in the American Psychiatric Association *Diagnostic and Statistical Manual of Mental Disorders* Version 5 (DSM-V), save that it excludes dementias, developmental disabilities, and tobacco use.

According to the DSM-V, BH disorders differ from "normal" feelings, thoughts, moods, and behaviors when they are intense, long lasting, and/or frequent and interfere with functioning and health. For example, unlike normal feelings of sadness, common symptoms of depression include an inability to concentrate and carry out usual activities, disrupted sleep and eating, and thoughts of suicide.

From a population perspective, identifying what *is* and is *not* an MH/SUD is complex. No biological markers or tests can determine if someone has a mental illness, as is possible in diabetes, hypertension, or HIV, for example. When thinking, feelings, moods, and behavior should be determined to be "pathological" as opposed to "normal" is not clear cut. Epidemiologic surveys use different assessments and criteria to determine whether someone has an MH/SUD. For example, the 2022 Substance Abuse and Mental Health Administration (SAMHSA) National Survey of Drug Use and Health (NSDUH) used three measures of mental illness: "any mental health illness," "serious mental illness," "major depressive episode" (SAMHSA, 2023a). SMI is a subset of mental illness. The 2022 NSDUH classified someone with SMI based on their degree of impairment as measured by the Sheehan Disability Scale. Earlier versions of the NSDUH did not have a measure of "serious mental illness" and instead used the K6 questionnaire to measure "serious psychological distress." Other national epidemiologic surveys, such as the Centers for Disease Control and Prevention (CDC) Behavioral Risk Factor Surveillance System (BRFSS), CDC National Health Interview Survey, and Census Pulse Survey, use different questionnaires and criteria to measure mental illness. A final challenge in determining population-level MH/SUD is that the NSDUH only captures mental health and substance use among individuals age 12 and older. In young children, mental health conditions often present as behavioral and emotional symptoms that differ from those in adults and therefore require different diagnostic criteria.

Unlike mental illness, laboratory tests can determine whether someone is using substances. Furthermore, epidemiologic surveys, such as the NSDUH, have a longer track record of measuring population SUDs. Long-running surveys, such as Monitoring the Future, have been used to track youth use of and attitudes toward substances and can identify precursors to future SUD epidemics. Nothing similar exists for early indicators of emerging mental disorders.

> **Examples of Risk Factors for MH/SUDs**
>
> Childhood sexual abuse, parental divorce, parental MH/SUD, single parenthood, parental incarceration, childhood media exposure, parenting harshness, family disruption, bullying, frequent moves during childhood, food insecurity, access to substances, cultural norms about substance use, chronic physical illnesses, traumatic brain injury, poor sleep, loneliness, peer, and parent substance use behavioral and attitudes, lack of physical activity, cigarette smoking, housing disadvantage, job loss, poverty neighborhood crime, exposure to violence, depressogenic cognitive style, social competence, self-regulation/impulsivity, academic failure

This paper does not conceive of MH/SUD as global "happiness" or "well-being" as described in the World Happiness Report, for example (Helliwell et al., 2024). If BH is broadly defined as general population *well-being*, then it could be argued that most of federal, state, and local government spending constitutes BH prevention, such as income transfers, housing supports, public education, violence protection, and sustainability initiatives.

Defining MH/SUD Prevention Interventions

National Academies of Sciences, Engineering, and Medicine reports have called out the challenge of defining BH prevention. This paper focuses on programs that were clearly identified as aiming to prevent MH/SUD or described as preventing adverse childhood experiences (ACEs). Tertiary prevention (e.g., SUD harm reduction, such as needle exchanges and naloxone distribution) was excluded, to the extent feasible. Programs focused on preventing suicide were included, although this is arguably often tertiary prevention because it can be achieved by identifying and treating MH/SUDs. This paper's definition of MH/SUD prevention is acknowledged to be too narrow in that it was not feasible to capture the financing for all effective programs or policies that can reduce the risk factors, given definitional ambiguities and research gaps. Risk factors are numerous and complex (see box). Genes, biology, childhood and subsequent life experiences, relationships, and what is broadly called "environment" interact in complex ways to increase the risk for developing a MH/SUD.

MH/SUDs often have their foundation in childhood experiences. ACEs have been shown across a large body of research to be major risk factors for MH/SUD (Danielsdottir et al., 2024; Gu et al., 2022; Solmi et al., 2021; Claussen et al, 2024; Beatty et al., 2024; Norman et al, 2012). "ACEs include child abuse (emotional, physical, or sexual), child neglect (emotional or physical), and household dysfunction (domestic violence, substance abuse, mental illness, criminal activity, or parental absence)" (Gu et al. 2022). Studies are beginning to highlight possible mechanisms of action whereby trauma and ACEs increase the risk for psychiatric illness and SUD later in life, such as through alteration of immune functioning (Maayan and Maayan, 2024). Evidence-based interventions that prevent ACEs have been developed, although more research is needed (Lorenc et al., 2020). Therefore, in addition to a focus on spending on programs that are clearly described as aimed at preventing SUD, mental illness, suicide, this paper also focuses on interventions aimed at reducing the crosscutting risk factor of childhood ACEs.

Children and adults across all income levels experience MH/SUDs and ACEs (Camacho and Henderson, 2022). However, poverty places children at higher risk for ACEs, and financial shocks are associated with an increase in suicide. Therefore, reducing poverty and financial shocks could reduce ACEs and MH/SUD. Programs that subsidize low-income families and individuals (e.g., Temporary Assistance to Needy Families (TANF)) and programs that protect against financial shocks (e.g., Medicare, Medicaid, employment insurance) are highlighted in this paper but not included in the funding estimates because of the challenge in drawing a causal direct line between these programs and MH/SUD prevalence rates.

It was nearly impossible to separate spending on prevention from spending on treatment. Most federal MH/SUD prevention programs are discretionary grant programs that allow spending on a combination of prevention and treatment with no requirements or accounting for how much funding was allocated to either. If a program appeared to be primarily for treatment, it was excluded from the spending estimates, but this determination was often difficult.

As noted in the 1994 Institute of Medicine Report *Reducing Risks for Mental Disorders: Frontiers for Preventive Intervention Research*, sometimes, treatment can also be prevention. For example, "psychotherapy for an anxious mother of a healthy child can be conceptualized as treatment of the mother as well as prevention of later difficulties [for] the child, [and] effective treatment of a physical illness may prevent a secondary mental disorder and vice versa" (p. 24).

In general, it was easier to identify financing for substance use than MH disorder prevention for several reasons. First, the federal government has one agency that oversees its efforts to prevent and treat SUDs, the Office of National Drug Control Policies (ONCDP). Second, as noted, population surveys to monitor SUD are longer running than those to monitor MH. Third, programs described as substance use prevention generally comprised interventions that (1) reduce the availability of substances, (2) change social norms and attitudes toward substance use, (3) provide information about the effect of substances, or (4) provide skills to reduce substance use in oneself or others.

Because of resource constraints and the availability of information, this paper focuses on federal spending on prevention to a greater extent than spending by states and the private sector. Few existing resources summarize states spending on mental health treatment or prevention.

Data Sources

The primary sources were budget documents of federal agencies and summary analyses of state, private insurance, charitable, and employer spending.

FEDERAL SPENDING ON BH PREVENTION

Federal Spending Overview

As context for understanding the size of federal investment in MH/SUD prevention, it is useful to first describe total federal spending. In fiscal year 2023, outlays were approximately $6 trillion in total (23 percent of the nation's gross domestic product) (see Table 1) (Ready, Salazar, and Verboon,

TABLE 1 Federal government total outlays, fiscal year 2023

Spending Category	Amount (billions)	Percent of Total
Non-Defense Discretionary	$917	15 percent
Medicare/Medicaid	$1,455	24 percent
Other	$502	8 percent
Income security programs	$448	7 percent
Social Security	$1,300	21 percent
Defense	$805	13 percent
Net Interest	$659	11 percent
Total	$6,086	100 percent

Source: CBO (Congressional Budget Office). *The Federal Budget in Fiscal Year 2023: An Infographic.* (Second graphic) https://www.cbo.gov/publication/59727

2024; Department of the Treasury, n.d.a.). Medicare and Medicaid programs comprised 24 percent of 2023 total federal outlays ($1.4 trillion). The remaining main components were Social Security (21 percent), national defense (13 percent), net interest (11 percent), income security programs (7 percent), and other (8 percent) (CBO, 2024).

Table 2 describes total federal outlays by federal agency for fiscal year 2023. The Department of Health and Human Services has the largest because it oversees Medicare and Medicaid.

Discretionary Versus Mandatory Funding

About 63 percent of the federal budget is mandatory spending, 30 percent is discretionary spending, and 8 percent is interest payments on debt (Department of the Treasury, n.d.b). *Primary prevention services are funded largely though discretionary mechanisms, such as block grants, as opposed to mandatory funding streams, such as Medicaid and Medicare entitlement programs.* This has limited their sustainability. Funding for mandatory programs is provided directly in authorizing legislation that establishes eligibility criteria or benefit formulas and usually not limited by the annual

TABLE 2 Federal Agency's Total Outlays, FY 2023 (millions)

Department	Amount
Department of Health and Human Services	$2,475,673
Department of the Treasury	$1,644,766
Social Security Administration	$1,506,843
Department of Defense	$1,330,544
Department of Veterans Affairs	$324,410
Department of Agriculture	$296,599
Department of Education	$254,914
Office of Personnel Management	$234,222
Department of Transportation	$139,004
Department of Homeland Security	$133,715
Department of Housing and Urban Development	$84,501
Department of Energy	$71,587
Department of Labor	$58,389
Department of Justice	$55,576
Department of the Interior	$43,363
Other	$645,886

Source: USA spending.gov https://www.usaspending.gov/explorer/agency (USASpending.gov, 2023)

appropriations process. Other examples of mandatory funding programs are child nutrition programs, State and Tribal Assistance Grants, Children's Health Insurance Program (CHIP), and TANF. The advantage of mandatory funding is that it provides a sustainable funding stream, which is sometimes perceived as a disadvantage because spending can grow rapidly and be difficult to contain without legislative changes.

Funding for discretionary grant programs is determined annually through appropriations acts. Examples of among the largest discretionary programs include federal-aid highways programs, Tenant Based Rental Assistance, Education for the Disadvantaged, and the Disaster Relief Fund (White House, 2023). Discretionary grant programs vary in the extent to which the federal government directs the way the funding must be spent.

Prevention and Public Health Fund

The Prevention and Public Health Fund was established in the Patient Protection and Affordable Care Act (ACA. P.L. 111-148, as amended) to provide for expanded and sustained national investment in prevention and public health programs that were not subject to the annual congressional approval process. Fund appropriations are mandatory, meaning that the amount of funding spent each year is set in the authorizing law, which requires that it be spent on prevention, wellness, and public health activities, including prevention research, health screenings, and prevention programs.

The Prevention and Public Health Fund budget was $1 billion in 2023, a reduction from the $2 billion in the original authorizing legislations. Amendments over the years also shifted the authority for authorizing the spending from the Secretary of Health and Human Services (HHS) to Congress.

In recent years, most Prevention and Public Health Fund resources went to CDC, with smaller amounts for SAMHSA and the Administration for Community Living (ACL). In the FY 2023 appropriations, $903.3 million went to CDC (for programs addressing breastfeeding, diabetes, health care–associated infections, heart disease and stroke prevention, smoking, immunization, and lead poisoning, early child care collaboratives, epidemiology and laboratory grants, and preventive services and health care services block grants), $27.7 million went to the ACL (for programs for Alzheimer's disease, falls prevention, and chronic disease self-management), and $12 million went to SAMHSA (for youth suicide prevention).

A Congressional Research Service analysis found that the Prevention and Public Health Fund did not result in an increase in CDC funding (a proxy for public health prevention funding in general) (CRS, 2024). The analysis noted that to increase prevention funding, Congress could consider statutorily describing what programs are eligible and creating greater oversight mechanisms to ensure the fund was achieving intended policy goals.

Total Federal Spending on Prevention

The Centers for Medicare & Medicaid Services (CMS) estimated in its National Health Expenditure Accounts that federal public health spending in 2022 was $92 billion ($208.4 billion overall with $116.4 from state sources) (CMS, 2024a). That includes disease prevention programs, epidemiological surveillance, immunization, and public health laboratories. CMS assumed that most public health spending was by the U.S. Food and Drug Administration and CDC.

Total Federal Spending on SUD Prevention

The Office of National Drug Control Policy (ONDCP), established by the Anti-Drug Abuse Act of 1988 and reauthorized by the SUPPORT for Patients and Communities Act (Public Law 115-271), is charged with developing policies, objectives, and priorities for the nation's drug policy and coordinating across federal agencies as part of a whole-of-government approach to substance misuse, addiction, and overdose. Under 21 U.S.C. § 1701(11), "National Drug Control Program Agency" means any agency that is responsible for implementing any aspect of the National Drug Control Strategy (except for those focused on drug control activities under the National Intelligence Program or Joint Military Intelligence Program). In addition to ONDCP, these agencies include the departments of Agriculture, Defense, Education, HHS, Homeland Security, Housing and Urban Development, Interior, Justice, Labor, State, Transportation, Treasury, and Veterans Affairs and the Court Services and Offender Supervision Agency for the District of Columbia, federal judiciary, U.S. Postal Inspection Service, and AmeriCorps. In FY 2023, ONCDP oversaw a $42.5 billion budget (GAO, 2022).

The ONDCP Office of Public Health develops and oversees the federal government's overall strategy for substance use prevention, including providing budget guidance to ensure adherence to evidence-based public health approaches (ONDCP, 2023a).

ONDCP reported that in 2023, the federal government budget for SUD prevention was $2.7 billion. Its definition of prevention includes education (e.g., programs proven to reduce the risk factors related to drug use), drug-free workplace programs, drug testing in various settings (e.g., athletics, schools, and workplaces), and other programs (e.g., family-based treatment) to prevent substance misuse and its consequences. The definition excludes screening for MH/SUD.

Table 3 describes how SUD prevention spending was allocated across federal agencies and adjusted estimates after removing spending for research, drug interdiction, and treatment and adding funding for SUD screening. ONDCP estimates that total SUD prevention funding was **$2,732 million**. This paper estimates that it was **$1,808 million**.

TABLE 3 Federal substance use disorder prevention funding, fiscal year 2023 (millions)

National Drug Control Program Agency	ONCDP Est. Funding Amount	Adjusted Est. Funding Amount
AmeriCorps	$13.1	$13.1
Court Services and Offender Supervision Agency	$27.9	$27.9
Department of Defense		
Drug Interdiction and Counterdrug Activities	$130.1	
Department of Education	$108.7	$108.7
Department of Health and Human Services		
Administration for Children and Families	$20	$20
Centers for Disease Control and Prevention	$528.6	$528.6
Centers for Medicare and Medicaid Services		$41.0
Food and Drug Administration	$12.5	$12.5
Health Resources and Services Administration	$142	$142
Indian Health Service	$34.8	$34.8
National Institute on Alcohol Abuse and Alcoholism	$66.4	
National Institute on Drug Abuse	$621.8	
Substance Use and Mental Health Services Administration	$785.1	$638.4
Department of Justice		
Bureau of Alcohol, Tobacco, and Firearms	$0.1	$0.1
Bureau of Prisons	$0.3	$0.3
Drug Enforcement Administration	$4.7	$4.7
Federal Bureau of Investigation	$0.1	$0.1
Office of Justice Programs	$34.1	$34.1
Department of Labor		
Employment and Training Administration	$6	$6
Office of Workers' Compensation Programs	$7.8	$7.8
Department of the Interior		
Bureau of Indian Affairs	$1	$1
Department of Transportation		
Federal Aviation Administration	$17.8	$17.8
National Highway Traffic Safety Administration	$17.6	$17.6
Office of National Drug Control Policy	$151.8	$151.8
TOTAL	**$2,732**	**$1,808**

Source: Office of National Control Policy. National Drug Control Budget, FY 2024 Funding Highlights, March 2023. https://www.whitehouse.gov/wp-content/uploads/2023/03/FY-2024-Budget-Highlights.pdf (ONDCP, 2023a).

Approximately 80 percent of the $1.8 billion in prevention spending was for HHS, with most spending by SAMHSA and CDC. The other 20 percent was for SUD prevention programs delivered by the Departments of Defense, Education, Interior, Justice, Labor, and Transportation.

Total Federal Spending on MH Disorder Prevention

There was no equivalent estimate for MH prevention, which reflects the fact that no agency is dedicated to a "whole-of-government" response to preventing mental illness. This paper estimates that federal agencies spent **$2,766 million** on MH prevention (see Table 4).

Approximately 40 percent of the MH prevention spending occurred under the direction of the Administration for Children and Families (ACF) for programs aimed at preventing child maltreatment ($1,126 million). The next largest amount was spent by SAMHSA ($919 million), of which $617 million was for suicide prevention and the rest mainly aimed at children and youth. The Health Resources and Services Administration (HRSA) MH prevention spending ($517 million) went toward the Maternal, Child, and Home Visiting Program ($500 million). CDC had a variety of programs aimed at preventing suicide, domestic and sexual violence, ACES, firearm injury, and student emotional health.

Total Federal Spending on BH (MH/SUD) Prevention

Combining the $1,808 million spent on federal SUD prevention programs with the $2,766 million spent on MH prevention programs yields $4,574 million *for BH prevention (see Table 5).*

TABLE 4 Federal mental health disorder prevention funding, fiscal year 2023 (millions)

Agency	Funding Amount
Substance Abuse and Mental Health Services Administration	$919
U.S. Centers for Disease Control and Prevention	$204
Centers for Medicaid and Medicare Services	Not known
Administration for Children and Families	$1,126
Health Resources and Services Administration	$517
Total	$2,766

Source: Author calculation based on Department of Health and Human Services fiscal year, 2024, justification of estimates for Appropriations Committees.

TABLE 5 Federal substance use and mental health disorder prevention funding, fiscal year 2023 (millions)

National Drug Control Program Agency	Substance Use Prevention Spending	Mental Health Prevention Spending	Combined Mental Health and Substance Use Disorder Spending
AmeriCorps	$13.10		$13
Court Services and Offender Supervision Agency	$27.90		$28
Department of Defense			$0
Drug Interdiction and Counterdrug Activities			$0
Department of Education	$108.70		$109
Department of Health and Human Services			$0
Administration for Children and Families	$20	$1,126	$1,146
Centers for Disease Control and Prevention	$528.6	$204	$732.6
Centers for Medicare and Medicaid Services	$41.00		$41
Food and Drug Administration	$12.50		$13
Health Resources and Services Administration	$142	$517	$659
Indian Health Service	$34.80		$35
National Institute on Alcohol Abuse and Alcoholism			$0
National Institute on Drug Abuse			$0
Substance Use and Mental Health Services Administration	$638.40	$919	$1,557
Department of Justice			$0
Bureau of Alcohol, Tobacco, and Firearms	$0.10		$0
Bureau of Prisons	$0.30		$0
Drug Enforcement Administration	$4.70		$5
Federal Bureau of Investigation	$0.10		$0
Office of Justice Programs	$34.10		$34
Department of Labor			$0
Employment and Training Administration	$6		$6
Office of Workers' Compensation Programs	$7.80		$8

TABLE 5 Continued

National Drug Control Program Agency	Substance Use Prevention Spending	Mental Health Prevention Spending	Combined Mental Health and Substance Use Disorder Spending
Department of the Interior			$0
Bureau of Indian Affairs	$1		$1
Department of Transportation			$0
Federal Aviation Administration	$17.80		$18
National Highway Traffic Safety Administration	$17.60		$18
Office of National Drug Control Policy	$151.80		$152
TOTAL	$1,808	$2,766	$4,574

Source: Agency Justifications for Estimates for Appropriations Committee; ONDCP, 2023 https://www.whitehouse.gov/wp-content/uploads/2023/03/FY-2024-ONDCP-CONGRESSIONAL-BUDGET-SUBMISSION-FINAL.pdf

As further context for the MH/SUD prevention spending estimates, Table 6 describes FY 2023 outlays across all HHS agencies. The total budget was $1,733 billion, with the majority ($1,593 billion) allocated to CMS. Thus, federal BH prevention spending was 0.2 percent of all HHS agencies' budgets in 2023 (4.574/1,733).

TABLE 6 Department of Health and Human Services total outlays, fiscal year 2023 (millions)

HHS Agency	Funding
Centers for Medicare & Medicaid Services	$1,593,907
Administration for Children and Families	$8,977
National Institutes of Health	$48,952
Health Resources and Services Administration	$14,705
Centers for Disease Control and Prevention	$10,979
Indian Health Service	$7,994
Substance Abuse and Mental Health Services Administration	$7,574
Public Health and Social Services Emergency Fund Authority	$3,792
Food and Drug Administration	$3,644
Administration for Community Living	$2,525
Agency for Healthcare Research and Quality	$485
Total	$1,773,525

Source: https://www.hhs.gov/sites/default/files/fy-2024-budget-in-brief.pdf

MEDICAID

Medicaid and CHIP are mandatory (entitlement) programs funded jointly by the federal and state governments to provide health coverage to low-income families and individuals. As of December 2023, 85,094,448 individuals were enrolled in Medicaid and CHIP, or 25 percent of the U.S population and 39 percent of all children (MACPAC, 2023). In FY 2022, Medicaid and CHIP spending was $853 billion.

Because of its size, flexibility, and focus on low-income children and families, Medicaid could be a robust tool for financing BH prevention interventions. However, it has been structured to only fund the delivery of narrowly defined health care services at the individual level. The federal government and states define the set of covered services within the broad outlines of Medicaid law and regulations. These services are typically defined by billing taxonomies, such as Current Procedural Terminology and revenue codes, and the credentials of the relevant professionals or health care providers. For providers to bill Medicaid, they must also be enrolled in the program. Moreover, services can only be delivered to Medicaid beneficiaries, with few exceptions described next. These legislative restrictions drive spending on health care services to people who are acutely or chronically ill and limit the ability of Medicaid to finance a broader array of effective population-based, primary MH/SUD prevention interventions. It reimburses for some prevention services if delivered by appropriately credentialed providers. "Preventive services are a benefit specified in section 1905(a)(13) of the [Medicaid law]. Medicaid regulations at 42 C.F.R. § 440.130(c) generally define [these] as recommended by a physician or other licensed practitioner of the healing arts, within the scope of authorized practice under state law, to prevent disease, disability, and other health conditions or their progression; prolong life; and promote mental and physical health and efficiency" (CMS, 2023a). To encourage coverage of preventive services, section 4106 of the ACA established a 1 percentage point increase in the Medicaid federal medical assistance applied to such expenditures to states that cover all U.S. Preventive Services Task Force Grade A and B preventive services. Health education or "counseling/anticipatory guidance/risk factor reduction interventions" are also covered if from a participating provider. Health education and counseling can be provided in a variety of settings such as clinics, homes, and schools.

States can optionally reimburse for screening, brief intervention, and referral to treatment (SBIRT) for drugs and alcohol. Federal and state agencies have made concerted efforts to increase coverage and use of SBIRT. As of 2023, 38 states covered SBIRT. Other examples of covered health education services include counseling concerning problems related to lifestyle (V69.0–V69.9), parental concerns about a child (V61.60), and spouses and partners (V61.10).

In 2020, Medicaid spent approximately $43 million on SUD screening and brief interventions. No equivalent estimate for MH screening and brief interventions was available.

The challenges of financing health education and counseling under Medicaid include that primary care clinicians only see patients sporadically (e.g., children and adolescents once during annual visits) and have limited time during visits to provide extensive counseling. Additionally, because counseling must be billed by Medicaid-participating clinicians, it is more expensive than if Medicaid allowed it to be provided by uncredentialed individuals, such as community health workers or teachers, or through public health campaigns.

Medicaid's Early and Periodic Screening, Diagnostic and Treatment (EPSDT)

This benefit covers MH and development preventive health care screening and health education services for children under age 21 (Medicaid.gov, n.d.b.). In 2021, 34 million individuals were screened under EPSDT, or about 69 percent of those eligible (Medicaid.gov, n.d.b.). Data are not available on Medicaid spending attributable to EPSDT. In 2022, CMS issued guidance to states on how to better leverage Medicaid in general, and EPSDT specifically, to reduce BH disorders among children (CMS, 2022). CMS described in the guidance, for example, how the Massachusetts Medicaid program implemented universal BH screening of MassHealth members under the age of 21 during well-child visits, directing all primary care clinicians seeing such youth to use one of several approved screening tools (CMS, 2013).

Health Services Initiatives (HSIs)

CHIP allows states to use a limited amount of funding to implement HSIs focused on improving the health of eligible children under (§2105(a)(1)(D)(ii) of the Social Security Act. HSIs can be a broad community-wide public health initiatives that serve children regardless of income, as long as they improve the health of low-income children under 19 years who are eligible for CHIP or Medicaid (MACPAC, 2019). Eight states have established HSIs to deliver parenting education and supports, six have HSIs focused on MH/SUD services, and one has an HSI-focused on violence prevention (MACPAC, 2019). For example, New Jersey funded the Pediatric Psychiatry Collaborative to promote universal MH/SUD screening in pediatric settings and referral to services (Medicaid.gov., n.d.c.). *States could expand their HSIs to include social marketing campaigns on alcohol and drug use and other population-level BH prevention interventions.*

Social Determinants of Health (SDOH)

Recently, CMS provided more flexibility to states to cover health-related social needs (HRSNs, also known as SDOH) under Medicaid (Medicaid.gov, 2023). For example, as of November 2023, CMS has approved Section 1115 demonstrations in seven states that cover certain evidence-based housing and nutritional services. CMS requires that Medicaid-covered HSRN services not supplant the funding of another federal or state non-Medicaid agency and be complementary to existing social services, such as those provided by the Department of Housing and Urban Development and Department of Agriculture Supplemental Nutrition Assistance Program (SNAP). CMS also restricts the amount and type of HSRN services that can be covered under Medicaid (Medicaid.gov, 2023). For example, it can cover finding and securing housing, security deposits, application and inspection fees, utilities activation, tenancy and sustaining services, benefit program application assistance and fees, eviction prevention, and tenant rights education. However, it cannot pay for room and board. Similarly, nutrition services paid for under Medicaid may only include grocery provisions to high-risk individuals required to avoid unnecessary acute care admission or institutionalization or foods identified as "evidence-based" for persons with diabetes.

Medicaid in Lieu of Services

Medicaid managed care organizations can cover services or settings that are substitutes for services or settings covered under the state plan (known as In Lieu of Services and Settings). This is permitted if they are medically appropriate and cost effective compared with standard care (NCSL, 2023). Since 2019, states have used this flexibility to cover a variety of services, such as chiropractic treatment in lieu of physiotherapy and mobile crisis services as an alternative to inpatient psychiatric treatment (NCSL, 2023). This can only be used in Medicaid managed care if it is a coverable service or setting in the state plan or Section 1915 waiver. Therefore, it cannot be used for primary prevention activities, such as social marketing campaigns to prevent overdoses.

BH Prevention Focused on Parents

MH/SUD conditions can profoundly interfere with parenting. Children of parents with untreated MH/SUD are at higher risk for developing MH/SUD (Klaman et al., 2017; Morales et al., 2023). Medicaid covers a wide array of effective MH/SUD treatments. States have used various Medicaid program flexibilities to deliver parenting skills training and other BH-focused interventions in homes, such as stress management, intimate partner screening, and education (Thompson and Hasan, 2023). Some states require the use of recognized, evidence-based models to receive in-home BH reimbursement, such as Nurse-Family Partnership, Parents as Teachers, and Healthy Families America (Thompson and Hasan, 2023).

Congress and federal agencies are encouraging greater coordination between Medicaid and child welfare to prevent family separations and child maltreatment and neglect (MACPAC, 2015). However, recent research finds large gaps in receipt of Medicaid funding BH services among parents with MH/SUD involved in the child welfare program (Mark, 2024b). It has also shown large racial disparities in receipt of Medicaid-financed MH/SUD services among caregivers of children identified by child protective services (Mark, 2024a). For example, an analysis of data from two states found that White versus Black caregivers with SUD and Medicaid who were involved child protective services were much more likely to have received Medicaid-funded counseling (43 vs. 20 percent) or an SUD medication (43 vs. 11 percent).

Because of the known connection between perinatal maternal depression and children's MH, there has also been a growing focus on identifying and treatment postpartum depression among Medicaid beneficiaries. (Mandl et al., 2024). Some states cover maternal depression screening as part of a Medicaid well-child visit (Wachino, 2016).

School-Based Medicaid Funding

States and schools have long relied on Medicaid to fund covered services provided to children with disabilities under the Individuals with Disabilities Education Act (IDEA). Although schools can deliver Medicaid-funded MH/SUD screening and treatment services to all students with Medicaid, not just children eligible under IDEA, only 16 states have plans that allow for reimbursing services to other Medicaid-eligible students (ED, 2024; Medicaid.gov, n.d.). CMS and the Education Department are encouraging states and schools to expand their offering of school-based Medicaid services (Tsai, 2023). CMS recently provided schools with a new flexibility on billing and documentation to help ease the administration of Medicaid services for local education agencies, such as billing on a per-enrolled-student per-month bundled "capitated" rate rather than per service. The new flexibility also allows states to establish qualifications for school-based providers that differ from those of non-school-based providers of the same services. For example, if a school-based provider is qualified under state or local law to counsel any child, the state cannot impose additional requirements as a condition for reimbursement for a Medicaid beneficiary. The recent CMS guidance also notes that allowable administrative activities can include any cost of general public health initiatives made available to all persons, as long as the activities related to assisting Medicaid-eligible students are specifically identified (CMS, 2023a, p. 74). Research demonstrates that school-based interventions can prevent drug use, depression, and anxiety, although the effect sizes may be small, and questions remain about how best to target these (Faggiano et al., 2014; Werner-Seidler et al., 2021). *Encouraging more states to expand their Medicaid programs to take advantage of the new flexibilities to provide school services to all children could increase the financing for BH prevention.*

Population-Based Quality Measures

One way to incentivize Medicaid managed care organizations and providers to focus on preventing BH conditions is to create and hold them accountable for population-level BH measures (CMS, 2021a). CMS requires state Medicaid programs to report on approximately 35 adult measures, including 11 focused on BH (CMS, n.d.), which all address service delivery. To encourage greater focus on MH/SUD prevention by Medicaid managed care plans, *CMS could create quality measures that focus on population health, such as the percentage of a state's population that died by suicide or had depression.* Population-based MH/SUD measures are already collected in the NSDUH and BRFSS. Using these measures could shift Medicaid program focus to preventing BH disorders rather than just delivering treatment (CMS, 2023a; Wong, 2024). *States could encourage Medicaid managed care plans to track the health of their populations and provide incentives for reducing the incidence of or risk factors for MH/SUD.*

1115 Demonstration Programs

CMS successfully reduced heart attacks and strokes in its Million Hearts demonstration program, in which providers received supports and incentives to reduce cardiac risk among high-risk Medicare beneficiaries (CMS, 2023b). *A similar model could be piloted to prevent BH conditions, such as offering managed care plans flexibilities and incentives to prevent youth from developing anxiety and depression.*

Medicare

Medicare covers medical care services to those aged 65+ and disabled persons, including those with end-stage renal disease. Medicare will reimburse for preventive services determined to be effective by its National Coverage Determination process. For BH prevention coverage, Medicare will reimburse for alcohol and drug misuse screening and counseling and once-a-year depression screening (CMS, 2021; Jacques et al., 2011; CMS,

2024b). It does not cover primary prevention, such as social marketing campaigns. Medicare spending was $944.3 billion in 2022 and approximately $1.4 million on SUD screening in 2020 (Mark, 2024). *As noted for Medicaid, Congress could mandate that CMS conduct a demonstration to allow Medicare greater flexibility to offer a greater range of primary prevention interventions aimed at preventing BH conditions, using population-based quality measures, such as the percentage of Medicare beneficiaries with depression, anxiety, or alcohol use disorders.*

SAMHSA

SAMHSA is the HHS agency that leads public health efforts to advance the BH of the nation and improve the lives of individuals living with MH/SUD and their families. It has five priority areas: (1) preventing substance use and overdose, (2) enhancing access to suicide prevention and mental health services; (3) promoting resilience and emotional health for children, youth, and families; (4) integrating behavioral and physical health care; and (5) strengthening the BH workforce.

SAMHSA is organized into four main divisions: the Center for Mental Health Services, Center for Substance Abuse Treatment (CSAT), Center for Substance Abuse Prevention (CSAP), and Center for Behavioral Health Statistics and Quality. In FY 2023, SAMHSA's total budget outlays were $7.567 billion.

Substance Use Prevention

In 2023, SAMHSA's budget for CSAP was $236 million. Additionally, states are required to allocated 20 percent of the CSAT Substance Use Prevention, Treatment, and Recovery Services Block Grant to SUD prevention. In FY 2020, it equaled $2.008 billion; 20 percent of that is $401 million. Thus, total SAMHSA SUD prevention spending in 2023 was approximately $638 million (Table 7). This calculation assumes that none of the funding

TABLE 7 SAMHSA substance use disorder prevention funding, fiscal year 2023 (millions)

Program	Funding Amount
Substance Use Prevention, Treatment, and Recovery Services Block Grant (2020 = 2.008B) (assume 20 percent)	$401
Center for Substance Abuse Prevention (2023)	$236
TOTAL	$638

Source: SAMHSA, Justification for Estimates for Appropriations Committee, FY 2024, p. 352. https://www.samhsa.gov/sites/default/files/samhsa-fy-2024-cj.pdf

for $1,575 million budgeted for State Opioid Response grants was allocated for primary or secondary prevention.

Examples of SAMHSA SUD Prevention Programs One of CSAP's largest SUD prevention programs—*Strategic Prevention Framework Partnership for States*—allocates grants to develop and deliver state and community substance misuse prevention and MH promotion services (SAMHSA, 2023b). Another relatively large SAMHSA SUD prevention program is the *Strategic Prevention Framework for Prescription Drugs*—which raises awareness about the dangers of sharing medications and works with pharmaceutical and medical communities on the risks of overprescribing to young adults. SAMHSA also provides *Sober Truth on Preventing Underage Drinking* grants that aim to prevent and reduce alcohol use among those aged 12–20. Its *Federal Drug-Free Workplace* programs aim to eliminate illicit drug use within executive branch agencies and federally regulated industries. Its *Tribal Behavioral Health Grants* program focuses on substance use, misuse, and suicide among American Indian/Alaskan Native populations. CSAP's Center for the Application of Prevention Technologies provides prevention training and technical assistance through cooperative agreements.

MH Disorder Prevention

Unlike for substance use, SAMHSA has no office of MH disorder prevention. Drawing the line between SAMHSA funding for prevention and treatment is challenging. **Table 8** displays SAMHSA's total FY 2023 budget in the second column; the third column lists the programs that this paper estimated to be primarily for prevention. This paper estimates that in FY 2023, $919 million of SAMHSA's total MH funding of $2,788 million was for programs identified as being primarily for prevention.

SAMHSA MH Disorder Prevention Programs The majority of SAMHSA's prevention funding went toward preventing suicide and developing the crisis system ($617 million of $912 million, or 67 percent). The remainder primarily focused on preventing mental illness among youth. *The Project AWARE* discretionary grant program focuses on promoting MH in school. The *Project LAUNCH* discretionary grant program promotes the wellness of young children, from birth to age 8, by addressing the social, emotional, cognitive, and behavioral aspects of their development. The *Infant and Early Childhood Mental Health* grant program aims to improve outcomes for children from birth through 12 by developing, maintaining, or enhancing infant and early childhood MH promotion, intervention, and treatment services.

Some excluded programs might be considered prevention, broadly defined. For example, SAMHSA budgeted $22 million for Criminal and Juvenile Justice Programs providing grants and technical assistance to divert

TABLE 8 SAMHSA total mental health funding and mental health disorder prevention funding, fiscal year 2023 (millions)

Programs	All Programs Funding Amount	Specific Programs of Regional and National Significance	Prevention Programs
Programs of Regional and National Significance	$1,044		
Project AWARE		$140	$140
Mental Health Awareness Training		$27	
Healthy Transitions		$30	
Children and Family Programs		$7	$7
Consumer and Family Network Grants		$4	
MH System Transformation and Health Reform		$3	
Project LAUNCH		$25	$25
Primary and Behavioral Health Care Integration		$55	
Suicide Prevention Programs		$617	$617
Homelessness Prevention Programs		$33	
Criminal and Juvenile Justice Programs		$22	
Assertive Community Treatment for Individuals with SMI		$9	
Minority Aids		$9	
Seclusion and Restraint		$1	
Tribal Behavioral Health Grants		$22	$22
Infant and Early Childhood Mental Health		$15	$15
Interagency Task Force on Trauma-Informed Care		$2	
Primary and Behavioral Health Care Integration TTA		$1	
Practice Improvement and Training		$7	
Consumer and Consumer Support TA Centers		$1	
Disaster Response		$1	
Homelessness Prevention Programs		$2	
MH Minority Fellowship Program		$11	

continued

TABLE 8 Continued

Programs	All Programs Funding Amount	Specific Programs of Regional and National Significance	Prevention Programs
National Child Traumatic Stress Network	$93		$93
Assisted Outpatient Treatment (AOT) for Individuals with SMI	$21		
Children's Mental Health Services	$130		
Projects for Assistance in Transitions from Homelessness	$66		
Protection and Advocacy for Individuals with Mental Illness	$40		
Certified Community Behavioral Health Clinics	$385		
Community Mental Health Services Block Grant	$1,007		
TOTAL	**$2,788**		**$919**

Source: Department of Health and Human Services Fiscal Year 2024, Substance Abuse and Mental Health Services Administration, Justification of Estimates for Appropriations Committees. https://www.samhsa.gov/sites/default/files/samhsa-fy-2024-cj.pdf

adults and/or youth with mental illness from the criminal or juvenile justice systems to community-based MH and SUD and other supports before arrest and booking. **Table 9** provides a brief description of the purpose of the programs listed in Table 8.

CDC

CDC is a "federal public health agency that develops and supports community-based and population-wide programs and systems to promote health and prevent the leading causes of disease, injury, disability, and death, both domestically and globally" (CRS, 2023). CDC activities include "developing expertise and best practices in disease prevention and control; conducting and supporting public health research; supporting and conducting public health surveillance and data collection; developing public health laboratory capacity; supporting health education and promotion efforts; coordinating and providing technical assistance to public health programs at the state and local level; supporting some preventive health services programs (e.g., some vaccination and cancer screening programs); and supporting public health emergency preparedness and response efforts." (CRS,

TABLE 9 Description of SAMHSA's major mental health programs (treatment and prevention focused)

Program Name	Brief Description of Purpose
Project Advancing Wellness and Resiliency in Education (AWARE)	Project AWARE is made up of three components: Project AWARE; ReCAST (Resilience in Communities after Stress and Trauma); and Cooperative Agreements for School-Based Trauma-Informed Support Services and Mental Health Care for Children and Youth (Trauma-Informed Services in Schools).
Mental Health Awareness Training	The purpose is to (1) train individuals (e.g., school personnel and emergency services personnel including fire department and law enforcement personnel, veterans, armed services members and their families, etc.) to recognize the signs and symptoms of mental disorders and how to safely de-escalate crisis situations involving individuals with a mental illness and (2) provide education on resources available in the community for individuals with a mental illness and other relevant resources, including how to establish linkages with school and/or community-based mental health (MH) agencies.
Healthy Transitions	The purpose is to improve and expand access to developmentally, culturally, and linguistically appropriate services and supports for transition-aged youth and young adults (ages 16–25) who either have or are at risk of developing serious MH conditions.
Children and Family Programs	A 3-year infrastructure/planning grant provides tribes and tribal organizations with the tools and resources to plan and design a family-driven, community-based, and culturally and linguistically competent system of care.
Consumer and Family Network Grants	Provides consumers, families, and youth with opportunities to participate meaningfully in the development of policies, programs, and quality assurance activities related to U.S. MH.
MH System Transformation and Health Reform	Aims to increase employment among individuals with serious mental illness (SMI).
Project Linking Actions to Unmet Needs in Children's Health (LAUNCH)	Promotes the wellness of young children, from birth to 8 years of age, by addressing the social, emotional, cognitive, physical, and behavioral aspects of their development.
Primary and Behavioral Health (BH) Care Integration	Aims to promote integration and collaboration in clinical practice between BH care and primary/physical health care.
Suicide Prevention Programs	These include 988 Suicide and Crisis Lifeline and Behavioral Health Crisis Services; National Strategy for Suicide Prevention and Zero Suicide grant programs; and interventions that focus on youth suicide prevention, such as the Garrett Lee Smith and American Indian/Alaska Native (AI/AN) programs.

continued

TABLE 9 Continued

Program Name	Brief Description of Purpose
Homelessness Prevention Programs	Aims to develop and/or expand infrastructure that integrates BH treatment, peer support, recovery support services, and linkages to sustainable permanent housing.
Criminal and Juvenile Justice Programs	The purpose is to establish or expand programs that divert adults and/or youth with a mental illness or a co-occurring disorder from the criminal or juvenile justice system to community-based MH and substance use disorder services (SUD) and other supports before arrest and booking.
Assertive Community Treatment (ACT) for Individuals with SMI	Establishes or expands and maintains ACT programs for transition-aged youth and adults with an SMI or serious emotional disturbance.
Minority Aids	Provides resources to help reduce the co-occurring epidemics of HIV, hepatitis, and MH disorders through accessible, evidence-based, culturally appropriate mental and co-occurring disorder treatment that is integrated with HIV primary care and prevention services.
Seclusion and Restraint	The purpose is to disseminate and implement evidence-based practices for treating mental disorders into the field.
Tribal Behavioral Health Grants	The purpose is to prevent and reduce suicidal behavior and substance use, reduce the impact of trauma, and promote MH among AI/AN youth, through age 24, by building a healthy network of systems, services, and partnerships that impact youth.
Infant and Early Childhood Mental Health	Supports two programs: the Infant and Early Childhood Mental Health grant program and Center of Excellence for Infant and Early Childhood Mental Health Consultation. The purpose of the former is to improve outcomes using a prevention-based approach that pairs a MH consultant with adults who work with infants and young children in the different settings where they learn and grow, such as child care, preschool, home visiting, early intervention, and their home. The latter was established to provide technical assistance to communities, states, territories, tribal communities, its grantees, and professional development to individual MH consultants to increase access to high-quality MH consultation throughout the country.
Interagency Task Force on Trauma-Informed Care	The SUPPORT Act mandated that the Substance Abuse and Mental Health Services Administration lead a task force composed of 20 agencies in developing a National Strategy for Trauma-Informed Care and submit an operating plan that outlines its implementation.
National Child Traumatic Stress Network	A national network of grantees increases access to effective trauma- and grief-focused treatment and services systems for children, adolescents, and their families, who experienced traumatic events.

TABLE 9 Continued

Program Name	Brief Description of Purpose
Assisted Outpatient Treatment (AOT) for Individuals with SMI	Grant for technical assistance for AOT, the practice of delivering outpatient treatment under a civil court order to adults with SMI.
Children's Mental Health Services	Provides grants to assist states, local governments, tribes, and territories in their efforts to deliver services and supports to meet the needs of children and youth with serious emotional disturbances.
Projects for Assistance in Transitions from Homelessness	Funds community-based outreach, mental illness and SUD treatment, case management, assistance with accessing housing, and other supportive services for individuals with SMI or a co-occurring disorder who are experiencing homelessness.
Protection and Advocacy for Individuals with Mental Illness	Ensures that the most vulnerable individuals with SMI and significant emotional impairment, especially those in public and private residential care and treatment facilities, are free from abuse, including inappropriate restraint and seclusion, neglect, and rights violations while receiving appropriate SMI treatment and discharge planning services.

Source: Department of Health and Human Services Fiscal Year 2024, Substance Abuse and Mental Health Services Administration, Justification of Estimates for Appropriations Committees. https://www.samhsa.gov/sites/default/files/samhsa-fy-2024-cj.pdf

2023). CDC is organized into several centers, institutes, and offices, some of which focus on specific public health challenges (e.g., immunization and respiratory diseases, injury prevention), but none focus on BH prevention specifically.

CDC's core budget outlays were $10 billion in FY 2023. CDC's budget is primarily determined through annual appropriations rather than mandatory spending programs, although CDC administers several programs funded by mandatory spending authorities, such as the Vaccines for Children program. It also frequently receives one-time supplemental appropriations in response to specific incidents—such as infectious disease threats (CRS, 2023). Many of CDC's programs support public health activities at the state and local levels, and a substantial portion of CDC's annual budget is awarded as grants or cooperative agreements to state and local health departments (CRS, 2023).

CDC noted that its discretionary budget has grown increasingly complex, with 13 different Treasury accounts. This complexity may contribute to CDC's fragmented approach to BH prevention. **Table 10** describes CDC's total budget by the 13 divisions and the subset of funding determined in this paper to be for MH/SUD prevention.

TABLE 10 CDC total funding and mental health/substance use disorder prevention funding, fiscal year 2023 (millions)

Programs	All Funding	MH/SUD Prevention Funding
Immunization and Respiratory Diseases	$499	
HIV/AIDS, Viral Hepatitis, STI and TB Prevention	$1,391	
School Health—HIV		$38
Emerging Zoonotic Infectious Diseases	$698	
Chronic Disease and Health Promotion	$1,175	
School Health		$19
Excessive Alcohol Use		$6
Social Determinants of Health		$8
Birth Defects, Developmental Disabilities, Disability and Health	$205	
Fetal Alcohol Syndrome		$11
Environmental Health	$229	
Injury Prevention and Control	$761	
Domestic Violence		$38
Youth and Community Violence Prevention		$18
Domestic Violence Community Projects		$7
Rape Prevention		$61
Suicide Prevention		$30
Adverse Childhood Experiences		$9
Opioid Abuse and Overdose Prevention and Surveillance		$505
Firearm Injury and Mortality Prevention Research		$12
Public Health Scientific Services	$754	
Occupational Safety and Health	$362	
Global Health	$692	
Public Health Preparedness and Response	$905	
Crosscutting Activities and Program Support	$563	
Buildings and Facilities	$40	
TOTAL	**$8,274**	**$762**

Sources: Department of Health and Human Services Fiscal Year 2024, Centers for Disease Control and Prevention, Justification of Estimates for Appropriations Committees. https://www.cdc.gov/budget/documents/fy2024/FY-2024-CDC-congressional-justification.pdf

TABLE 11 CDC substance use prevention funding, fiscal year 2023 (millions)

Program	Funding Amount
Opioid abuse and overdose prevention and surveillance	$505.6
Excessive alcohol use	$6
Fetal Alcohol Syndrome	$11
Misc.	$6
TOTAL	**$528.6**

Source: Department of Health and Human Services Fiscal Year 2024, Centers for Disease Control and Prevention, Justification of Estimates for Appropriations Committees. https://www.cdc.gov/budget/documents/fy2024/FY-2024-CDC-congressional-justification.pdf

According to ONDCP, in FY 2023, CDC budgeted $528.6 million on drug abuse prevention. According to CDC, the majority of this ($505 million) was for opioid abuse and overdose prevention and surveillance (see **Table 11**). Examples of programs and products funded with the $505 million include information systems to collect and report on overdoses; ACEs data collection; syringe services programs cooperative agreements; guidelines on safely prescribing pain medications; research on the opioid epidemic; and public health campaigns about opioid overdoses. The majority of CDC's drug use prevention funding is allocated toward surveillance and research rather than primary prevention interventions.

CDC budgeted approximately $17.5 million toward preventing alcohol use and fetal alcohol syndrome. One example of how this funding is used to encourage primary care providers to screen women of reproductive age for risky alcohol use and provide pregnant women appropriate, evidence-based interventions to reduce alcohol use.

As shown in **Table 12**, CDC budgeted $204 million for a variety of other programs that influence risk factors for developing MH conditions, such as those aimed at preventing childhood adverse events, firearm injury, rape, and domestic violence. CDC budgeted $30 million for suicide prevention through grants to a variety of state, territorial, tribal, and nongovernmental organizations (CDC, n.d.b). CDC budgeted $19 million for programs to support students' emotional well-being (i.e., school health).

> As part of CDC's *What Works in Schools* program, CDC developed guidance and curricula to reduce risk behaviors, experience of violence, substance use, and poor mental health among students.

TABLE 12 CDC budget for mental health disorder prevention funding, fiscal year 2023 (millions)

Program	Funding Amount
Suicide prevention	$30
Domestic violence and sexual violence	$38
Youth violence prevention	$18
Domestic violence community projects	$7
Rape prevention	$61
Social determinants of health	$8
Adverse Childhood Experiences (ACES)	$9
Firearm injury and mortality prevention research	$12
What works in schools	$2
School health	$19
TOTAL	**$204**

Source: Department of Health and Human Services Fiscal Year 2024, Centers for Disease Control and Prevention, Justification of Estimates for Appropriations Committees. https://www.cdc.gov/budget/documents/fy2024/FY-2024-CDC-congressional-justification.pdf

ACF

ACF "promotes the economic and social well-being of families, children, youth, individuals, and communities with funding, strategic partnerships, guidance, training, and technical assistance . . . ACF administers more than 60 programs with 2023 outlays of more than $78 billion, making it the second largest agency in HHS" (ACF, 2024a). Approximately 54 percent of spending is for mandatory programs, and the remaining 46 percent is for discretionary programs.

ACF's FY 2023 largest programs included TANF (25 percent of outlays), Head Start (17 percent), Foster Care (15 percent), Child Care and Development Block Grant (16 percent), Child Support (6 percent), Low Income Home Energy Assistance Program (2 percent), and Refugee/Entrant Assistance (12 percent) (ACF, n.d.-a).

Many ACF programs are focused on promoting well-being and aim to reduce risk factors that contribute to the development of MH/SUD conditions, such as poverty, economic stress, and ACEs. For example, the Community Services Block Grant "provides funds to states, territories, and tribes to administer to support services . . . [such as] housing, nutrition, utility, and transportation assistance; employment, education, and other income and asset building services; crisis and emergency services; and community asset building initiatives" (ACF, 2024b).

As shown in **Table 13**, this paper estimates that ACF spent **$1.126 billion** on preventing MH/SUD conditions. The largest MH/SUD programs are the *Promoting Safe and Stable Families Program (PSSF)*; *Child Welfare Services*; *Family Violence and Prevention Services*; and *Child Abuse Prevention and Treatment Act (CAPTA) State Grant program*.

The PSSF is a mandated program that aims to enable states and tribes to operate community-based services to "(1) ensure children's safety within the home and preserve intact families in which children have been maltreated when the family's problems can be addressed effectively (family preservation services), (2) prevent child maltreatment among families at risk by providing supportive family services (family support services); (3) address the problems of families whose children have been placed in foster care so that reunification may occur in a safe and stable manner (family reunification services); and (4) support adoptive families by providing support services so that they can make a lifetime commitment to their children (adoption promotion and support services)" (Capacity Building Center for States, 2023, p.1). Mandatory PSSF funds are distributed to states, territories, and tribes through formula grants based on the jurisdiction's share of children receiving benefits through SNAP. The law requires that states and tribes provide 25 percent.

Child Welfare Services The Social Security Act of 1935 created the Child Welfare Services Program, which provides formula grants to state and tribal public child welfare agencies to promote and protect the welfare of all children; prevent neglect, exploitation, and abuse of children; and support

TABLE 13. Administration on Children and Families mental health prevention funding, fiscal year 2023 (millions)

Program	Funding Amount
Promoting Safe and Stable Families	$325
Child Welfare Services	$268
Family Violence Prevention and Services	$240
Child Abuse Prevention and Treatment Act State Grants	$105
Child Abuse Discretionary Activities	$38
Community-Based Child Abuse Prevention	$70
Native American Programs	$60
National Domestic Violence Hotline	$20
Total	$1,126

Source: Department of Health and Human Services Fiscal Year 2024, Administration for Children and Families, Justification of Estimates for Appropriations Committees. https://www.acf.hhs.gov/sites/default/files/documents/olab/fy-2024-congressional-justification.pdf

at risk families through services that allow children to remain in home when appropriate. Services are available to children and families regardless of income. States are required to match federal funding by 25–35 percent.

Family Violence and Prevention Services This is a congressionally authorized discretionary program to support programs and projects to prevent family, domestic, and dating violence and provide shelter and immediate services for adult and youth survivors of domestic violence. Eighty percent of the funding goes to states and tribes based on formula grants. States then distribute the funding to local public and nonprofit organizations.

The CAPTA State Grant Program This was created by the Child Abuse and Treatment Act (P.L. 93-247) to provide formula grants to states to improve child protective services. It assists states in such services, such as providing training and investigating child abuse and neglect reports. "States perform a range of prevention activities, including addressing the needs of infants born with prenatal drug exposure, referring children not at risk of imminent harm to community services, implementing criminal record checks for prospective foster and adoptive parents and other adults in their homes, training child protective services workers, protecting the legal rights of families and alleged perpetrators, and supporting citizen review panels," (ACF, n.d.-b, p. 167).

HRSA

HRSA is an HHS agency whose mission is to "enhance the health and well-being of all Americans by providing for effective health and human services" (HRSA, n.d.a.). Its "strategic goals are to take actionable steps to achieve health equity and improve public health, improve access to quality health services, foster a health workforce and health infrastructure able to address current and emerging needs, optimize its operations, and strengthen program engagement" (HRSA, n.d.-b).

HRSA's budgetary outlays in FY 2023 were $14.795 billion, $9.487 billion of which is discretionary. The largest programs by funding amount were health centers (e.g., federally qualified health centers) ($1.737 billion); workforce innovations ($1,820 million); Maternal, Child, and Home Visiting Program ($1,677 million); and the Maternal and Child Block Grant ($815 million).

I estimate that HRSA spending was **$142 million** on SUD prevention (see **Table 14**); $88 million was for the Rural Communities Opioid Response Program, which issues competitive and cooperative grants "to reduce the morbidity and mortality associated with SUD . . . in high-need rural communities by establishing, expanding, and sustaining prevention, treatment, and recovery services"; $54 million was for SUD prevention delivered through HRSA's health center program (ONDCP, 2023c, p. 103).

TABLE 14 HRSA substance use disorder prevention funding, fiscal year 2023 (millions)

Program	Funding Amount
Health Center Program	$54
Rural Communities Opioid Response Program	$88
TOTAL	$142

Source: Health Resources and Services Administration, Fiscal Year 2024, Justification of Estimates for Appropriations Committee.

I categorized HRSA's Early Childhood Home Visiting Program as an MH prevention program (see **Table 15**). HRSA funds states, jurisdictions, and tribes to develop and conduct home-visiting programs. States and jurisdictions must use evidence-based home-visiting models approved by the Home Visiting Evidence of Effectiveness review. The latest list of approved models includes the Family Check-Up for children and Nurse-Family Partnership.

ACL

ACL is a department within HHS whose mission is to maximize the independence, well-being, and health of older adults with disabilities across the life span and their families and caregivers. ACL's FY 2023 outlays were about $2.526 billion, which were mostly discretionary. ACL "funds services and supports provided primarily by networks of community-based organizations; advocates to ensure the needs of disabled people and older adults are reflected in federal policy and programs; and invests in research, education, and innovation" (ACL, 2022, p.5). "ACL focuses on two categories of performance measures: (1) supporting people's ability to remain independent and live in the community and (2) generating new knowledge about what works for older adults and people with disabilities" (ACL, 2022, p.11).

TABLE 15 HRSA mental health disorder prevention funding, fiscal year 2023 (millions)

Program	Funding Amount
Maternal, Child, and Home Visiting Program	$500
Maternal Mental Health Hotline	$7
Screening and Treatment for Maternal Depression	$10
TOTAL	$517

Source: Health Resources and Services Administration, Fiscal Year 2024, Justification of Estimates for Appropriations Committee

ACL has specific programs focused on prevention; however, no programs in its FY 2023 enacted budget specifically call out MH/SUD prevention. Some relevant activities are scattered within its programs. For example, *National Technical Assistance Center on Kinship and Grandfamilies* describes one of its activities as engaging "experts to stimulate the development of new, and identify existing evidence-based, evidence-informed, and exemplary practices or programs related to health promotion (including mental health and substance use disorder treatment)" (ACL, 2023; p. 274). ACL's nutrition service programs deliver "dietary interventions, combined with educational, social, and behavioral interventions; and enhancing the identification of, and support for, older adults with elevated suicide risk or in mental health distress" (ACL, 2023; p. 65).

The main source of ACL funding for prevention services is Title III-D of the Older Americans Act, established in 1987 to provide formula grants to states to support healthy lifestyles and promote healthy behaviors among older adults (age 60 and older). Priority is given to those living in medically underserved areas of the state and with greatest economic need (ACL, n.d.-a). States that receive funds under Title III-D must spend those funds on evidence-based programs that have been proven to improve health and well-being and reduce disease and injury. Title III-D funding does not appear to be used to focus on preventing MH/SUD but could be used to expand ACL's focus on BH prevention in older adults.

DEPARTMENT OF EDUCATION

In 2023, the Department of Education reported budgeting $108.7 million for SUD prevention, allocated to implement "evidence-based, multi-tiered behavioral frameworks" for "improving behavioral outcomes and learning conditions for students" (ONDCP, 2023b).

The Department of Education provides funding for programs that may contribute to preventing mental disorders, such as preschool readiness programs. However, I excluded these estimates from the financial totals. I also excluded programs that were described as primarily to increase the number of MH professionals in schools.

STATE SPENDING BH PREVENTION

State Financing Overview

Total state spending in FY 2023 was $2.96 trillion, including federal transfers (NASBO, 2023). The largest portion of spending went to Medicaid (29.6 percent) and education (27.3 percent) (NASBO, 2023). Approximately $1.04 trillion was transfers from the federal government (35 percent); $1.24 trillion (38 percent) came from general funds through broad-based state taxes and 0.74 trillion (25 percent) from other state funding sources that are restricted by law to a particular government activity, such as tuition and fees for higher education and provider fees under Medicare. The remaining 1.5 percent came from bonds.

In 2021, total state tax revenue comprised "15 percent from property taxes, 13 percent from individual income taxes, 12 percent from general sales taxes and gross receipts taxes, 5 percent from selective sales taxes on purchases such as alcohol, motor fuel, and tobacco products, 2 percent from corporate income taxes, and 3 percent from all other taxes, such as license, estate, and severance taxes" (Urban Institute and Brookings Institution, 2024).

State Spending on BH Prevention

States reporting to SAMHSA spending approximately $1,464 million on SUD prevention in 2022 (see **Table 16**). It requires states to report spending on primary substance use prevention funding directed by the state agency in charge of substance use treatment and prevention as part of states' maintenance of effort requirements. The largest source of state SUD prevention spending was the SAMHSA block grant, followed by Medicaid, other federal funds, and state funds. Direct funding from the state and local governments, excluding federal funds and Medicaid, was $124 million.

States reported spending approximately $196 million on primary MH disorder prevention (see **Table 17**). This was defined as funds for prevention under the direction of the state's MH agency. The largest source was state funds, other federal funds, and local funds. Direct funding from the state and local governments, excluding federal funds and Medicaid, was $145 million.

TABLE 16 State primary substance use disorder prevention spending, 2023 (millions)

Source	Funding Amount
Substance Use Prevention, Treatment, and Recovery Services Block Grant Funds	$364
Medicaid	$721
Other federal funds	$255
State funds	$118
Local funds	$3
Other funds	$3
Total	$1,464

Source: SAMHSA: WebBGAS (samhsa.gov)

TABLE 17 State mental health disorder prevention spending, 2023 (millions)

Source	Funding Amount
MH Block Grant funds	$9
Medicaid	$0.9
Other Federal Funds	$39
State Funds	$125
Local Funds	$19
Other	$0.7
Total	$196

Source: SAMHSA: WebBGAS (samhsa.gov)

State departments of education provide funding for school counselors, social workers, and psychologists. This spending is described as primarily aimed at treating MH conditions, rather than prevention, so it was not included in these estimates. However, some portion of their time may consist of prevention activities. A few states, such as California and Arkansas, target tax dollars for student MH, including MH disorder prevention (Rafa et al., 2021).

Combined, state spending on MH/SUD prevention, excluding federal funds and Medicaid, was $269 million.

State Laws and Regulations to Prevent Substance Use

CDC recommends that states and local communities use regulations to reduce the availability of alcohol, such as zoning and licensing rules that limit where and when it can be sold (CDC, n.d.-a). The National Institute on Alcohol Abuse and Alcoholism has a database that tracks the variety of state laws pertaining to the sale of alcohol and recreational cannabis (NIAAA, 2023). States must finance the enforcement of these regulations, which is an unrecognized cost of prevention.

Expanding State Spending on BH Prevention Through Earmarked Taxes

One option for expanding MH/SUD prevention spending is earmarked taxes. A 2023 study found that "approximately 30 percent of the U.S. population lives in a jurisdiction with a tax earmarked for MH, and these taxes generate over $3.57 billion annually" (Purtle et al., 2023, p. 458). Some taxes include the option to fund prevention services, whereas some are only focused on treatment. The nature of the taxes varies: on income, property, and specific goods/services. A growing potential source of revenue are excise taxes on cannabis and gambling (Purtle, Brinson and Stadnick, 2022). As with many prevention funding sources, there is a need to ensure that the taxes are being used to fund evidence-based prevention activities.

Expanding State Spending on BH Prevention Through Settlement Funds

Settlements from several lawsuits of manufacturers and distributors of opioid pain medications has resulted in approximately $55 billion in funding going to states and localities (Minhee, n.d.). The settlements restrict the funding to focus primarily on abatement of the opioid epidemic and explain that this includes prevention, such as media campaigns to prevent opioid use, evidence-based prevention programs in schools, medical provider outreach and education regarding opioid prescribing best practices, and community drug disposal programs (Attorney General, 2021). Various efforts are underway to try to track how states and localities are using their opioid settlement funds, but there is no comprehensive accounting on how much is being allocated to prevention rather than treatment or other activities. However, a high-level review of some of the states that are reporting how they are using their funds indicate that a small share is going to prevention of opioid use disorder rather than treatment or harm reduction (e.g., Massachusetts, Florida). States may be able to require that a larger proportion of opioid use disorder settlement funds go to primary prevention.

PRIVATE SPENDING ON BH PREVENTION

Private actors, such as charities/foundations, health care providers, nonprofit and for-profit businesses, and employers, also contribute directly to funding BH preventions and could increase their contributions.

Charitable/Nonprofit Organizations

One estimate is that approximately $150 billion in private foundation funding goes to public health, including BH (Shaw-Taylor, 2016). In 2022, the largest private foundations focused on public health include the Robert Woods Johnson Foundation ($705 million in total charitable disbursements), Bill and Melinda Gates Foundation ($7,043 million), Bloomberg Philanthropies ($1,700 million), and California Endowment ($249 million). No accounting exists of how much of their funding goes to primary MH/SUD prevention.

Private Insurance

The ACA requires "that most private insurance plans provide zero-dollar coverage for the preventive services recommended by four ACA designated organizations, specifically: U.S. Preventive Services Task Force, Advisory Committee on Immunization Practices, Women's Preventive Services Initiative, [and] Bright Futures" (AMA, 2024).

Employers

Employers fund workplace wellness programs and employee assistance programs that can be targeted at reducing MH/SUD. CDC has a registry of effective workplace health promotion interventions that include those focused on alcohol and substance use and depression (CDC, 2024). According to CDC, key principles to develop a well-defined alcohol- and drug-free workplace policy include publicizing the policies and ensuring that employees are know that substance misuse is never permitted in the workplace; implementing workplace health promotion programs, including education on substance misuse; and offering employee assistance programs, which provide assessment, counseling, and referral for employees regarding substance misuse. Surveys of employers find 46 percent of small, and 68 percent of large firms offer some other lifestyle or behavioral coaching program, such as stress management and substance use counseling (KFF, 2023). The U.S. corporate wellness market size was estimated to be $20.05 billion in 2022 (Fortune Business Insights, 2024).

CONCLUSIONS

I estimate that the federal government spent **$4,574 million** on BH prevention and states and localities spent **$269 million** on BH prevention. No data were available to estimate total spending on BH prevention by the private sector.

As explained in the method section of this paper, this estimate is both too large and too small. It is too large, for example, because programs often do not separate out funding for treatment and tertiary prevention from that for primary and secondary prevention. In recent years, the federal government has increased spending on tertiary prevention (also known as "harm reduction") to reduce deaths caused by drug overdoses.

This estimate is also too small because it excludes funding on social safety-net programs that may reduce the risk of developing MH/SUD conditions, particularly among low-income families, such as nutrition programs, Head Start, CHIP, TANF, Tenant Based Rental Assistance, and Education for the Disadvantaged.

APPENDIX C

The range and complexity of the risk factors that may increase the odds that an individual will develop an MH/SUD make it challenging to neatly define the BH prevention infrastructure and financing landscape.

Based on this paper, I presented information to the committee about potential opportunities to improve financing for prevention of mental, emotional, and behavioral disorders. Together with presentations at public information-gathering meetings, this contributed to the committee's deliberations and the development of its recommendations.

REFERENCES

ACF (Administration for Children & Families). n.d.-a. *ACF 2024 budget*. https://www.acf.hhs.gov/about/budget (accessed October 17, 2024).

ACF. n.d.-b. FY 2024 Administration for Children and Families Justification of Estimates for Appropriations Committees. https://acf.gov/sites/default/files/documents/olab/fy-2024-congressional-justification.pdf (accessed May 27, 2025).

ACF. 2024a. *About*. https://www.acf.hhs.gov/about (accessed January 13, 2025).

ACF. 2024b. *Community Services Block Grant (CSBG)* https://www.acf.hhs.gov/ocs/programs/community-services-block-grant-csbg (accessed January 17, 2025).

ACL (Administration for Community Living). n.d.-a. *Health promotion*. https://acl.gov/programs/health-wellness/disease-prevention (accessed January 6, 2025).

ACL. n.d.-b. *ACL's budget request*. https://acl.gov/about-acl/budget (accessed January 6, 2025).

ACL. 2022. FY 2023 Justification of Estimates for Appropriations Committees https://acl.gov/sites/default/files/about-acl/2022-02/FY2023_ACL-BudgetJustification.docx (accessed January 13, 2025).

AMA (American Medical Association). 2024. *Preventive services coding guides*. https://www.ama-assn.org/health-care-advocacy/access-care/preventive-services-coding-guides (accessed January 3, 2025).

Arias, E., T. V. Betzaida, K. D. Kochanek, and F. B. Ahmad. 2022. Provisional life expectancy estimates for 2021. Hyattsville, MD: National Center for Health Statistics. https://dx.doi.org/10.15620/cdc:118999

Attorney General. 2021. List of opioid remediation uses. https://www.attorneygeneral.gov/wp-content/uploads/2021/12/Exhibit-E-Final-Distributor-Settlement-Agreement-8-11-21.pdf (accessed January 3, 2025).

BEA (Bureau of Economic Analysis). n.d. *Health satellite account. Health care*. https://www.bea.gov/data/special-topics/healthcare (accessed September 29, 2022).

Beatty, A., E. Shepard, E. Bickford, and L. Weyandt. 2024. Adverse childhood experiences and prescription stimulant use in adults: A systematic review. *Pharmacy (Basel)* 12(2).

Camacho, S., and S. C. Henderson. 2022. The social determinants of adverse childhood experiences: An intersectional analysis of place, access to resources, and compounding effects. *International Journal of Environmental Research and Public Health* 19(17). https://doi.org/10.3390/ijerph191710670.

Capacity Building Center for States. 2023. *Promoting safe and stable families program: Children's Bureau, Administration for Children and Families, U.S. Department of Health and Human Services*. https://capacity.childwelfare.gov/states/resources/promoting-safe-stable-families (accessed January 3, 2024).

CDC (Centers for Disease Control and Prevention) n.d.-a. *Alcohol use*. https://www.cdc.gov/alcohol/index.html (accessed October 17, 2024).

CDC. n.d.-b. *Injury center suicide prevention funding.* https://www.cdc.gov/injury/budget-funding/suicide-prevention-funding.html?CDC_AAref_Val=https://www.cdc.gov/injury/budget/suicidepreventionpolicy/SuicidePreventionInvestment.html (accessed October 17, 2024).

CDC. 2024. *CDC workplace health promotion.* https://www.cdc.gov/workplace-health-promotion/php/model/index.html (accessed October 17, 2024).

Claussen, A. H., J. R. Holbrook, H. J. Hutchins, L. R. Robinson, J. Bloomfield, L. Meng, R. H. Bitsko, B. O'Masta, A. Cerles, B. Maher, M. Rush, and J. W. Kaminski. 2024. All in the family? A systematic review and meta-analysis of parenting and family environment as risk factors for attention-deficit/hyperactivity disorder (ADHD) in children. *Prevention Science* 25(Suppl 2):249–271.

CMS (Centers for Medicare & Medicaid Services). 2013. *Prevention and early identification of mental health and substance use conditions* https://www.medicaid.gov/federal-policy-guidance/downloads/cib-03-27-2013.pdf (accessed January 3, 2025).

CMS. 2021a. *Population health measures.* https://www.cms.gov/sites/default/files/2021-09/Population-Health-Measures.pdf (accessed January 3, 2025).

CMS. 2021b. Screening, brief intervention, & referral to treatment (SBIRT) services. https://www.qualityhealth.org/bree/wp-content/uploads/sites/8/2021/03/CMS-MLN-SBIRT.pdf (accessed May 27, 2025).

CMS. 2022. *Leveraging Medicaid, CHIP, and other federal programs in the delivery of behavioral health services for children and youth.* https://sss.usf.edu/resources/topic/medicaid/cms_guidance/CMS_Informational_Bulletin_2022Leveraging.pdf (accessed June 1, 2024).

CMS. 2023a. *Delivering services in school-based settings: A comprehensive guide to Medicaid services and administrative claiming.* https://www.cms.gov/newsroom/fact-sheets/delivering-service-school-based-settings-comprehensive-guide-medicaid-services-and-administrative (accessed January 3, 2025).

CMS. 2023b. Million Hearts® cardiovascular disease risk reduction model (Million Hearts® model): Findings at a glance evaluation of period January 2017 to December 2021. https://www.cms.gov/priorities/innovation/data-and-reports/2023/mhcvdrrm-finalannevalrpt-fg (accessed October 7, 2024).

CMS. 2024a. *Historical.* https://www.cms.gov/data-research/statistics-trends-and-reports/national-health-expenditure-data/historical (accessed January 3, 2025).

CMS. 2024b. *Medicare prevention services.* https://www.cms.gov/Medicare/Prevention/PrevntionGenInfo/medicare-preventive-services/MPS-QuickReferenceChart-1.html (accessed January 3, 2025).

CMS. n.d. *Adult health quality measures.* https://www.medicaid.gov/medicaid/quality-of-care/performance-measurement/adult-and-child-health-care-quality-measures/adult-health-care-quality-measures/index.html (accessed October 7, 2024).

CRS (Congressional Research Service). 2023. *Centers for disease control and prevention (CDC) funding overview.* https://crsreports.congress.gov/product/pdf/R/R47207/4 (accessed October 7, 2024).

CRS. 2024. Prevention and Public Health Fund. In Brief. January 8, 2024. https://crsreports.congress.gov/product/pdf/R/R47895 (accessed May 27, 2025).

Daly, M. 2022. Prevalence of depression among adolescents in the U.S. From 2009 to 2019: Analysis of trends by sex, race/ethnicity, and income. *Journal of Adolescent Health* 70(3):496–499.

Danielsdottir, H. B., T. Aspelund, Q. Shen, T. Halldorsdottir, J. Jakobsdottir, H. Song, D. Lu, R. Kuja-Halkola, H. Larsson, K. Fall, P. K. E. Magnusson, F. Fang, J. Bergstedt, and U. A. Valdimarsdottir. 2024. Adverse childhood experiences and adult mental health outcomes. *JAMA Psychiatry* 81(6):586–594. https://doi.org/10.1001/jamapsychiatry.2024.0039.

Department of the Treasury. n.d.-a. *Fiscal data.* https://fiscaldata.treasury.gov/americas-finance-guide/federal-spending/ (accessed October 17, 2024).

Department of the Treasury. n.d.-b. *Fiscal data.* https://fiscaldata.treasury.gov/americas-finance-guide/federal-spending/ (accessed October 17, 2024).

ED (Department of Education). 2024. *Medicaid funding for school-based services* https://www.ed.gov/sites/ed/files/about/offices/list/osers/docs/medicaid-funding-for-school-based-services-03-08-2024.pdf (accessed October 9, 2024).

Ehlman, D. C., E. Yard, D. M. Stone, C. M. Jones, and K. A. Mack. 2022. Changes in suicide rates - united states, 2019 and 2020. *MMWR Morbidity and Mortality Weekly Report* 71(8):306–312. https://doi.org/10.15585/mmwr.mm7108a5

Faggiano, F., S. Minozzi, E. Versino, and D. Buscemi. 2014. Universal school-based prevention for illicit drug use. *Cochrane Database Systematic Reviews* 2014(12):CD003020. https://doi.org/10.1002/14651858.CD003020.

Fortune Business Insights, 2024. *Health IT/U.S. Corporate wellness market.* https://www.fortunebusinessinsights.com/u-s-corporate-wellness-market-108770 (accessed May 27, 2025).

GAO (Government Accountability Office). 2022. *Drug policy. Preliminary observations on the 2022 national drug control policy.* https://www.gao.gov/assets/gao-22-106087.pdf (accessed June 1, 2024).

Goodwin, R. D., A. H. Weinberger, J. H. Kim, M. Wu, and S. Galea. 2020. Trends in anxiety among adults in the United States, 2008-2018: Rapid increases among young adults. *Journal of Research* 130:441–446.

Gu, W., Q. Zhao, C. Yuan, Z. Yi, M. Zhao, and Z. Wang. 2022. Impact of adverse childhood experiences on the symptom severity of different mental disorders: A cross-diagnostic study. *General Psychiatry* 35(2):e100741.

Hedegaard, H., A. M. Miniño, and W. Warner. 2020. Drug overdose deaths in the United States, 1999–2018. https://www.cdc.gov/nchs/data/databriefs/db329-h.pdf (accessed May 27, 2025).

Helliwell, J. F., R. Layard, J. D. Sachs, J.-E. De Neve, L. B. Aknin, and S. Wang. 2024. *World happiness report 2024.* University of Oxford: Wellbeing Research Centre.

HRSA (Health Resources and Services Administration). n.d. *Justification of estimates for appropriations committees. Fiscal year 2024.* https://www.hrsa.gov/sites/default/files/hrsa/about/budget/budget-justification-fy2024.pdf (accessed October 17, 2024).

IOM (Institute of Medicine). 1994. *Reducing risks for mental disorders: Frontiers in preventive intervention research.* Patricia J. Mrazek and Robert J. Haggerty, Editors; Committee on Prevention of Mental Disorders. Washington, DC: The National Academies Press. https://doi.org/10.17226/2139.

Jacques, L., T. Syrek Jensen, J. Schafer, S. Caplan and L. Schott. 2011. Screening for depression in adults (cag-00425n) - decision memo: CMS. https://www.cms.gov/medicare-coverage-database/view/ncacal-decision-memo.aspx?proposed=N&NCAId=251 (accessed January 6, 2025).

Johnston, L. D., R. A. Miech, P. M. O'Malley, J. G. Bachman, J. E. Schulenberg, and M. E. Patrick. 2021. *Monitoring the future national survey results on drug use 1975–2020: Overview, key findings on adolescent drug use.* Ann Arbor: Institute for Social Research, University of Michigan. https://monitoringthefuture.org/wp-content/uploads/2022/08/mtf-overview2020.pdf (accessed January 3, 2025).

KFF (Kaiser Family Foundation). 2023. *2023 employer health benefits survey: Section 12 health screening and health promotion and wellness programs and disease management.* KFF.

Klaman, S. L., K. Isaacs, A. Leopold, J. Perpich, S. Hayashi, J. Vender, M. Campopiano, and H. E. Jones. 2017. Treating women who are pregnant and parenting for opioid use disorder and the concurrent care of their infants and children: Literature review to support national guidance. *Journal of Addiction Medicine* 11(3):178–190.

Lorenc, T., S. Lester, K. Sutcliffe, C. Stansfield, and J. Thomas. 2020. Interventions to support people exposed to adverse childhood experiences: Systematic review of systematic reviews. *BMC Public Health* 20(1):657.

Maayan, L., and M. Maayan. 2024. Inflammatory mediation of the relationship between early adversity and major depressive disorder: A systematic review. *Journal of Psychiatric Research* 169:364–377.

MACPAC (Medicaid and CHIP Payment and Access Commission). 2015. *The intersection of Medicaid and child welfare. In report to congress on Medicaid and CHIP*. https://www.macpac.gov/wp-content/uploads/2015/03/Intersection-of-Medicaid-and-Child-Welfare-March-2015-Presentation.pdf (accessed January 3, 2025).

MACPAC. 2019. CHIP health services initiatives: What they are and how states use them. https://www.macpac.gov/publication/chip-health-services-initiatives-what-they-are-and-how-states-use-them/ (accessed January 3, 2025).

MACPAC. 2023. MACPAC releases 2023 edition of MACStats: Medicaid and CHIP data book. https://www.macpac.gov/news/macpac-releases-2023-edition-of-macstats-medicaid-and-chip-data-book/ (accessed May 27, 2025).

Mandl, S., J. Alexopoulos, S. Doering, B. Wildner, R. Seidl, and L. Bartha-Doering. 2024. The effect of prenatal maternal distress on offspring brain development: A systematic review. *Early Human Development* 192:106009.

Mark, T. 2024. Author analysis of Medicare physician & other practitioners - by provider and service database totaling Medicare spending on billing codes g2011, g0396, and g0397.

Mark, T. L., M. Dolan, B. Allaire, W. Parish, C. Strack, D. Poehler, E. Madden, and V. Butler. 2024b. Untreated psychiatric and substance use disorders among caregivers with children reported to child protective services. *JAMA Health Forum* 5(4):e240637.

Mark, T. L., M. Dolan, B. Allaire, W. Parish, D. Poehler, C. Strack, E. Madden, and V. Butler. 2024a. Linked child welfare and Medicaid data in Kentucky and Florida highlights racial disparities in access to care. *Child Maltreatment*:10775595241234569.

Medicaid.gov. 2023. *Coverage of health-related social needs (HRSN) services in Medicaid and the children's health insurance program (CHIP)*. https://www.medicaid.gov/health-related-social-needs/downloads/hrsn-coverage-table.pdf (accessed January 3, 2025).

Medicaid.gov. n.d.-a. *Medicaid & school-based services*. https://www.medicaid.gov/resources-for-states/medicaid-state-technical-assistance/medicaid-and-school-based-services/index.html (accessed January 3, 2025).

Medicaid.gov. n.d.-b. *Early and periodic screening, diagnostic, and treatment*. https://www.medicaid.gov/medicaid/benefits/early-and-periodic-screening-diagnostic-and-treatment/index.html (accessed January 6, 2025).

Medicaid.gov. n.d.-c. *New Jersey CARTS FY2021 report*. https://www.medicaid.gov/CHIP/downloads/nj-2021chipannualreport.pdf (accessed January 6, 2025).

Minhee, C. n.d. *Will opioid settlements be spent in ways that bolster the public health response to drug use?* https://www.opioidsettlementtracker.com/ (accessed January 3, 2025).

Morales, M. F., L. C. Girard, A. Raouna, and A. MacBeth. 2023. The association of different presentations of maternal depression with children's socio-emotional development: A systematic review. *PLOS Global Public Health* 3(2):e0001649.

NASBO (National Association of State Budget Officers). 2023. State expenditure report. https://www.nasbo.org/reports-data/state-expenditure-report (accessed October 7, 2024).

APPENDIX C

NCSL (National Conference of State Legislatures) 2023. *Leveraging in lieu of services in Medicaid managed care.* https://www.ncsl.org/health/leveraging-in-lieu-of-services-in-medicaid-managed-care (accessed October 7, 2024).

NIAAA (National Institute on Alcohol Abuse and Alcoholism). 2023. *Alcohol Policy Information System.* https://alcoholpolicy.niaaa.nih.gov/ (accessed January 6, 2025).

Norman, R. E., M. Byambaa, R. De, A. Butchart, J. Scott, and T. Vos. 2012. The long-term health consequences of child physical abuse, emotional abuse, and neglect: A systematic review and meta-analysis. *PLoS Med* 9(11):e1001349.

ONDCP (Office of National Drug Control Policy). 2023a. *National drug control budget: FY 2024 funding highlights.* https://www.whitehouse.gov/wp-content/uploads/2023/03/FY-2024-Budget-Highlights.pdf (accessed January 3, 2025).

ONDCP. 2023b. *National drug control assessment.* https://bidenwhitehouse.archives.gov/wp-content/uploads/2023/06/2023-National-Drug-Control-Assessment_Final_20230531.pdf (accessed May 27, 2025).

ONDCP. 2023c. National Drug Control Strategy FY 2024 Budget Summary. https://www.whitehouse.gov/wp-content/uploads/2023/05/FY-2024-Budget-Summary.pdf (accessed January 13, 2025).

Purtle, J., K. Brinson, and N. A. Stadnick. 2022. Earmarking excise taxes on recreational cannabis for investments in mental health: An underused financing strategy. *JAMA Health Forum* 3(4):e220292.

Purtle, J., M. Wynecoop, M. E. Crane, and N. A. Stadnick. 2023. Earmarked taxes for mental health services in the United States: A local and state legal mapping study. *Milbank Quarterly* 101(2):457–485.

Rafa, A., M. McCann, C. Francies, and A. Evans. 2021. State funding for student mental health: Education Commission of the States. https://www.ecs.org/wp-content/uploads/State-Funding-for-Student-Mental-Health.pdf (accessed January 6, 2025).

Ready, D., J. Salazar, and C. Verboon. 2024. The federal budget in fiscal year 2023: An infographic: Congressional Budget Office. https://www.cbo.gov/system/files/2024-03/59727-Federal-Budget.pdf (accessed May 27, 2025).

SAMHSA (Substance Abuse and Mental Health Services Administration). 2023a. *Key substance use and mental health indicators in the United States: Results from the 2022 national survey on drug use and health.* HHS Publication No. PEP23-07-01-006, NSDUH Series H-58 https://www.samhsa.gov/data/report/2022-nsduh-annual-national-report (accessed October 7, 2024).

SAMHSA. 2023b. Strategic prevention framework – partnerships for success for states. Notice of funding opportunities. NOFO Number: SP-23-003. https://www.samhsa.gov/grants/grant-announcements/sp-23-003 (accessed October 7, 2024).

Saunders, H., and R. Rudowitz. 2024. A Look at the Latest Alcohol Death Data and Change Over the Last Decade *KFF.* May 23, 2024. https://www.kff.org/mental-health/issue-brief/a-look-at-the-latest-alcohol-death-data-and-change-over-the-last-decade/ (accessed October 7, 2024).

Shaw-Taylor, Y. 2016. Nongovernment philanthropic spending on public health in the United States. *American Journal of Public Health* 106(1):58–62.

Solmi, M., J. Radua, B. Stubbs, V. Ricca, D. Moretti, D. Busatta, A. F. Carvalho, E. Dragioti, A. Favaro, A. M. Monteleone, J. I. Shin, P. Fusar-Poli, and G. Castellini. 2021. Risk factors for eating disorders: An umbrella review of published meta-analyses. *Brazilian Journal of Psychiatry* 43(3):314–323. https://doi.org/10.1590/1516-4446-2020-1099.

Thompson V., and A. Hasan. 2023. *Medicaid reimbursement for home visiting.* NASHP. https://eadn-wc03-8290287.nxedge.io/wp-content/uploads/2023/05/NASHP_State-Medicaid-Reimbursement-for-Home-Visiting_Brief_FINAL.pdf (accessed January 3, 2025).

Tsai, D. 2023. *Information on school-based services in Medicaid: Policy flexibilities and guide on coverage, billing, reimbursement, documentation and school-based administrative claiming.* https://www.medicaid.gov/media/156331 (accessed January 3, 2025).

Urban Institute and Brookings Institution. 2024. *Tax Policy Center's briefing book: State and local tax policies.* https://taxpolicycenter.org/briefing-book/what-are-sources-revenue-state-and-local-governments#:~:text=In%202021%2C%2037%20%%20of,100%20%%20because%20of%20rounding (accessed January 3, 2025).

USASpending.gov. 2023. *FY2023 spending by agency.* https://www.usaspending.gov/explorer/agency (accessed October 7, 2024).

Wachino, V. 2016. *Maternal depression screening and treatment: A critical role for Medicaid in the care of mothers and children.* https://www.medicaid.gov/federal-policy-guidance/downloads/cib051116.pdf (accessed May 27, 2025).

Werner-Seidler, A., S. Spanos, A. L. Calear, Y. Perry, M. Torok, B. O'Dea, H. Christensen, and J. M. Newby. 2021. School-based depression and anxiety prevention programs: An updated systematic review and meta-analysis. *Clinical Psychology Review* 89:102079. https://doi.org/10.1016/j.cpr.2021.102079

White House. 2023. *Aid to state and local governments.* https://www.whitehouse.gov/wp-content/uploads/2024/03/ap_8_state_and_local_fy2025.pdf (accessed October 7, 2024).

Wong, C. A., D. Houry, and M. K. Cohen. 2024. Integrating public health and health care - protecting health as a team sport. *New England Journal of Medicine* 390(19):1739–1742.

Appendix D

Public Session Agendas

MEETING 1, PART 1

December 11, 2023

Virtual Meeting

3:00 pm ET	Welcome and Introduction *Marcella Alsan, Ph.D., M.D., and Marthe Gold, M.D., committee cochairs*
3:15 pm ET	Presentation of the Statement of Task and Background *Nora Volkow, M.D., National Institute on Drug Abuse (NIDA), National Institutes of Health (NIH)*
3:35 pm ET	Discussion with Committee Members
4:00 pm ET	Remarks on the Statement of Task and Background *CAPT Christopher Jones, Pharm.D., Dr.P.H., M.P.H., Substance Abuse and Mental Health Services Administration*
4:15 pm ET	Discussion with Committee Members
4:30 pm ET	Adjourn Open Session

MEETING 1, PART 2

January 25, 2024

National Academy of Sciences Building
2101 Constitution Ave NW, Washington, DC 20418

10:00 am ET   Welcome and Introduction
Marcella Alsan, Ph.D., M.D., and Marthe Gold, M.D., committee cochairs

Sponsor Remarks
Amy Goldstein, Ph.D., National Institute on Drug Abuse, National Institutes of Health

10:20 am ET   Panel 1: Current Landscape of State and Federal Efforts
Robert Morrison, National Association of State Alcohol and Drug Abuse Directors
Tequila Terry, M.B.A., M.P.H., Centers for Medicare and Medicaid Services
Shari M. Ling, M.D., Centers for Medicare and Medicaid Services (CMS)
Kirsten Beronio, J.D., CMS

Questions from the Committee

12:00 pm ET   Break

1:00 pm ET   Panel 2: A Sampling of Perspectives and Evidence on Interventions and Optimal Characteristics of the Infrastructure

Scaling up Evidence-Based Interventions in U.S. Public Systems to Prevent Behavioral Health Problems
Abigail Fagan, Ph.D., University of Florida

A National Strategy for Preventing Substance and Opioid Use Disorders Through Evidence-Based Prevention
Zili Sloboda, Sc.D., Applied Prevention Science
Diana (Denni) Fishbein, Ph.D., UNC Frank Porter Graham Child Development Institute

APPENDIX D 313

     A Registry of Evidence-Based Youth Development Programs
     Pamela Buckley, Ph.D., Blueprint for Healthy Youth Development

     Questions from the Committee
     Moderator: Joshua Breslau, Sc.D., RAND Corporation

2:25 pm ET Break

2:40 pm ET Panel 2 Continued

     Opportunities for Promoting Behavioral Health in Older Adults (e.g., addressing loneliness and social isolation)
     Nancy J. Donovan, M.D., Brigham and Women's Hospital; Massachusetts General Hospital; Harvard Medical School

     A Perspective on Preventing Behavioral Health Disorders in Veterans
     Rani Hoff, M.P.H., Ph.D., Northeast Program Evaluation Center; National Center for PTSD

     Perspectives on Prevention and Behavioral Health Across the Life Cycle: Challenges and Opportunities
     Robert Ursano, M.D., Uniformed Services University of Health Sciences

     Questions from the Committee

3:40 pm ET Public Comment

4:00 pm ET Adjourn

MEETING 2

February 22, 2024

Virtual Meeting

10:00 am ET **Welcome and Introduction**
     Marcella Alsan, Ph.D., M.D., and Marthe Gold, M.D., committee cochairs

10:10 am ET	**Social and Economic Policy Effects on Behavioral Health** *Lisa Gennetian, Ph.D., Duke Center for Child and Family Policy* Questions from Committee
10:45 am ET	**The Bidirectional Relationship Between Firearm Violence and Behavioral Health** *Therese S. Richmond, Ph.D., RN, FAAN, University of Pennsylvania* Questions from Committee
11:20 am ET	Break
11:25 am ET	**Implementation Processes** *Jonathan Purtle, Dr.P.H., M.P.H., M.Sc., New York University* Questions from Committee
12:00 pm ET	**Large Scale Roll-Out of Evidence-Based Practices Through the IAPT Program (United Kingdom)** *David M. Clark, D.Phil., CBE, FBA, FMedSci, FAcSS, University of Oxford* Questions from the Committee
12:45 pm ET	Break
1:15 pm ET	**Community, Local, and State Efforts to Build Prevention Infrastructure for Behavioral Health** *Sue Thau, M.C.R.P., CADCA* *Brian Hepburn, M.D., National Association of State Mental Health Program Directors* *Deepa Avula, M.P.H., NYC Department of Health and Mental Hygiene* Questions from the Committee
2:25 pm ET	Break

2:30 pm ET — Other Perspectives to Inform a National Prevention Infrastructure

The Community Guide's Role in a National Infrastructure to Prevent Behavioral Health Disorders
Amy Lansky, Ph.D., M.P.H., Centers for Disease Control and Prevention

HRSA's Approaches to Supporting Behavioral Health Preventive Interventions
Patsy Cunningham, M.A., LCPC, Health Resources and Services Administration

Looking Ahead at the Federal Role in Behavioral Health Prevention
Nathaniel Counts, J.D., Commonwealth Fund

Questions from the Committee

3:35 pm ET — Public Comment

4:00 pm ET — Adjourn

MEETING 3

April 4, 2024

National Academy of Sciences Building
2101 Constitution Ave NW, Washington, DC 20418

9:00 am ET — Welcome and Introduction
Marcella Alsan, Ph.D., M.D., and Marthe Gold, M.D., committee cochairs

9:10 am ET — State-Level Infrastructure to Support Prevention
Chinazo Cunningham, M.D., New York State Office of Addiction Services and Supports
Sarah Mariani, CPP, Washington State Health Care Authority; National Prevention Network

Q&A with Committee

9:55 am ET Local-Level and Community Infrastructure to Support Prevention
Jonah C. Cunningham, M.P.P., National Association of County Behavioral Health and Developmental Disability Directors; National Association for Rural Mental Health
Rev. Dr. Que English, HHS Office of Faith-Based and Neighborhood Partnerships
Zeke Cohen, 1st District of Baltimore, MD

Q&A with Committee

10:55 am ET Break

11:00 am ET Infrastructure Supporting Prevention Among Older Adults
Kari Benson, HHS Administration for Community Living
Namkee G. Choi, Ph.D., University of Texas at Austin Steve Hicks School of Social Work

Q&A with Committee

11:45 am ET Infrastructure Supporting Prevention Among Children and Adolescents
Kym Ahrens, M.D., M.P.H., Washington State's Juvenile Justice System; Seattle Children's
Joe Neigel, CPP, Monroe School District, Washington

Q&A with Committee

12:30 pm ET Break

1:15 pm ET CDC Policies and Approaches to Prevention
Greta Massetti, Ph.D., M.A., National Center for Injury Prevention and Control, Centers for Disease Control and Prevention

Q&A with Committee

1:45 pm ET International Comparisons of Public Policies Related to Prevention and Behavioral Health
Jody Heymann, M.D., Ph.D., UCLA Fielding School of Public Health
Reginald D. Williams, II, The Commonwealth Fund

Q&A with Committee

APPENDIX D   *317*

2:30 pm ET   Break

2:40 pm ET   **Data Resources, Challenges, and Opportunities**
              Katie McLaughlin, Ph.D., University of Oregon
              Kristine McCoy, M.D., M.P.H., Two Oceans, LLC
              & Stewards of Change Institute

              Q&A with Committee

3:25 pm ET   **Decision-Making to Support the Prevention Infrastructure**
              Sara Whaley, M.P.H., M.S.W., M.A., Johns Hopkins
              Bloomberg School of Public Health; Bloomberg
              Overdose Prevention Initiative
              Stephanie Lee, Washington State Institute for
              Public Policy
              David Hughes, Ph.D., Human Services Research Institute

              Q&A with Committee

4:30 pm ET   Adjourn

LISTENING SESSION 1

May 31, 2024

Virtual

11:00 am ET   Welcome and Introduction

11:05 am ET   **Public Comments**
               Sally Manninen
               Michael Mumper
               Angela Kimball
               Benjamin Miller

               Discussion with Committee

12:30 pm ET   Adjourn

LISTENING SESSION 2

June 5, 2024

Virtual

11:00 am ET   Welcome and Introduction

11:05 am ET   Public Comments
David Willis
Rahil Briggs

Discussion with Committee

12:30 pm ET   Adjourn

LISTENING SESSION 3

June 6, 2024

Virtual

11:00 am ET   Welcome and Introduction

11:05 am ET   Public Comments
Erin Jamieson Day
Jeanette Ickovics
Sarah Chilenski
Brenda Blasingame

Discussion with Committee

12:30 pm ET   Adjourn

Appendix E

Related Reports of the National Academies of Sciences, Engineering, and Medicine

This appendix is a list of recent report recommendations relevant to preventing mental, emotional, and behavioral (MEB) disorders and promoting MEB health and well-being, including those related to interventions and the broader infrastructure for delivering interventions. This table adapts and expands a similar appendix that can be found in *Fostering Healthy Mental, Emotional, and Behavioral Development in Children and Youth* (2019).

TABLE E-1 Select Relevant Recommendations, Conclusions, and Messages

Reducing Suicide: A National Imperative (2002)

Recommendation 1. The National Institute of Mental Health (in collaboration with other agencies) should develop and support a national network of suicide research Population Laboratories devoted to interdisciplinary research on suicide and suicide prevention across the life cycle

Recommendation 2: National monitoring of suicide and suicidality should be improved. Steps toward improvement should include the following:
- Funding agencies (including NIMH, NIA, NICHD, NIDA, NIAAA, CDC, SAMHSA, and DVA) should encourage that measures of suicidality (e.g., attempts) be included in all large and/or long-term studies of health behaviors, mental health interventions, and genetic studies of mental disorder. Funding agencies should issue program announcements for supplements to ongoing longitudinal studies to include the collection and analysis of these additional measures.
- Suicidal patients should be included in clinical trials when appropriate safeguards are in place.
- A national suicide attempt surveillance system should be developed and coordinated through the CDC.
- Federal funding should be provided to support a surveillance system such as the National Violent Death Reporting System that includes data on mortality from suicide.

Recommendation 3: Because primary care providers are often the first and only medical contact of suicidal patients, tools for recognition and screening of patients should be developed and disseminated.

Recommendation 4: Programs for suicide prevention should be developed, tested, expanded, and implemented through funding from appropriate agencies including NIMH, DVA, CDC, and SAMHSA.

Community Programs to Promote Youth Development (2002)

Recommendation 1: Community programs for youth should be based on a developmental framework that supports the acquisition of personal and social assets in an environment, and through activities, that promote both current adolescent well-being and future successful transitions to adulthood.

Recommendation 2: Communities should provide an ample array of program opportunities that appeal to and meet the needs of diverse youth, and should do so through local entities that can coordinate such work across the entire community. Particular attention should be placed on programs for disadvantaged and underserved youth.

Recommendation 3: To increase the likelihood that an ample array of program opportunities will be available, communities should put in place some locally appropriate mechanism for monitoring the availability, accessibility, and quality of programs for youth in their community.

Recommendation 4: Private and public funders should provide the resources needed at the community level to develop and support community- wide programming that is orderly, coordinated, and evaluated in reasonable ways. In addition to support at the community level, this is likely to involve support for intermediary organizations and collaborative teams that include researchers, practitioners, funders, and policy makers.

TABLE E-1 Continued

Recommendation 5: Federal agencies that fund research on adolescent health, development, and well-being, such as the Department of Health and Human Services, the Department of Justice, and the Department of Education, should build into their portfolios new or more comprehensive longitudinal and experimental research on the personal and social assets needed to promote the healthy development and well-being of adolescents and to promote the successful transition from childhood through adolescence and into adulthood.

Recommendation 6: Public and private funders should support research on whether the features of positive developmental settings identified in this report are the most important features of community programs for youth. This research should encourage program design and implementation that meets the diverse needs of an increasingly heterogeneous population of youth.

Recommendation 7: All community programs for youth should undergo evaluation—possibly multiple evaluations—to improve design and implementation, to create accountability, and to assess outcomes and impacts. For any given evaluation, the scope and the rigor should be appropriately calibrated to the attributes of the program, the available resources, and the goals of the evaluation.

Recommendation 8: Funders should provide the necessary funds for evaluation. In many cases, this will involve support for collaborative teams of researchers, evaluators, theoreticians, policy makers, and practitioners to ensure that programs are well designed initially and then evaluated in the most appropriate way.

Recommendation 10: Public and private funders should support collaboration between researchers and the practice community to develop social indicator data that build understanding of how programs are implemented and improve the ability to monitor programs. Collaborative efforts would further the understanding of the relationship between program features and positive developmental outcomes among young people.

Recommendation 11: Public and private funders should provide opportunities for individual programs and communities to increase their capacity to collect and use social indicator data. This requires better training for program staff and more support for national and regional intermediaries that provide technical assistance in a variety of ways, including Internet-based systems.

Reducing Underage Drinking: A Collective Responsibility (2004)

Recommendation 10-2: The U.S. Department of Health and Human Services and the U.S. Department of Education should fund only evidence-based education interventions, with priority given both to those that incorporate elements known to be effective and those that are part of comprehensive community programs.

Preventing Mental, Emotional, and Behavioral Disorders Among Young People: Progress and Possibilities (2009)

Recommendation 13-1: The federal government should make the healthy mental, emotional, and behavioral development of young people a national priority, establish public goals for the prevention of specific [mental, emotional, and behavioral] MEB disorders and for the promotion of healthy development among young people, and provide needed research and service resources to achieve these aims.

continued

TABLE E-1 Continued

Recommendation 13-2: The White House should create an ongoing mechanism involving federal agencies, stakeholders (including professional associations), and key researchers to develop and implement a strategic approach to the promotion of mental, emotional, and behavioral health and the prevention of MEB disorders and related problem behaviors in young people. The U.S. Departments of Health and Human Services, Education, and Justice should be accountable for coordinating and aligning their resources, programs, and initiatives with this strategic approach and for encouraging their state and local counterparts to do the same.

Recommendation 13-3: States and communities should develop networked systems to apply resources to the promotion of mental health and prevention of MEB disorders among their young people. These systems should involve individuals, families, schools, justice systems, health care systems, and relevant community-based programs. Such approaches should build on available evidence-based programs and involve local evaluators to assess the implementation process of individual programs or policies and to measure community-wide outcomes.

Recommendation 13-4: Research funders should establish parity between research on preventive interventions and treatment interventions.

Recommendation 13-5: The National Institutes of Health, with input from other funders of prevention research, should develop a comprehensive 10-year research plan targeting the promotion of mental health and prevention of both single and comorbid MEB disorders. This plan should consider current needs, opportunities for cross-disciplinary and multi-institute research, support for the necessary research infrastructure, and establishment of a mechanism for assessing and reporting progress against 10-year goals.

Funding and Implementation

Recommendation 12-1: Congress should establish a set-aside for prevention services and innovation in the Community Mental Health Services Block Grant, similar to the set-aside in the Substance Abuse Prevention and Treatment Block Grant.

Recommendation 12-2: The U.S. Departments of Health and Human Services, Education, and Justice should braid funding of research and practice so that the impact of programs and practices that are being funded by service agencies (e.g., the Substance Abuse and Mental Health Services Administration, the Office of Safe and Drug Free Schools, the Office of Juvenile Justice and Delinquency Prevention) are experimentally evaluated through research funded by other agencies (e.g., the National Institutes of Health, the Institute of Education Sciences, the National Institute of Justice). This should include developing appropriate infrastructure through which evidence-based programs and practices can be delivered and evaluated.

Recommendation 12-3: The U.S. Departments of Health and Human Services, Education, and Justice should fund states, counties, and local communities to implement and continuously improve evidence-based approaches to mental health promotion and prevention of MEB disorders in systems of care that work with young people and their families.

TABLE E-1 Continued

Recommendation 8-2: The U.S. Departments of Health and Human Services, Education, and Justice should develop strategies to identify communities with significant community-level risk factors and target resources to these communities.

Recommendation 11-4: Researchers and community organizations should form partnerships to develop evaluations of (1) adaptation of existing interventions in response to community-specific cultural characteristics; (2) preventive interventions designed based on research principles in response to community concerns; and (3) preventive interventions that have been developed in the community, have demonstrated feasibility of implementation and acceptability in that community, but lack experimental evidence of effectiveness.

Recommendation 12-4: Federal and state agencies should prioritize the use of evidence-based programs and promote the rigorous evaluation of prevention and promotion programs in a variety of settings in order to increase the knowledge base of what works, for whom, and under what conditions. The definition of evidence-based should be determined by applying established scientific criteria.

Data Collection and Monitoring

Recommendation 2-1: The U.S. Department of Health and Human Services should be required to provide (1) annual data on the prevalence of MEB disorders in young people, using an accepted current taxonomy (e.g., the Diagnostic and Statistical Manual of Mental Disorders, the International Statistical Classification of Diseases) and (2) data that can provide indicators and trends for key risk and protective factors that serve as significant predictors for MEB disorders.

Recommendation 2-2: The Substance Abuse and Mental Health Services Administration should expand its current data collection to include measures of service use across multiple agencies that work with vulnerable populations of young people.

Workforce Development

Recommendation 12-6: Training programs for relevant health (including mental health), education, and social work professionals should include prevention of MEB disorders and promotion of mental, emotional, and behavioral health. National certifying and accrediting bodies for training should set relevant standards using available evidence on identifying and managing risks and preclinical symptoms of MEB disorders.

Recommendation 12-7: The U.S. Departments of Health and Human Services, Education, and Justice should convene a national conference on training in prevention and promotion to (1) set guidelines for model prevention research and practice training programs and (2) contribute to the development of training standards for certifying trainees and accrediting prevention training programs in specific disciplines, such as health (including mental health), education, and social work.

Recommendation 12-8: Once guidelines have been developed, the U.S. Departments of Health and Human Services, Education, and Justice should set aside funds for competitive prevention training grants to support development and dissemination of model interdisciplinary training programs. Training should span creation, implementation, and evaluation of effective preventive interventions.

continued

TABLE E-1 Continued

Continuing a Course of Rigorous Research

Recommendation 4-3: Research funders* should fund preventive intervention research on (1) risk and protective factors for specific disorders; (2) risk and protective factors that lead to multiple mental, emotional, and behavioral problems and disorders; and (3) promotion of individual, family, school, and community competencies. (*The term "research funders" is used to refer to federal agencies and foundations who fund research on mental health promotion or prevention of MEB disorders.)

Recommendation 10-1: Research funders should invest in studies that (1) aim to replicate findings from earlier trials, (2) evaluate long-term outcomes of preventive interventions across multiple outcomes (e.g., disorders, academic outcomes), and (3) test the extent to which each prevention program is effective in different race, ethnic, gender, and developmental groups.

Recommendation 12-5: The National Institutes of Health and other federal agencies should increase funding for research on prevention and promotion strategies that reduce multiple MEB disorders and that strengthen accomplishment of age-appropriate developmental tasks. High priority should be given to increasing collaboration and joint funding across institutes and across federal agencies that are responsible for separate but developmentally related outcomes (e.g., mental health, substance use, school success, contact with justice).

Recommendation 7-2: Research funders should strongly support research to improve the effectiveness of current interventions and the creation of new, more effective interventions with the goal of wide-scale implementation of these interventions.

Screening Linked to Interventions

Recommendation 8-1: Research funders should support a rigorous research agenda to develop and test community-based partnership models involving systems such as education (including preschool), primary care, and behavioral health to screen for risks and early mental, emotional, and behavioral problems and assess implementation of evidence-based preventive responses to identified needs.

Implementatione. Programs focused on preventing suicide were included, although this is arguably often tertiary prevention because it can be achieved by identifying and treating MH/SUD

Recommendation 10-2: The National Institutes of Health should be charged with developing methodologies to address major gaps in current prevention science approaches, including the study of dissemination and implementation of successful interventions.

Recommendation 11-1: Research funders should fund research and evaluation on (1) dissemination strategies designed to identify effective approaches to implementation of evidence-based programs, (2) the effectiveness of programs when implemented by communities, and (3) identification of core elements of evidence-based programs, dissemination, and institutionalization strategies that might facilitate implementation.

Recommendation 11-2: Research funders should fund research on state- or community-wide implementation of interventions to promote mental, emotional, or behavioral health or prevent MEB disorders that meet established scientific standards of effectiveness.

TABLE E-1 Continued

Adaptation

Recommendation 11-3: Research funders should prioritize the evaluation and implementation of programs to promote mental, emotional, or behavioral health or prevent MEB disorders in ethnic minority communities. Priorities should include the testing and adoption of culturally appropriate adaptations of evidence-based interventions developed in one culture to determine if they work in other cultures and encouragement of adoption when they do.

Neuroscience Linkages

Recommendation 5-1: Research funders, led by the National Institutes of Health, should dedicate more resources to formulating and testing hypotheses of the effects of genetic, environmental, and epigenetic influences on brain development across the developmental span of childhood, with a special focus on pregnancy, infancy, and early childhood.

Recommendation 5-2: Research funders, led by the National Institutes of Health, should dedicate resources to support collaborations between prevention scientists and basic and clinical developmental neuroscientists. Such collaborations should include both basic science approaches and evaluations of the effects of prevention trials on neurobiological outcomes, as well as the use of animal models to identify and test causal mechanisms and theories of pathogenesis.

Recommendation 5-3: Research funders, led by the National Institutes of Health, should fund research consortia to develop multidisciplinary teams with expertise in developmental neuroscience, developmental psychopathology, and preventive intervention science to foster translational research studies leading to more effective prevention efforts.

Economic Analyses

Recommendation 9-1: The National Institutes of Health, in consultation with government agencies, private-sector organizations, and key researchers, should develop outcome measures and guidelines for economic analyses of prevention and promotion interventions. The guidelines should be widely disseminated to relevant government agencies and foundations and to prevention researchers.

Recommendation 9-2: Funders of intervention research should incorporate guidelines and measures related to economic analysis in their program announcements and provide supplemental funding for projects that include economic analyses. Once available, supplemental funding should also be provided for projects with protocols that incorporate recommended outcome measures.

Competencies

Recommendation 4-1: Research funders, led by the National Institutes of Health, should increase funding for research on the etiology and development of competencies and healthy functioning of young people, as well as how healthy functioning protects against the development of MEB disorders.

Recommendation 4-2: The National Institutes of Health should develop measures of developmental competencies and positive mental health across developmental stages that are comparable to measures used for MEB disorders. These measures should be developed in consultation with leading research and other key stakeholders and routinely used in mental health promotion intervention studies.

continued

TABLE E-1 Continued

Technology

Recommendation 7-3: Research funders should support research on the effectiveness of mass media and Internet interventions, including approaches to reducing stigma.

Other Research Gaps

Recommendation 7-4: Research funders should address significant research gaps, such as preventive interventions with adolescents and young adults, in certain high-risk groups (e.g., children with chronic diseases, children in foster care), and in primary care settings; interventions to address poverty; approaches that combine interventions at multiple developmental phases; and approaches that integrate individual, family, school, and community-level interventions.

For Researchers

Recommendation 3-1: Research and interventions on the prevention of MEB disorders should focus on interventions that occur before the onset of disorder but should be broadened to include promotion of mental, emotional, and behavioral health.

Recommendation 7-1: Prevention researchers should broaden the range of outcomes included in evaluations of prevention programs and policies to include relevant MEB disorders and related problems, as well as common positive outcomes, such as accomplishment of age-appropriate developmental tasks (e.g., school, social, and work outcomes). They should also adequately explore and report on potential iatrogenic effects.

Recommendation 9-3: Researchers should include analysis of the costs and cost-effectiveness (and whenever possible cost-benefit) of interventions in evaluations of effectiveness studies (in contrast to efficacy trials).

Recommendation 11-4: Researchers and community organizations should form partnerships to develop evaluations of (1) adaptation of existing interventions in response to community-specific cultural characteristics; (2) preventive interventions designed based on research principles in response to community concerns; and (3) preventive interventions that have been developed in the community, have demonstrated feasibility of implementation and acceptability in that community, but lack experimental evidence of effectiveness.

Adolescent Health Services: Missing Opportunities (2009)

RECOMMENDATION 3: Providers of adolescent primary care services and the payment systems that support them should make disease prevention, health promotion, and behavioral health—including early identification, management, and monitoring of current or emerging health conditions and risky behavior—a major component of routine health services.

RECOMMENDATION 4: Within communities—and with the help of public agencies—health care providers, health organizations, and community agencies should develop coordinated, linked, and interdisciplinary adolescent health services.

TABLE E-1 Continued

RECOMMENDATION 11: The Federal Interagency Forum on Child and Family Statistics should work with federal agencies and, when possible, states to organize and disseminate data on the health and health services, including developmental and behavioral health, of adolescents. These data should encompass adolescents generally, with subreports by age, selected population characteristics, and other circumstances.

Accounting for Health and Health Care: Approaches to Measuring the Sources and Costs of Their Improvement (2010)

RECOMMENDATION 1.1: Work should proceed on two projects that are distinct but complementary in nature. One accounts for inputs and outputs in the medical care sector; the other involves developing a data system designed to track current population health and coordinate information on the determinants of health (including but not limited to medical care).

For the Public's Health: The Role of Measurement in Action and Accountability (2011)

RECOMMENDATION 2: The committee recommends that the Department of Health and Human Services support and implement the following to integrate, align, and standardize health data and health-outcome measurement at all geographic levels:

- A core, standardized set of indicators that can be used to assess the health of communities.
- A core, standardized set of health-outcome indicators for national, state, and local use.
- A summary measure of population health that can be used to estimate and track health-adjusted life expectancy for the United States.

RECOMMENDATION 3: The committee recommends that the Department of Health and Human Services produce an annual report to inform policy makers, all health system sectors, and the public about important trends and disparities in social and environmental determinants that affect health.

RECOMMENDATION 7: The committee recommends that the Department of Health and Human Services work with relevant federal, state, and local public-sector and private-sector partners and stakeholders to facilitate the development of a performance measurement system that promotes accountability among governmental and private-sector organizations that have responsibilities for protecting and improving population health at local, state, and national levels.

Primary Care and Public Health: Exploring Integration to Improve Population Health (2012)

RECOMMENDATION 1: To link staff, funds, and data at the regional, state, and local levels, HRSA and CDC should join efforts to undertake an inventory of existing health and health care databases and identify new data sets, creating from these a consolidated platform for sharing and displaying local population health data that could be used by communities.

continued

TABLE E-1 Continued

Priorities for Research to Reduce the Threat of Firearm-Related Violence (2013)

Priority: Improve understanding of risk factors that influence the probability of firearm violence in specific high-risk physical locations.

Examples of topics that could be examined:

- What are the characteristics of high- and low-risk physical locations?
- Are the locations stable or do they change?
- What factors in the physical and social environment characterize neighborhoods or subneighborhoods with higher or lower levels of gun violence?
- Which characteristics strengthen the resilience of specific community locations?
- What is the effect of stress and trauma on community violence, especially firearm-related violence?
- What is the effect of concentrated disadvantage on community violence, especially firearm-related violence?

Priority: Improve understanding of whether interventions intended to diminish the illegal carrying of firearms reduce firearm violence.

Examples of research questions that could be examined:

- What is the degree to which background checks at the point of sale are effective in deterring acquisition of firearms by those who are legally disqualified from owning one?
- What is the public health impact of removing firearms from persons who develop a disqualifying characteristic, for example, mental illness, with potential for violence?
- Do programs that focus on changing norms in a community decrease illegal gun carrying?

Priority: Improve understanding of whether reducing criminal access to legally purchased guns reduces firearm violence.

Examples of topics that could be examined:

- Are there methods to enhance the reporting of stolen guns in order to reduce illegal access?
- To what degree would mandatory reporting of transfer of private ownership of guns be effective in reducing illegal access?
- To what extent do focused interventions (for example, "server training," straw-purchase stings) targeted at high-risk retailers found to be disproportionately associated with gun crimes reduce illegal access?
- How do firearms move from federal firearms licensed dealers to high-risk/criminal possessors? How can we develop detailed analyses of this illegal area of firearm distribution?

Priority: Improve understanding of the effectiveness of actions directed at preventing access to firearms by violence-prone individuals.

Examples of topics that could be examined:

- What would be the effects of altering environmental alcohol availability, such as reducing the number of off-premise alcohol outlets, on firearm violence?
- How effective are policies and enforcement of laws preventing gun sales to people with specific psychiatric diagnoses?
- To what extent does enforcement of laws requiring removal of firearms from the homes of people with a history of intimate partner violence reduce homicide and injury?

TABLE E-1 Continued

Priority: Determine the degree to which various childhood education or prevention programs reduce firearm violence in childhood and later in life.

Examples of topics that could be examined:

- Are school-, family-, and community-based risk-reduction and health-promotion programs effective in reducing firearm violence?
- Are gun safety programs effective in reducing unintentional injury to children from firearms?
- Are school personnel (for example, nurses, resource officers, teachers) effective at detecting students at risk of causing firearm violence?

Priority: Do programs to alter physical environments in high-crime areas result in a decrease in firearm violence?

Examples of topics that could be examined:

- Is there a correlation between alcohol sales for off-premises consumption and firearm violence in high-risk neighborhoods? Do laws and enforcement regarding sales of alcohol affect gun violence? What are the effects on firearm violence of community engagement programs to improve the physical environment? Is there a reduction in firearm violence among youth living in neighborhoods where community policing is practiced?
- For community programs that are considered to have sufficient effectiveness in reducing gun violence, what are the factors that affect adoption, fidelity vs. adaptation, and sustainability or scale-up of programs so that they have a public health impact?

Capturing Social and Behavioral Domains and Measures in Electronic Health Records: Phase 2 (2014)

FINDING 5-1: Four social and behavioral domains of health are already frequently collected in clinical settings. The value of this information would be increased if standard measures were used in capturing these data.

FINDING 7-1: Standardized data collection and measurement are critical to facilitate use and exchange of information on social and behavioral determinants of health. Most of these data elements are experienced by an individual and are thus collected by self-report. Currently, EHR vendors and product developers lack harmonized standards to capture such domains and measures.

RECOMMENDATION 7-2: The Office of the Director of the National Institutes of Health (NIH) should develop a plan for advancing research using social and behavioral determinants of health collected in electronic health records. The Office of Behavioral and Social Science Research should coordinate this plan, ensuring input across the many NIH institutes and centers.

RECOMMENDATION 7-3: The Secretary of Health and Human Services should convene a task force within the next 3 years, and as needed thereafter, to review advances in the measurement of social and behavioral determinants of health and make recommendations for new standards and data elements for inclusion in electronic health records. Task force members should include representatives from the Office of the National Coordinator for Health Information Technology, the Center for Medicare & Medicaid Innovation, the Agency for Healthcare Research and Quality, the Patient-Centered Outcomes Research Institute, the National Institutes of Health, and research experts in social and behavioral science.

continued

TABLE E-1 Continued

Implementing Juvenile Justice Reform: The Federal Role (2014)

RECOMMENDATION 3-3: OJJDP should take a leadership role in local, state, and tribal jurisdictions with respect to the development and implementation of administrative data systems by providing model formats for system structure, standards, and common definitions of data elements. OJJDP should also provide consultation on data systems as well as opportunities for sharing information across jurisdictions.

RECOMMENDATION 5-2: OJJDP should initiate and support collaborative partnerships at the federal, state, local, and tribal levels and should use them strategically to advance the goal of a developmentally appropriate juvenile justice system.

Vital Signs: Core Metrics for Health and Health Care Progress (2015)

This report provides a detailed analysis of measurement of individual and population health outcomes and costs, identifying fragilities and gaps in available systems, and considering approaches and priorities for developing the measures necessary for a continuously learning and improving health system. It notes, "Substantial disparities exist among and within subpopulations in the United States with respect to the relative impact of each of the domains of influence on health and health care, including disparities by race, ethnicity, income, education, gender, geography, and urban or rural populations. In the aggregate, this issue represents one of the greatest health and health care challenges faced by the nation."

RECOMMENDATION 4: With the engagement and involvement of the Executive Office of the President, the Secretary of the Department of Health and Human Services should develop and implement a strategy for working with other federal and state agencies and national organizations to facilitate the use and application of the core measure set.

RECOMMENDATION 5: The Secretary of the Department of Health and Human Services should establish and implement a mechanism for involving multiple expert stakeholder organizations in efforts to develop as necessary, maintain, and improve each of the core measures and the core measure set as a whole over time.

Mental Disorders and Disabilities Among Low-Income Children (2015)

Poverty is a risk factor for child disability, including disability associated with mental disorders. At the same time, child disability is a risk factor for family poverty. In times of economic hardship in the United States, more children with mental disorder–related disabilities will qualify for benefits because they meet the income eligibility threshold.

Children living in poverty are more likely than other children to have mental health problems, and these conditions are more likely to be severe. Low-income families containing a child with a disability may be particularly vulnerable in times of economic hardship. Access to Medicaid and income supports via the SSI disability program may improve long-term outcomes for both children with disabilities and their families.

Investing in the Health and Well-Being of Young Adults (2015)

RECOMMENDATION 6-1: State and local public health departments should establish an office to coordinate programs and services bearing on the health, safety, and well-being of young adults. If a separate office is not established for young adults, these responsibilities should be assigned to the adolescent health coordinator.

TABLE E-1 Continued

RECOMMENDATION 6-2: Each community should establish a multi-stakeholder private-public coalition on "Healthy Transitions to Adulthood," with the goal of promoting the education, health, safety, and wellbeing of all young adults. State or local public health agencies should take the lead in convening these coalitions.

RECOMMENDATION 8-2: Federal and state governments should continue encouraging programs that serve marginalized populations to make better use of administrative data for describing the overlap of populations across service systems and young adults' trajectories into and out of these systems, and for evaluating policies and programs affecting young adults.

Advancing the Power of Economic Evidence to Inform Investments in Children, Youth, and Families (2016)

This committee assessed available means of establishing economic evidence to support investments in health and well-being interventions and promotion. The report details methods and makes recommendations to program developers, funders, policy makers, etc. about the use of this economic evidence.

Parenting Matters: Supporting Parents of Children Ages 0–8 (2016)

RECOMMENDATION 1: The U.S. Department of Health and Human Services, the U.S. Department of Education, state and local agencies, and community-based organizations responsible for the implementation of services that reach large numbers of families (e.g., health care, early care and education, community programs) should form a working group to identify points in the delivery of these services at which evidence-based strategies for supporting parents can be implemented and referral of parents to needed resources can be enhanced. Based on its findings, the working group should issue guidance to service delivery organizations on increasing parents' access to evidence-based interventions.

RECOMMENDATION 2: The U.S. Department of Health and Human Services, the Institute of Education Sciences, the Patient-Centered Outcomes Research Institute, and private philanthropies should fund research focused on developing guidance for policy makers and program administrators and managers on how to scale effective parenting programs as widely and rapidly as possible. This research should take into account organization-, program-, and system-level factors, as well as quality improvement. Supports for scaling efforts developed through this research might include cost tools, measurement toolkits, and implementation guidelines.

Ending Discrimination Against People with Mental and Substance Use Disorders: The Evidence for Stigma Change (2016)

RECOMMENDATION 2: The U.S. Department of Health and Human Services should evaluate its own service programs and collaborate with other stakeholders, particularly the criminal justice system and government and state agencies, for the purpose of identifying and eliminating policies, practices, and procedures that directly or indirectly discriminate against people with mental and substance use disorders.

Communities in Action: Pathways to Health Equity (2017)

CONCLUSION 3-2: Based on its review of the evidence, the committee concludes that health inequities are the result of more than individual choice or random occurrence. They are the result of the historic and ongoing interplay of inequitable structures, policies, and norms that shape lives.

continued

TABLE E-1 Continued

RECOMMENDATION 4-1: A public–private consortium should create a publicly available repository of evidence to inform and guide efforts to promote health equity at the community level. The consortium should also offer support to communities, including technical assistance.

RECOMMENDATION 6-4: Through multi-sectoral partnerships, hospitals and health care systems should focus their community benefit dollars to pursue long-term strategies (including changes in law, policies, and systems) to build healthier neighborhoods, expand access to housing, drive economic development, and advance other upstream initiatives aimed at eradicating the root causes of poor health, especially in low-income communities. Hospitals and health systems should also advocate for the expansion of efficient and effective services responding to health-related social needs for vulnerable populations and people living in poverty.

Transforming the Financing of Early Care and Education (2018)

RECOMMENDATION 10: The federal government should align its data collection requirements across all federal early care and education (ECE) funding streams to collect comprehensive information about the entire ECE sector and sustain investments in regular, national, data collection efforts from state and nationally representative samples that track changes in the ECE landscape over time to better understand the experiences of ECE programs, the ECE workforce, and the developmental outcomes of children who participate in ECE programs.

A Roadmap for Reducing Child Poverty (2019)

CONCLUSION 4-6: The Earned Income Tax Credit, the Child Tax Credit, the Supplemental Nutrition Assistance Program (SNAP), and to a lesser extent Social Security are the most important programs for reducing Supplemental Poverty Measure (SPM)based child poverty. SNAP and Social Security are the most important programs for reducing deep poverty among children. Tax credits are the most important means of keeping children above near-poverty. Health care programs account for more than one-third of total federal expenditures on children but are not properly accounted for in the SPM poverty measure.

CONCLUSION 7-3: Evidence suggests that paid family and medical leave increases parents' ability to continue in employment and has positive impacts on children's health, although it might also reduce employment among women potentially eligible for such leave.

RECOMMENDATION 9-4: Relevant federal departments and agencies should prioritize research and experimentation designed to find ways to mitigate the effects of contextual factors that impair the effectiveness of current programs to combat child poverty. These contextual factors include (1) detrimental neighborhood conditions, (2) racial and social discrimination, and (3) adverse consequences of the criminal justice system.

RECOMMENDATION 9-8: The Bureau of Labor Statistics and the U.S. Census Bureau should move expeditiously to evaluate a health-inclusive poverty measure of the kind illustrated in this report.

RECOMMENDATION 9-9: Federal and state executive agencies and legislatures should ensure that child anti-poverty assistance programs require and include adequate resources for regular monitoring of program operations and child outcomes, as well as for rigorous program evaluation and research on ways to improve program effectiveness.

TABLE E-1 Continued

Fostering Healthy Mental, Emotional, and Behavioral Development in Children and Youth: A National Agenda (2019)

Recommendation 1: Relevant federal agencies should lead and collaborate with agencies at the state and local levels, as well as private partners, including national and local foundations and the business community, in coordinating a highly visible national effort to make the promotion of healthy mental, emotional, and behavioral (MEB) development a national priority, such as by designating a Decade of Children and Youth. These agencies should:

- articulate specific national goals and objectives in support of healthy MEB development throughout the life cycle, encompassing health promotion and disorder prevention;
- develop an integrated plan for longitudinal data collection and coordination and analysis of federal surveys, administrative data, and vital statistics that provides a comprehensive approach to measuring and tracking child and adolescent MEB health; and
- encourage and support the integration and coordination of new and existing efforts to pursue those goals and objectives at the federal, state, and local levels, using coordinating and convening capacities, pooling of resources, funding of outcomes analyses, regulatory options, and other powers and incentives.

Recommendation 2: Relevant federal agencies should use their program creation, regulatory, and other policy capabilities to promote healthy mental, emotional, and behavioral (MEB) development and mitigate risks to MEB health by, for example:

- developing and disseminating guidance for use by states and local jurisdictions in delivering effective promotion and prevention interventions—including preconception, prenatal, and postnatal care services; two-generation (including parent MEB health and parenting) interventions; preschool and school interventions; and universal screening for risk and protective factors—and in ensuring access to affordable treatment for parents and children to reduce risk;
- developing both guidance and targeted accountability measures for use by states and local jurisdictions to identify effective ways of reducing the exposure of children and families to risks—such as lead and air particulate matter; ineffective and inequitable disciplinary practices; unsafe sex and unintended pregnancies; use of tobacco, alcohol, and other drugs; traumatic experiences; and negative living conditions, including exposure to violence, unstable housing, food insufficiency, and underemployment—that can contribute to unhealthy MEB development;
- promoting coverage of behavioral health services for children and caregivers, especially those needed during pregnancy and the postpartum period and those offered by parenting programs, in reimbursement for private health insurance and Medicaid, encompassing both behavioral health promotion and risk prevention;
- setting expectations for the adoption and evaluation of programs known to enhance social and emotional development in schools, in health care settings, and in communities;
- supporting consistent polices on accreditation, certification, and licensing requirements for a multidisciplinary workforce oriented toward healthy MEB development in children and youth; and
- supporting and collaborating with local and state initiatives that contribute to healthy MEB development.

continued

TABLE E-1 Continued

Recommendation 3: Relevant federal agencies should support rapid progress in the development and dissemination of effective mental, emotional, and behavioral (MEB) interventions for delivery to large populations by providing funding and other resources to, for example:
- support research and demonstration projects to determine the effectiveness of promising interventions for MEB health promotion, prevention of MEB disorders, and population screening at large scales, including the implementation of effective in-person and digital interventions;
- support states and local jurisdictions in developing cross-sector partnerships among schools, employers, the health care system, community-based organizations, and others to advance the scale-up of effective promotion and prevention interventions;
- support states and local jurisdictions in developing innovative funding mechanisms that can be sustained through changes in political leadership or funding shortfalls;
- use economic evaluation tools and other methods to analyze such factors as costs and availability of funding, benefit/cost ratio, level of complexity, and need for supportive infrastructure; and
- document needs and develop strategies for sustainability over time.

The Promise of Adolescence: Realizing Opportunity for All Youth (2019)

RECOMMENDATION 7-2: Improve access to comprehensive, integrated, coordinated health services for adolescents.

RECOMMENDATION 7-5: Improve federal and state data collection on adolescent health and wellbeing, and conduct adolescent-specific health services and disseminate the findings.

RECOMMENDATION 8-5: Foster greater collaboration between the child welfare, juvenile justice, education, and health systems.

Strengthening the Military Family Readiness System for a Changing American Society (2019)

RECOMMENDATION 3: The U.S. Department of Defense should more fully identify, analyze, and integrate existing data to longitudinally track population-based military child risk and adversity, while also ensuring the privacy of individual family member information.

RECOMMENDATION 10: To enhance the effectiveness and efficiency of the Military Family Readiness System, the U.S. Department of Defense should investigate innovations in big data and predictive analytics to improve the accessibility, engagement, personalization, and effectiveness of policies, programs, practices, and services for military families.

Monitoring Educational Equity (2019)

RECOMMENDATION 4: Governmental and philanthropic funders should work with researchers to develop indicators of the existence and effectiveness of systems of cross-agency integrated services that address context-related impediments to student success, such as trauma and chronic stress created by adversity. The indicators and measures should encompass screening, intervention, and supports delivered not only by school systems, but also by other child-serving agencies.

TABLE E-1 Continued

Vibrant and Healthy Kids: Aligning Science, Practice, and Policy to Advance Health Equity (2019)

CONCLUSION 5-1: The current health care system focuses mainly on clinical goals and addresses the multiple other determinants of health in fragmented and highly variable ways. Despite high-quality clinical care, the health status of America's children and young families is far worse than in comparable developed countries. U.S. health care provides only limited attention to integration of health care for the whole family, health care across the life course, or integration of mental and behavioral health with the rest of health care.

CONCLUSION 6-1: Increasing the economic resources families have available to meet basic needs when children are young (including prenatally) will improve children's health and has the potential to reduce health and developmental disparities in early childhood.

RECOMMENDATION 4-2: Federal, state, local, tribal, and territorial agencies, along with private foundations and philanthropies that invest in research, should include in their portfolios research on the development of interventions that are culturally sensitive and tailored to meet the needs of subgroups of children known to be vulnerable, such as those living in chronic poverty, children from immigrant backgrounds, children in foster care, and children with incarcerated parents.

RECOMMENDATION 4-3: To strengthen and expand the impact of evidence-based home visiting programs federal, state, local, tribal, and territorial agencies overseeing program implementation should continue to strengthen programmatic coordination and policy alignment between home visiting, other early care and education programs, and medical homes.

RECOMMENDATION 5-3: The U.S. Department of Health and Human Services, state, tribal, and territorial government Medicaid agencies, health systems leaders, and state and federal policy makers should adopt policies and practices that improve the organization and integration of care systems, including promoting multidisciplinary team-based care models that focus on integrating preconception, prenatal, and postpartum care with a whole-family focus, development of new practice and payment models that incentivize health creation and improve service delivery, and structures that more tangibly connect health care delivery systems to other partners outside of the health care sector.

RECOMMENDATION 8-1: Policy makers and leaders in the health care, public health, social service, criminal justice, early care and education/education, and other sectors should support and invest in cross-sector initiatives that align strategies and operate community programs and interventions that work across sectors to address the root causes of poor health outcomes. This includes addressing structural and policy barriers to data integration and cross-sector financing and other challenges to cross-sector collaboration.

continued

TABLE E-1 Continued

Integrating Social Care into the Delivery of Health Care: Moving Upstream to Improve the Nation's Health (2019)

Goal 1. Design health care delivery to integrate social care into healthcare.

Recommendation 1. Health care organizations should take steps to integrate social care into health care. Specific steps include

a. Make and communicate an organizational commitment to addressing health-related social needs and health disparities at the community and individual levels.
b. Recognize that comprehensive health care should include understanding an individual's social context. Evidence is rapidly accumulating concerning the most effective strategies for screening and assessing for social risk factors and social needs. Such strategies should include standardized and validated questions, as available, and should use interoperable data systems to document results.
c. Use patient-centered care models to more routinely incorporate social risk data into care decisions.
d. Design and implement integrated care systems using approaches that engage patients, community partners, frontline staff, social care workers, and clinicians in planning and evaluation and that incorporate the preferences of patients and communities. Include social care workers as being integral to a team-based approach to designing and delivering health care.
e. Establish linkages and communication pathways between health care and social service providers. This is important for personal care aides, home care aides, and others who provide care and support for seriously ill and disabled patients and who have extensive knowledge of patients' social needs.
f. Develop and finance referral relationships with selected social care providers when feasible, supported by operational integration such as co-location or patient information systems. Social care providers and health care providers should establish a formal understanding and accountability within their contracting and referral relationships.
g. Support the development of those infrastructure components needed to meet the goal of care integration, including the redesign and refinement of workflows, technical assistance and support, staff with the ability to support the redesign, champions of the redesign, information on best practices, health information technology to enhance integration, and support for community partners and their infrastructure needs.

Goal 2. Build a workforce to integrate social care into health care delivery.

Recommendation 2a: State legislatures, licensing boards, professional associations, and federal agencies should develop, expand, and standardize the scopes of practice of social workers, community health workers, gerontologists, and other social care workers.

Recommendation 2b: Social workers and other social care workers should be considered to be providers who are eligible for reimbursement by payers. Public and private payers should create standards for the reimbursement of social care, including assessment and such treatment as chronic care management, behavioral health integration, and transitional care management. Medicare/Medicaid payment advisory commissions should evaluate models in which social workers and other social care workers are reimbursement-eligible providers of social care services.

TABLE E-1 Continued

Recommendation 2c: Funders of health care workforce training (e.g., the U.S. Department of Health and Human Services, the U.S. Department of Veterans Affairs, and foundations) should include the social care workforce in their education, training, and practice initiatives.

Recommendation 2d: Schools for health professions (including schools of medicine and nursing) as well as continuing education programs should incorporate competency-based curricula on social care. Curricula should include evidence on the social determinants of health, protocols for working in interprofessional teams to address social needs in health care settings, interpersonal and organizational approaches to advancing health equity and decreasing health disparities, and competencies relating to collecting, securing, and using data and technology to facilitate social and health care integration. Schools of health professions should also engage social workers in instructional roles in order to model their participation in interprofessional teams and to provide information on social risk screening and social care resources and referrals.

Recommendation 2e: Credentialing organizations for medicine, nursing, and other health professions should incorporate knowledge about the social determinants of health and the importance of addressing social needs in licensing examinations and continuing education requirements.

Recommendation 2f: Schools of social work as well as continuing education programs should use competency-based curricula on social care. In addition to educating students about the social determinants of health and health disparities, the curricula should include information about effective models that integrate social care and health care delivery, the interprofessional workforce, technology, and payment models that facilitate implementation and competencies relating to collecting, securing, and using data and technology to facilitate social and health care integration.

Recommendation 2g: State agencies and academic institutions, including community colleges, should develop standards for training and advancement (e.g., career ladder programs) for community health workers and other emerging social care workers.

Recommendation 2h: Foundations and other funders should commission a follow-up comprehensive report on the role of social work in health care as social care and health care integration continues to evolve.

Recommendation 2i: Foundations and other funders should fund a campaign to raise awareness among the health care professions and others about the value and contributions of social workers and other social care workers in health care.

Goal 3. Develop a digital infrastructure that is interoperable between health care and social care organizations.

Recommendation 3a: The federal government should establish a 21st-century social care digital infrastructure on a scale similar to that described in the Health Information and Technology for Economic and Clinical Health Act of 2009,2 and it should identify and deploy policies and resources to build the internal capacity necessary for social care organizations and consumers to interoperate and interact with each other and the health care system.

continued

TABLE E-1 Continued

Recommendation 3b: The Office of the National Coordinator should be resourced to act on the Patient Protection and Affordable Care Act of 20103 Section 1561 recommendations, including the adoption of modern, secure, interoperable digital systems and processes that will allow all partners to share the administrative and other data necessary to enable consumers to seamlessly obtain and maintain the full range of available health care and social care services.

Recommendation 3c: The Office of the National Coordinator should support states and regions as they identify the appropriate interoperable platforms for their communities, based on open standards and a modern technical architecture that supports flexible interfaces to allow the health and social care systems and consumers to share the structured data necessary for care coordination, avoidance of error, and a reduced burden on organizations and people being served.

Recommendation 3d: The Federal Health Information Technology Coordinating Committee should facilitate data sharing at the community level across diverse domains such as health care, housing, and education so as to support social care and health care integration.

Recommendation 3e: Integrating social care and health care requires the sharing of new types of data between new partners, some of whom are covered by the privacy rule promulgated by the Health Insurance Portability and Accountability Act of 19964 and some of whom are not; therefore, the U.S. Department of Health and Human Services should work with the private sector to disseminate educational tools and guidance on the data security and privacy issues that arise when collecting and sharing personally identifiable information.

Recommendation 3f: The parts of the public and private sectors involved in developing and implementing analytic and technology resources, including cell and Internet access, should do so with an explicit focus on equity; the goal should be to avoid unintended consequences such as perpetuation or aggravation of discrimination and bias and the further marginalization of populations and to proceed with an appreciation of the impact on the existing social care system.

Goal 4. Finance the integration of health care and social care.

Recommendation 4a: The Centers for Medicare & Medicaid Services should clearly define which aspects of social care that Medicaid can pay for as covered services (e.g., in the context of providing care management, targeted case management, and home- and community-based long-term care services and supports as well as within the context of managed care).

Recommendation 4b: State Medicaid agencies should use the flexibility described by the U.S. Centers for Medicare & Medicaid Services in the social care that Medicaid pays for as a covered service and make the opportunities and limitations associated with that flexibility clear to health plans and health care and social care service providers.

Recommendation 4c: The Centers for Medicare & Medicaid Services (CMS) should accelerate learning about how the integration of health and social care can improve health and reduce health care costs by encouraging and approving waivers that support social care. Sustainable financing for effective interventions piloted in the waiver should be identified by the state and CMS as an outcome of the waiver.

TABLE E-1 Continued

Recommendation 4d: States should pursue policies of continuous program eligibility to, among other benefits, create stable pools of populations for which entities can be held accountable.

Recommendation 4e: The Centers for Medicare & Medicaid Services should consider additional Medicare reforms that can broaden Medicare coverage rules in a way that is consistent with lessons from Medicaid populations and the Creating High-Quality Results and Outcomes Necessary to Improve Chronic Care Act of 2018 (the CHRONIC Care Act).5 Health plans should take full advantage of the flexibility provided under the CHRONIC Care Act for supplemental benefits under Medicare.

Recommendation 4f: The Centers for Medicare & Medicaid Services and the states should coordinate the coverage and benefits administration of their Medicare and Medicaid dually eligible populations consistent with the emerging lessons of the financial alignment demonstrations. Efforts to improve alignment should be aggressively pursued over the short and long term, with an intentional focus on social care integration.

Recommendation 4g: The Centers for Medicare & Medicaid Services should develop incentives for health care organizations and the managed care programs that contract with Medicaid and Medicare to collaborate with community-based social services, such as area agencies on aging and centers for independent living.

Recommendation 4h: The Centers for Medicare & Medicaid Services, state Medicaid agencies, employers, and health plans should accelerate the movement to alternative payment models. The measurements aimed at assessing value in these models should include activity-based measures for social care integration and outcome measures that reflect social risk and protective factors. These value-based payment and outcome measurement models should incorporate social risk adjustment and stratification in a way that is consistent with previous recommendations (NASEM, 2016).

Recommendation 4i: The U.S. Department of Health and Human Services, payers, and other private organizations, such as foundations and institutions with community-benefit obligations, should provide funding and technical assistance to support formal contractual relationships between community-based organizations and health care entities.

Recommendation 4j: Federal and state policy makers, health plans, health systems, and private-sector investors should consider collective financing mechanisms to spread risk and create shared returns on investments in social care so that returns do not accrue to a single investor.

Recommendation 4k: Health systems subject to community benefit regulations should comply with those regulations by considering partnering in social care.

Recommendation 4l. States should pursue opportunities to align their hospital licensing requirements and public reporting with federal regulations regarding community benefits to ensure consistent obligations for health systems and to explicitly link their community benefits to the provision of social care.

continued

TABLE E-1 Continued

Goal 5. Fund, conduct, and translate research and evaluation on the effectiveness and implementation of social care practices in health care settings.

Recommendation 5a: Federal and state agencies, payers, providers, delivery systems, and foundations should contribute to advancing research on and the evaluation of the effectiveness and implementation of social care practices.

- The National Institutes of Health (NIH), the Agency for Healthcare Research and Quality (AHRQ), the Centers for Medicare & Medicaid Services (CMS), the Patient-Centered Outcomes Research Institute, the Health Resources and Services Administration (HRSA), and other funders of research and program evaluation should encourage payers, providers, and delivery systems to incorporate a range of study designs and methods that include rapid learning cycles and experimental trials.
- NIH, AHRQ, CMS, foundations, and other funders of research and program evaluation should cultivate and support researchers who have expertise in health services, social sciences, and cross-disciplinary research.
- CMS should fully finance (without state contributions) independent state waiver evaluations to ensure robust evaluation of social care and health care integration pilot programs and to facilitate the dissemination of findings.
- The U.S. Department of Health and Human Services should establish and support a clearinghouse containing information on the best and most promising practices for social care integration in order to provide "lessons learned" to health systems, community- based organizations, researchers, and others.

Recommendation 5b: Funders of health care workforce research (e.g., the Agency for Healthcare Research and Quality and foundations) should include the social care workforce in studies of the effect of the social care workforce on the health and financial outcomes of health care delivery organizations.

Recommendation 5c: The Health Resources and Services Administration and other funders should support studies of the contribution of the social care workforce, including additional workers such as gerontologists and public interest lawyers, to addressing the social determinants of health in health and community care settings.

Recommendation 5d: The Centers for Medicare & Medicaid Services, the U.S. Department of Health and Human Services, state Medicaid agencies, the National Quality Forum, and the National Committee for Quality Assurance should establish mechanisms that ensure that research on effective demonstrations informs more permanent health care reforms, including the development of accountability measures and payment models.

Recommendation 5e: To enable comparative research and evaluation, researchers, evaluators, and agencies that develop measures and standards (e.g., the National Quality Forum, the National Committee for Quality Assurance, and the Centers for Medicare & Medicaid Services) should develop a consensus on and use a common core of measures reflecting social risk and protective factors as well as key health and social outcome measures. These measures should not be limited to clinical or economic metrics, but should include patient-reported outcomes and other outcomes relevant to a range of stakeholders, including patients, families, caregivers, communities, social care organizations, health care organizations, and payers. The Agency for Healthcare Research and Quality should curate these measures in a publicly available item bank.

TABLE E-1 Continued

Promoting Positive Adolescent Health Behaviors and Outcomes: Thriving in the 21st Century (2020)
Recommendation 1: The U.S. Department of Health and Human Services should fund additional research aimed at identifying, measuring, and evaluating the effectiveness of specific core components of programs and interventions focused on promoting positive health behaviors and outcomes among adolescents.
Recommendation 2: The Division of Adolescent and School Health of the Centers for Disease Control and Prevention should • update and expand the Youth Risk Behavior Survey (YRBS) to include • out-of-school youth (e.g., homeless, incarcerated, dropped out), and • survey items that reflect a more comprehensive set of sexual risk behaviors with specific definitions; and conduct further research on the ideal setting and mode for administering the YRBS with today's adolescents.
Recommendation 5-3: The Office of the Assistant Secretary for Health within the U.S. Department of Health and Human Services should fund universal, holistic, multicomponent programs that meet all of the following criteria: • promote and improve the health and well-being of the whole person, • laying the foundation for specific, developmentally appropriate behavioral skills development; • begin in early childhood and are offered during critical developmental windows, from childhood throughout adolescence; • consider adolescent decision making, exploration, and risk taking as normative; • engage diverse communities, public policy makers, and societal leaders to improve modifiable social and environmental determinants • of health and well-being that disadvantage and stress young people and their families; and • are theory driven and evidence based.
Promising Approach 5-1: Programs can benefit from implementing and evaluating policies and practices that promote inclusiveness and equity so that all youth are able to thrive.
Promising Approach 5-2: Programs can benefit from including youth of diverse ages, racial/ethnic backgrounds, socioeconomic status, rurality/urbanity, sexual orientations, sexes/genders, and disability/ability status in their decision-making processes.
Mental Health, Substance Use, and Well-Being in Higher Education: Supporting the Whole Student (2021)
Recommendation 5-3: Institutions should ensure their leave of absence and reenrollment policies and practices will accommodate the needs of students experiencing mental health and substance use problems and the time needed for effective treatment and recovery.
Recommendation 5-4: Institutions of higher education and the government agencies that support them should increase the priority given to funding for campus and community mental health and substance use services.
Recommendation 5-5: Institutions of higher education should work with insurance companies and health plans and federal, state and local regulators to remove barriers to seeking reimbursement for student mental health and substance use costs for covered students.

continued

TABLE E-1 Continued

Recommendation 5-10: Institutions of higher education should recognize that there is no single approach to promoting wellbeing and dealing with mental health and substance use problems that will be appropriate for all student populations.

Federal Policy to Advance Racial, Ethnic, and Tribal Health Equity (2023)

Recommendation 1: To improve health equity, the president of the United States should create a permanent and sustainable entity within the federal government that is charged with improving racial, ethnic, and tribal equity across the federal government. This should be a standing entity, sustained across administrations, with advisory, coordinating, and regulatory powers. The entity would work closely with other federal agencies to ensure equity in agency processes and outcomes.

Recommendation 2: The president of the United States should appoint a senior leader within the Office of Management and Budget (OMB) who can mobilize assets within OMB to serve as the cochair of the Equitable Long-Term Recovery and Resilience Steering Committee.

Recommendation 3: The federal government should assess if federal policies address or exacerbate health inequities by implementing an equity audit and developing an equity scorecard. Specifically,

a) Federal agencies should engage in a retrospective review of federal policies that had a historical impact on racial and ethnic health inequities that exist today to address contemporary impacts.
b) The Office of Management and Budget should develop, and federal agencies should conduct, an equity audit of existing federal laws. The federal laws reviewed should be identified via public input obtained by a variety of means. The equity audit should include a review of how the laws are implemented and enforced by federal agencies and state and local governments. The audit should also include criteria related to equity in process, measurement, and outcomes.
c) Congress should develop and implement an equity scorecard that is applied to all proposed federal legislation, similar to the requirement of a Congressional Budget Office score.
d) The process and results from the equity audit and scorecard should be transparent and made publicly available.

Recommendation 4: The federal government should prioritize community input and expertise when changing or developing federal policies to advance health equity. Specifically,

1. The president of the United States should require federal agencies relevant to the social determinants of health to generate and sustain community representation and advisory practices that are integrated with accountability measures and enforcement mechanisms.
2. Congress should request a Government Accountability Office report to document across federal agencies whose work impacts the social determinants of health, as well as federal statistical agencies, that
    a) Assesses how community advisory boards are positioned within their agencies, whom they are composed of, how often they meet, how they report back, and how that work influences the agencies' policies and programs; and
    b) Identifies promising and evidence-based practices, gaps, and opportunities for community advisory boards that could be applied by other agencies.

TABLE E-1 Continued

Recommendation 5: The Office of Management and Budget (OMB) should require the Census Bureau to facilitate and support the design of sampling frames, methods, measurement, collection, and dissemination of equitable data resources on minimum OMB categories—including for American Indian or Alaska Native, Asian, Black or African American, Hispanic or Latino/a, and Native Hawaiian or Pacific Islander populations—across federal statistical agencies. The highest priority should be given to the smallest OMB categories—American Indian or Alaska Native and Native Hawaiian or Pacific Islander.

Recommendation 6: The Office of Management and Budget (OMB) should update and ensure equitable collection and reporting of detailed-origin and tribal affiliation data for all minimum OMB categories through data disaggregation by race, ethnicity, and tribal affiliation (to be done in coordination with meaningful tribal consultation), including populations who self-identify as American Indian or Alaska Native, Asian, Black or African American, Native Hawaiian or Pacific Islander, and Hispanic or Latino/a.

Recommendation 7: The Centers for Disease Control and Prevention should coordinate the creation and facilitate the use of common measures on multilevel social determinants of racial and ethnic health inequities, including scientific measures of racism and other forms of discrimination, for use in analyses of national health surveys and by other federal agencies, academic researchers, and community groups in analyses examining health, social, and economic inequities among racial and ethnic groups.

Recommendation 8: Congress should increase funding for federal agencies responsible for data collection on social determinants of health measures to provide information that leads to a better understanding of the correlation between the social environment and individual health outcomes.

Recommendation 9: The president of the United States should convert the Equitable Data Working Group, currently coordinated between the Office of Management and Budget (OMB) and the Office of Science and Technology Policy, into an Office of Data Equity under OMB with representation from the Domestic Policy Council, with an emphasis on small and underrepresented populations and with a scientific and community advisory commission, to achieve data equity in a manner that is coordinated across agencies and informed by scientific and community expertise.

Recommendation 10: Congress and executive agencies should leverage the full extent of federal authority to ensure equitable implementation of federal policies and access to federal programs.

   a) Relevant federal departments and agencies should design and implement policies to improve the administration of assistance programs to facilitate access to the benefits to which individuals and families are entitled. Such activities should include implementation and delivery processes, including administrative burden, eligibility, enrollment, enforcement, and client experience; and, where applicable, the creation of performance standards in federal programs administered by other (state, local, and tribal) governments.

   b) Congress should ensure that sufficient funding is made available to conduct these activities.

continued

TABLE E-1 Continued

Recommendation 11: The president of the United States should direct the Office of Management and Budget to review federal programs that exclude specific populations, such as immigrants and those with a criminal record and, in some cases, currently incarcerated people (e.g., Medicaid coverage), to assess the rationale and implications for equity of excluding these populations, including potential impacts on their families and communities. A report on the findings and suggested changes (when applicable) should be made publicly available.

Recommendation 12: The federal government should undertake the following actions to advance health equity for American Indian and Alaska Native communities in both urban and rural settings by raising the prominence of the agencies that have jurisdiction. Specifically,

a) The president of the United States and Congress should raise the level of the Director of Indian Health Service (IHS) to an Assistant Secretary.
b) Congress should authorize funding of IHS at need/parity with other health care programs. This funding should be made mandatory and include advance appropriations.
c) The House of Representatives should re-establish an Indian Affairs Committee.

Recommendation 13: The Departments of Health and Human Services, Defense, Veterans Affairs, Homeland Security, and Justice, as federal government purchasers and direct providers of health care, should undertake strategies to achieve equitable access to health care across the life span for the individuals and families they serve in every community. These strategies should prioritize access to effective, comprehensive, affordable, accessible, timely, respectful, and culturally appropriate care that addresses equity in the navigation of health care. While these strategies have a greater chance of success when everyone has adequate health insurance, there are ways the executive branch can improve and reinforce access to care for the adequately insured, the underinsured, and the uninsured.

Appendix F

Calculations for Recommendation 6-1

CURRENT FUNDING LEVEL: $4.57 BILLION

From Appendix C, about funding for prevention of substance use disorder (SUD) ($1.81 billion):

"Approximately 80 percent of the $1.8 billion in prevention spending was for prevention delivered by HHS, with most spending by SAMHSA and the CDC."

From Appendix C, about funding for prevention in mental health (MH) (total of $2.76 billion):

"Approximately 40 percent of the MH prevention spending occurred under the direction of the Administration for Children and Families (ACF) for programs aimed at preventing child maltreatment ($1,126 million). The next largest funding amount was spent by SAMHSA ($919 million), of which $617 million was for suicide prevention and the rest of the funding was mainly aimed at children and youth. The Health Resources and Services Administration (HRSA)'s MH prevention spending ($517 million) went toward the Maternal, Child, and Home Visiting Program ($500 million). The CDC had a variety of programs aimed at preventing suicide, domestic and sexual violence, ACEs, firearm injury, and two programs aimed at improving student emotional health."

OPTION 1: FROM A $1.8 BILLION INCREASE

The lower end estimate (i.e., increase by 40 percent main sources of funding for prevention of MEB disorders) would involve adding to the funding of agencies with a role in MEB disorder prevention (relevant rows highlighted in the table below). For some, this means adjust to inflation, for others, a justification for additional modest increases to expand capacity.

Table 5 from Appendix C (highlights on 4 major sources of funding for prevention of MEB disorders)

National Drug Control Program Agency	SU Prevention Spending	MH Prevention Spending	SU + MH Prevention Spending
AmeriCorps	$13.10		$13
Court Services and Offender Supervision Agency	$27.90		$28
Department of Defense			$0
Drug Interdiction and Counterdrug Activities			$0
Department of Education	$108.70		$109
Department of Health and Human Services			$0
Administration for Children and Families	$20	$1,126	$1,146
Centers for Disease Control and Prevention	$528.6	$204	$733
Centers for Medicare and Medicaid Services	$41.00		$41
Food and Drug Administration	$12.50		$13
Health Resources and Services Administration	$142	$517	$659
Indian Health Service	$34.80		$35
National Institute on Alcohol Abuse and Alcoholism			$0
National Institute on Drug Abuse			$0
Substance Use and Mental Health Services Administration	$638.40	$919	$1,557
Department of Justice			$0

APPENDIX F   347

Table 5 from Appendix C Continued

National Drug Control Program Agency	SU Prevention Spending	MH Prevention Spending	SU + MH Prevention Spending
Bureau of Alcohol, Tobacco, and Firearms	$0.10		$0
Bureau of Prisons	$0.30		$0
Drug Enforcement Administration	$4.70		$5
Federal Bureau of Investigation	$0.10		$0
Office of Justice Programs	$34.10		$34
Department of Labor			$0
Employment and Training Administration	$6		$6
Office of Workers' Compensation Programs	$7.80		$8
Department of the Interior			$0
Bureau of Indian Affairs	$1		$1
Department of Transportation			$0
Federal Aviation Administration	$17.80		$18
National Highway Traffic Safety Administration	$17.60		$18
Office of National Drug Control Policy	$151.80		$152
TOTAL	**$1,808**	**$2,766**	**$4,574**

The 4 main funding sources in Table 5. See below for calculations to fill in the "Shortfall" column.

Agency	2024 MH+SUD spending	Shortfall (e.g., not keeping up with inflation or TFAH, 2024, or with need)
A. ACF	$1,146 million	(inflation)
B. CDC	$733 million	(TFAH estimate)
C. HRSA	$659 million	(need)
D. SAMHSA	$1,557 million	(inflation)
(CMS, DOJ, Ed, etc.)	*$499 million*	n/a
TOTAL (Federal funding for prevention of MEB disorders)	$4.57 billion	

A. **Parts of ACF funding have not kept up with inflation (and in some cases decreased)—see blue highlights**

Program (ACF)	2024 Funding (adjusted for inflation from the 2007 figure)	2020	2019	2009	2008	2007
Promoting Safe and Stable Families	$325 (should be 477, so +152)	92.515	99.56	365	365	365
Child Welfare Services	$268 (should be 400M, so +132)	268	267	281	281	286
Family Violence Prevention and Services	$240	187	174	122	122	124
Child Abuse Prevention and Treatment Act (CAPTA) State Grants	$105	90	90	26.5	26.5	27
Child Abuse Discretionary Activities	$38 (should be 55)	35	35	41	37	26
Community-Based Child Abuse Prevention	$70	55	55	41.7	41.6	42
Native American Programs	$60	56	56	47	45	44
National Domestic Violence Hotline	$20	12	12	3.2	2.9	2.9
Total	**$1,126**					

Sources: ACF Congressional Budget Justifications for 2008, 2009, 2010, 2019, 2020, and 2024. The years 2021-23 were omitted due to the temporary increases due to COVID-19 related supplemental funding.

B. **CDC funding for MEB prevention could be increased in some key areas (according to TFAH 2024 recommendations); currently it's about $733M**

According to Appendix C, CDC spent $204M for MH prevention, including the following:

- Suicide $30M, ACEs $9M
- Domestic Violence and Sexual Violence: $38,200,000
- Youth and Community Violence Prevention: $18,100,000
- Domestic Violence Community Projects: $7,500,000
- Rape Prevention: $61,750,000

APPENDIX F

According to Appendix C, CDC spending for SUD prevention in 2024: $528.6M

TFAH's 2024 report on public health spending recommended increases in the following MEB related areas in the CDC budget:

Program	2024	TFAH 2025 recommendation
Division of Adolescent and School Health	$57 million	$100 million
Suicide Prevention	$30 million	$80 million
Adverse Childhood Experiences	$9 million	$33 million

(Source: TFAH, 2024, page 6)

C. **SAMHSA funding in several key areas has not kept up with inflation, or does not include sufficient support for SU prevention**

NASADAD (2018) shows - Substance Use Prevention, Treatment, and Recovery Services Block Grant (SUBG) was $1.779 billion in 2009, and SAMHSA budget request was $2.0 billion in 2024; adjusting 2009 amount for inflation (x0.47) = $2.6 billion.

D. **HRSA** – main contribution to MEB prevention is MIECHV (Maternal, Infant, and Early Childhood Home Visiting) programs. Funding has increased over the years, not quite keeping up with inflation. However, funding allows the evidence-based programs covered here to only reach approximately 15 percent of the more than 465,000 families who are likely eligible at any given time and could benefit from MIECHV services (Zaid et al., 2022).

Based on the discussion above, the committee could recommend a minimum increase in the 4 key federal sources for MEB prevention (ACF, CDC, HRSA, and SAMHSA) as follows:

Agency	2024 MH+SUD prevention spending	Shortfall (e.g., not keeping up with inflation, TFAH recommendation, or ability to meet need)	Sources for additional funding
ACF	$1,146M	$301M	
CDC	$709M	$117M (increase per TFAH, 2024 recommendation)	
HRSA	$659M	$500M (double MIECHV to reach 30%, instead of 15% of eligible families)	

(continued)

Agency	2024 MH+SUD prevention spending	Shortfall (e.g., not keeping up with inflation, TFAH recommendation, or ability to meet need)	Sources for additional funding
SAMHSA	$1,557M	SUBG + $600M for inflation (incl. + $120M for 20% prev. set-aside)	
		CSAP +$64M (inflation)	
		$250M to MHBG to allow 20% prev. set aside for MH, while keeping stable the $1B for treatment)	
DOJ, Ed, etc.	$499M	–	
TOTAL (Fed MH/SUD prevention)	$4.57B	$1.8B (40% increase)	Could include $700M from a restored Prevention and Public Health Fund

OPTION 2: TO A $14 BILLION INCREASE

Developing an estimate for preventive services for children

Why the focus on children? The onset for more than half of mental health conditions is before age 18 (Solmi et al., 2022). Also, intervening in early life offers best opportunities for prevention and associated benefits (NASEM, 2019).

The cost of mental health treatment in children has been estimated at approximately $4,361 (Loo et al., 2024). The public health and prevention portion of the 2021 National Health Expenditure Accounts (all health care spending) is approximately 5 percent (Martin et al., 2023). Five percent of $4,361 is $218 per individual.

If $218 were spent on each of 73.2 million US children[1] 0 to 18 years old for a package of interventions that met their needs (from nurse family partnership to family and school-based interventions), that would cost approximately $16 billion.

---

[1] https://www.childstats.gov/americaschildren/tables/pop1.asp (accessed January 2, 2025).

APPENDIX F

Subtract from $16 billion the current amount being spent on prevention in children by the primary federal agencies working on MEB health.

(1) Amounts from federal agencies prevention funding for MEB disorders that seems largely devoted to children (not including SAMHSA):

    a. $1,146 million for ACF
    b. $500 million for HRSA home visiting
    c. $57 million + $9 million for CDC (Division on Adolescent and School Health and Adverse Childhood Experiences program), and
    d. $109 million for Department of Education (Appendix C; TFAH, 2024).

That is $1.8 billion.

(2) SAMHSA funding for prevention efforts in children (some portion of $1,557 million SAMHSA prevention spending on BH disorders—see above), which is calculated below. Amounts that seem largely or entirely relevant to children and are either definitely prevention or very likely prevention:

    a. Substance Use Prevention, Treatment, and Recovery Services Block Grant proportion for children under 18: $16 million

    Calculated by using the demographics information from Fiscal Year 2022 reported in SAMHSA's Fiscal Year 2025 Justification of Estimates for Appropriations Committees (SAMHSA, 2024):

    - Children 17 years old and under: 3.89 percent, rounded up to 4 percent
    - The 20 percent set aside of the $2 billion SUBG = $400 million
    - 4 percent of the $400 million = $16 million of the prevention set-aside supports services for children

b.	Project AWARE	$190 million
c.	Project LAUNCH	$25 million
d.	Partnerships for Success	$135 million
e.	STOP Act	$14.5 million
TOTAL		**$380 million**

Assuming that includes much of prevention spending on children, $380 million is approximately 24 percent of the $1,577B.

(3) Estimated total spending on prevention in children:

- $1.8 billion + $380 million is the amount currently spent by federal agencies on prevention for children.
- $16 billion − $2.18 billion = $13.62 billion, or **approximately $14 billion more could be spent on prevention of MEB disorders in children under 18.**

This does not include the percentage of prevention spending out of the combined state funding for prevention in children (some small portion of the combined SUD and MH $45.8B [2014 figure] spent by states on all prevention and treatment) (SAMHSA, 2017).

REFERENCES

ACF (HHS Administration for Children and Families). 2008. Department of Health and Human Services Fiscal Year 2009 Administration for Children and Families Justification of Estimates for Appropriations Committees. https://www.acf.hhs.gov/olab/fy-2009-acf-congressional-justification (accessed January 2, 2025).

ACF. 2009. Department of Health and Human Services Fiscal Year 2010 Administration for Children and Families Justification of Estimates for Appropriations Committees https://www.acf.hhs.gov/sites/default/files/documents/olab/2010cj_comb.pdf (accessed January 2, 2025).

ACF. 2018. Department of Health and Human Services Fiscal Year 2019 Administration for Children and Families Justification of Estimates for Appropriations Committees. https://www.acf.hhs.gov/olab/budget/fy-2019-congressional-justification (accessed January 2, 2025).

ACF. 2019. Department of Health and Human Services Fiscal Year 2020 Administration for Children and Families Justification of Estimates for Appropriations Committees. https://www.acf.hhs.gov/olab/budget/acf-congressional-budget-justification-fy-2020 (accessed January 2, 2025).

ACF. 2023. Department of Health and Human Services Fiscal Year 2024 Administration for Children and Families Justification of Estimates for Appropriations Committees. https://www.acf.hhs.gov/sites/default/files/documents/olab/fy-2024-congressional-justification.pdf (accessed January 2, 2025).

HRSA (Health Resources and Services Administration). 2023. Department of Health and Human Services Fiscal Year 2024 Health Resources and Services Administration Justification of Estimates for Appropriations Committees. https://www.hrsa.gov/sites/default/files/hrsa/about/budget/budget-justification-fy2024.pdf (accessed January 2, 2025).

Loo, T. M, M. Altman, D. M. Bravata, and C. Whaley. 2024. Medical Spending Among US Households with Children with a Mental Health Condition Between 2017 and 2021. *JAMA Netw Open.* 2024;7(3):e241860. doi:10.1001/jamanetworkopen.2024.1860

Martin, A. B., M. Hartman, J. Benson, A. Catlin, and The National Health Expenditure Accounts. 2023. National health care spending in 2021: Decline in federal spending outweighs greater use of health care. Health Affairs (Millwood) 42(1):6–17. https://doi.org/10.1377/hlthaff.2022.01397.

NASADAD (National Association of State Alcohol and Drug Abuse Directors). 2018. Substance Abuse Prevention and Treatment (SAPT) Block Grant. https://nasadad.org/wp-content/uploads/2018/06/SAPT-Block-Grant-Fact-Sheet-5.2.2018.pdf (accessed January 2, 2025).

NASEM (National Academies of Sciences, Engineering, and Medicine). 2019. *Fostering Healthy Mental, Emotional, and Behavioral Development in Children and Youth: A National Agenda*. Washington, DC: The National Academies Press. https://doi.org/10.17226/25201.

SAMHSA (Substance Abuse and Mental Health Services Administration). 2017. Funding and Characteristics of Single State Agencies for Substance Abuse Services and State Mental Health Agencies, 2015. HHS Pub. No. (SMA) SMA-17-5029. Rockville, MD: Substance Abuse and Mental Health Services Administration. https://store.samhsa.gov/sites/default/files/sma17-5029.pdf (accessed October 5, 2024).

SAMHSA. Department of Health and Human Services Fiscal Year 2025 Substance Abuse and Mental Health Services Administration Justification of Estimates for Appropriations Committees 2024. https://www.samhsa.gov/sites/default/files/samhsa-fy-2025-cj.pdf

Solmi, M., Radua, J., Olivola, M. et al. 2022. Age at onset of mental disorders worldwide: large-scale meta-analysis of 192 epidemiological studies. *Mol Psychiatry* 27:281–295. https://doi.org/10.1038/s41380-021-01161-7.

TFAH (Trust for America's Health). 2024. The Impact of Chronic Underfunding on America's Public Health System 2024: Trends, Risks, and Recommendations. https://www.tfah.org/report-details/funding-2024/ (accessed January 2, 2025).

Zaid, S., K. McCombs-Thornton, K. Faucetta, L. Childress, P. Cachat, and J. Filene. 2022. Family Level Assessment and State of Home Visiting outreach and recruitment study report (OPRE Report No. 2022-110). Office of Planning, Research, and Evaluation; Administration for Children and Families; U.S. Department of Health and Human Services.